Error Reduction in Health Care

A Systems Approach to Improving Patient Safety

Second Edition

PATRICE L. SPATH, EDITOR

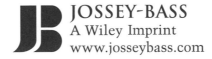

JOSSEY-BASS
A Wiley Imprint
www.josseybass.com

Published by Jossey-Bass

A Wiley Imprint

989 Market Street, San Francisco, CA 94103-1741—www.josseybass.com

Jossey-Bass books and products are available through most bookstores. To contact Jossey-Bass directly call our Customer Care Department within the U.S. at 800-956-7739, outside the U.S. at 317-572-3986, or fax 317-572-4002.

Jossey-Bass also publishes its books in a variety of electronic formats. Some content that appears in print may not be available in electronic books.

Library of Congress Cataloging-in-Publication Data
Error reduction in health care : a systems approach to improving patient safety / Patrice L. Spath, editor.— Second Edition.
    p. ; cm.
  Includes bibliographical references and index.
    ISBN 978-0-470-50240-2 (pbk.); 978-1-118-00151-6(ebk.); 978-1-118-00155-4 (ebk.); 978-1-118-00156-1 (ebk.)
1. Health facilities–Risk management. 2. Medical errors–Prevention. I. Spath, Patrice L., 1949- editor.
  [DNLM: 1. Medical Errors–prevention & control. 2. Quality Assurance, Health Care–methods.
3. Risk Management–methods. WB 100]
  RA971.38.E77 2011
  362.1–dc22

                                    2010047564

Printed in the United States of America

SECOND EDITION

PB Printing   10 9 8 7 6 5 4 3 2 1

CONTENTS

PART THREE: Reactive and Proactive Safety Investigations

PART FOUR: How to Make Health Care Processes Safer

PART FIVE: Focused Patient Safety Initiatives

FIGURES, TABLES, AND EXHIBITS

Figures

Tables

Exhibits

FOREWORD

Lucian L. Leape

It is hard to believe that it was only 11 years ago that the Institute of Medicine shocked the world with the revelation that hundreds of thousands of hospitalized patients are injured by medical errors and as many as 98,000 die annually as a result. In that relatively brief period the patient safety "movement" has grown exponentially, so that now every hospital has a patient safety officer and some kind of a safety program. There are very few providers—nurses, doctors, pharmacists, or technicians—who have not been involved in at least one systems change designed to improve safety.

Yet, most of us feel woefully ill-equipped to take on the patient safety challenge. For one reason, it is so complicated. In the increasing complex world of modern health care, there seems to be an infinite number of possibilities for things to go wrong. And, in response, there seems to be an infinite number of types of changes we are being called on to make. Where to start?

A good place to start is by getting a serious understanding not just of the extent of medical injury, but also of the theories of why people make mistakes and how you can prevent them. The next step is to learn what is available in terms of methods for understanding risk, analyzing mistakes, and designing care processes to make them difficult to make. *Error Reduction in Health Care* does just that. The first two chapters provide a succinct yet comprehensive description of what is known about the extent of medical errors and the current thinking about why people make mistakes and how to design systems to reduce risk. Then there are chapters on how to analyze accidents and how to use deductive methods to understand hazards before accidents occur, how to prioritize risks in order to know where to focus efforts at systems redesign. The chapter on the application of human factors principles in designing systems changes is especially valuable, and the chapter on performance measurement provides perhaps the most comprehensive list of measures available—a veritable treasure trove that can be used to assess safety and, equally important, progress in improvement.

But there is more to safety than measuring risk and redesigning processes using human factors concepts. In health care, more than any other industry, the processes are people processes. Although there are important examples where automation is being used effectively, for most patients, most of the time, health care is the result of human interactions. James Reason pointed out years ago that the essence of a safe culture is to be found in the interrelationships of the caregivers—how we work together, or don't. The power of this observation comes through in the several chapters in *Error Reduction in Health Care*. Implementing information technology, changing medication systems, creating "lean" systems, and, of course, functioning effectively in teams, all require that caregivers work well together. Creating a culture where that happens is proving to be the great challenge in patient safety. It requires knowledge, commitment, and leadership. But first it requires that you have a clear vision of where you want to go. *Error Reduction in Health Care* is a good place to start.

Medical accidents, near-miss situations, and recommendations for preventing these events are not new topics. For example, in 1886 Dr. Frank Hamilton wrote that "a few years ago a strong, healthy woman died in the dentist's chair in New York City while under the influence of nitrous oxide." Hamilton then goes on to describe how future events of this sort might be prevented, saying, "The danger to life would no doubt in these cases be diminished if the patient were in the recumbent position. Recent experiments and observations seem to have shown that the admixture of oxygen gas with the nitrous oxide in certain proportions averts the danger of asphyxia, while it does not diminish the anesthesia" (Hamilton, 1886, p. 946). In 1915 Gordon Christine, MD, wrote about problems related to ownership of patient records. According to Christine, "there is a widespread notion among nurses that bedside clinical records of a patient are the property of the attending nurse, and that they can therefore be rightfully removed by her from the home of the patient at the conclusion of her services" (Christine, 1915, p. 22). Christine relates an incident in which the nurse took a patient's chart and refused to return it even though the continuity of care was being compromised. In two other instances Christine notes that records were removed "because the nurses wished to cover up some of their mistakes."

Safe health care is recognized by the Institute of Medicine as one of the key dimensions of health care quality. In *Crossing the Quality Chasm*, safe health care is defined as, "avoidance of unintended patient injuries" (IOM, 2001). Since publication of this report, much has been done to improve patient safety. We've learned a lot and have made progress toward achieving the safe health care goal, yet there's still much more learning and work to be done.

Patient safety improvement is what this book is all about. In the pages that follow you'll find out why errors occur at the front lines of patient care and what is needed to prevent these errors. Some of the fixes are fairly simple—use checklists to remind caregivers of required actions. Some of the fixes are costly—to implement computerized order entry systems. Some of the fixes challenge our traditions—to break down professional silos. All of the fixes require systems thinking—problems must be viewed as parts of the overall system and solutions must address the underlying causes.

The basics of patient safety are covered in Part One of the book. These chapters provide a foundation for further learning. In Chapter One, McClanahan, Goodwin, and Perlin present an overview of issues surrounding health care accidents. Using a real-life case study, the authors describe how our system of care actually fosters mistakes. And although errors are often attributed to the action of an individual, there are usually a set of external forces and preceding events that lead up to the error. Quality experts agree that the most common cause of performance problems is the system itself, not the individuals functioning within the system. Though a human error may have occurred, the root cause is likely to be found in the design of the system that permitted such an error to be made. The professionals who work together to provide patient care do not function in isolation. The activities of caregivers are influenced by multiple factors, including personal characteristics, attitudes, and qualifications; the composition of teams, organizational culture, and climate; physical resources; and the condition of the patient. These factors affect performance as well as influence decision making, task prioritization, and conflict resolution.

A fundamental understanding of the kinds of errors that health care professionals make can help us design better systems. In Chapter Two Ternov draws from work in the cognitive sciences and analyses of human performance to provide an in-depth review of the causes of medical mistakes. Ternov's previous work as principal investigator of medical accidents for the Board of Health and Welfare in Sweden has offered a unique insight into the causes of mistakes. He describes several medical accidents and near-miss events and provides commentary as to why they occurred and ways to keep them from recurring.

Is health care reliable? What is the probability that a health care process will adequately perform its intended purpose? Are health care professionals mindful of the safety risks associated with patient care? These questions, and more, are addressed in Chapter Three. To further advance patient safety, senior leaders must create an environment where everyone is aware of the error potential in operations and safe behaviors and attitudes are rewarded. In addition, work processes must be designed to perform as expected a high proportion of the time. Dlugacz and Spath detail what must be done by health care organizations if they are to become highly reliable.

The chapters in Part Two of the book address measurement and evaluation of patient safety performance data. Accident investigators have found that most disasters in complex organizations had long incubation periods characterized by a number of discrete events signaling danger that were often overlooked or misinterpreted during the incubation period. This observation has important implications for health care organizations. Patient safety can be enhanced with the introduction of measures that continually evaluate risk-prone processes. By monitoring the performance of these processes, health care professionals can detect impending problems before an undesirable event occurs. Included in Chapter Four is advice on how to select the important tasks that should be regularly evaluated. The authors offer a scoring matrix that can be used to identify safety-critical patient care activities. More than 100 patient safety measures are included in this chapter.

Collecting measurement data is just the first step toward making improvements. The information gathered must be analyzed for danger signals needing further investigation. Chapter Five describes techniques for evaluating the results of patient safety measurement, starting with effective data display. Statistical process control tools can be used to judge performance as well as comparison data from other health care organizations. In Chapter Six Latino illustrates how performance data can be used to select the process failures most in need of fixing. This involves gathering and analyzing data to make the business case for improvement projects.

In Part Three of the book you'll find chapters describing how health care organizations use retrospective and prospective investigation techniques to uncover root causes and latent failures. Feldman began studying the causes of sentinel events in the early 1960s. In Chapter Seven, he and Roblin of Kaiser Permanente show how the private industry model of root cause analysis can be applied to untoward patient care events to find the underlying causes. You'll learn how to identify the root causes of adverse events and fix the latent failures that contribute to medical accidents. In addition, Feldman and Roblin introduce anticipatory failure analysis—prospective risk assessment techniques designed to identify and resolve process failures before an accident occurs. It is not enough to wait for an accident to happen and then start improving patient care tasks. Better system reliability cannot be achieved by acting only on what is learned from yesterday's mistakes—proactive patient safety initiatives should be used to keep ahead of the accidents.

In Chapter Eight Ternov describes methods used in Sweden to retrospectively analyze medical accidents and proactively study high-risk health care processes so that preventive measures can be taken before an adverse event occurs. A deductive analysis approach to analyzing adverse event is favored by Latino, author of Chapter Nine. Deductive analysis is an investigation technique that explores from the general to the specific to determine how the system failed and why wrong decisions were made. He details the advantages of using a deductive analysis tool to identify failures and appropriate corrective actions.

Once the decision is made to improve the safety of a process, how should the work be redesigned? Much has been learned about improving the reliability and safety of health care processes in the past ten years and this learning is detailed in Part Four of the book. In Chapters Ten and Eleven readers learn how to design patient care processes to be more resistant to error occurrence and more accommodating of error consequences. When errors cannot be completely eliminated, then clinicians must learn how to quickly recognize the mistake and take appropriate actions to mitigate the consequences. Many of the techniques used to create more efficient health care processes also help to make them safer. In Chapter Twelve Lavallee shows how lean techniques borrowed from private industry can be used to reduce the likelihood of harmful mistakes during the delivery of health care services.

Targeted patient safety improvement recommendations are found in Part Five. An often-cited suggestion for improving patient safety is technology—tools that automate or mechanize clinical and administrative processes. In Chapter Thirteen, Slovensky and Menachemi describe how automation can reduce human errors in health care work processes but not without some challenges. The current state of the art in information technology and patient safety, as well as recommendations for avoiding common automation-induced hazards are covered in Chapter Thirteen.

The aviation industry has discovered that faulty teamwork among crew members is a frequent causal factor in airline accidents. Many scientists involved in improving airline crew performance are now applying the same concepts to health care teams. By adopting structured teamwork improvement strategies, caregivers are finding that medical accidents can be prevented. Tactics for enhancing teamwork and communication among health care professionals are included in Chapter Fourteen. In this chapter readers will find a checklist that can be used to identify the teamwork and communication problems that lead to an adverse patient event as well as a teamwork improvement action plan.

It is estimated that each year medication errors injure approximately 1.3 million people in the United States. In a study of fatal medication errors from 1993 to 1998, improper dosing of medicine accounted for 41% of fatal errors. Giving the wrong drug and using the wrong route of administration each accounted for 16% of the errors (Institute of Medicine, 2006). The important topic of how to reduce the incidence of medication errors is covered by Dlugacz in Chapter Fifteen.

Following publication in 2000 of the first edition of *Error Reduction in Health Care* there was considerable national attention on the problem of patient safety and this focus has not subsided. We hope that some of the progress we've made toward the goal of safe patient care can be attributed to what readers learned in the first edition. Eleven years later we know more about what works and what doesn't work. We know errors cannot be eliminated by simply disciplining the people who make the mistakes. Quick fixes must give way to systems thinking and adoption of reliability principles that have improved safety in other complex, high-risk industries. We should seek to prevent errors, but also design systems that more readily catch and mitigate the effects of errors. Most important is maintaining an organizational culture of safety and reliability.

Patrice L. Spath, MA, RHIT
Health Care Quality Specialist
Forest Grove, Oregon

Patrice L. Spath, MA, RHIT, is a health information management professional with broad experience in health care quality and safety improvement. She is president of Brown-Spath & Associates (www.brownspath.com), a health care publishing and training company based in Forest Grove, Oregon. During the past twenty-five years, Patrice has presented more than 350 educational programs on health care quality and patient safety topics and has completed numerous quality program consultations for health care organizations.

Ms. Spath has authored and edited many books and peer-reviewed articles for Health Administration Press, AHA Press, Jossey-Bass, AHC Media LLC, Brown-Spath & Associates, and other groups. Her recent books include *Engaging Patients as Safety Partners* (AHA Press, 2008) and *Leading Your Health Care Organization to Excellence* (Health Administration Press, 2005) for which she received the James A. Hamilton Book of the Year Award. This award is given annually to the author of a management or health care book judged outstanding by the American College of Healthcare Executives' Book of the Year Committee.

Ms. Spath is an adjunct assistant professor in the Department of Health Services Administration at the University of Alabama, Birmingham, where she teaches online quality management courses. She has also had teaching responsibilities in the health information technology program at Missouri Western State University in St. Joseph and the graduate health administration program at Montana State University in Billings.

Ms. Spath currently serves as consulting editor for Hospital Peer Review and is an active member of the advisory board for WebM&M (http://webmm .ahrq.gov), an online case based journal and forum on patient safety and health care quality that is supported by a contract from the Agency for Healthcare Research and Quality.

This book is dedicated to everyone involved in improving the safety of health care services.

Richard J. Croteau, MD, is a senior patient safety advisor at Joint Commission International with a principal focus on international patient safety activities in collaboration with the WHO's World Alliance for Patient Safety. For the past twenty years, he has held several positions with The Joint Commission including executive director for patient safety initiatives and vice president for accreditation services. Earlier activities include chief of surgery at South County Hospital in Rhode Island and rocket systems analyst for NASA's Lunar Module program, Project Apollo. He currently splits his time between international patient safety activities and woodworking.

Yosef D. Dlugacz, PhD, is the senior vice president and chief of clinical quality, education and research of the Krasnoff Quality Management Institute, a division of the North Shore-Long Island Jewish Health System which was the recipient of the National Quality Forum's 2010 National Quality Healthcare Award. Dr. Dlugacz was instrumental in designing the impressive and sophisticated quality management structure that integrates quality management methods into every level of care within the vast 15-hospital system. His latest book, *Value Based Health Care: Linking Finance and Quality* (Jossey-Bass, 2010), explores the relationship between quality care and organizational efficiency.

Sanford E. Feldman, MD, FACS, a general surgeon in private practice in San Francisco, was a pioneer in the area of medical peer review. He was a founder and first director of the San Francisco Medical Peer Review Organization and became director of the California Medical Review Organization. After retirement from surgery Dr. Feldman continued to work for the improvement of patient care. He was an expert in the assurance of quality care by hospitals and wrote about physician and hospital error for various medical journals. Dr. Feldman passed away in 2008 at the age of 93.

Karen Ferraco was a risk management consultant at ProNational Insurance Company in Okemos, Michigan, and at PHICO Insurance Company in Pennsylvania. She specialized in risk management with an emphasis on professional and hospital liability. Ms. Ferraco was frequently involved in training and educational presentations for medical professionals and medical staff and hospital boards. In addition to her strengths in analyzing high-risk exposures, she practiced as a registered nurse for 10 years. Ms. Ferraco passed away in 2002 at the age of 55.

Susan T Goodwin, RN, MSN, CPHQ, FNAHQ, FACHE, is assistant vice president in the Clinical Services Group for the Hospital Corporation of America (HCA) and currently concentrating on the development and redesign of credentialing, privileging, and peer review systems and processes for HCA affiliates. Ms. Goodwin is the 2011 president of the National Association of Healthcare Quality (NAHQ), and most recently served as chairman and NAHQ representative for the Joint Commission's Professional and Technical Advisory Committee for the Hospital Accreditation Program.

Robert J. Latino is CEO of Reliability Center, Inc. (RCI) (www.reliability .com). RCI is a reliability consulting firm specializing in improving equipment, process, and human reliability. He has facilitated root cause analyses and failure mode and effect analyses with his clientele in more than 20 countries around the world for 25 years and has taught more than 10,000 students in the PROACT® methodology. Mr. Latino is the author of *Root Cause Analysis: Improving Performance for Bottom Line Results* (2006, Taylor & Francis) and *Patient Safety: The PROACT Root Cause Analysis Approach* (2008, Taylor & Francis) as well as coauthor on several other patient safety articles and publications.

Danielle Lavallee, PharmD, PhD, is the senior health care consultant for Lean Hospitals, LLC (www.leanhospitals.org). Her work and research focuses on improving the efficiency of health care practices through the incorporation of lean principles and she is a Lean Hospitals Certified Six Sigma Black Belt. Dr. Lavallee holds degrees of doctor of pharmacy from the University of Kansas and doctor of philosophy from the Department of Pharmaceutical Health Services Research at the University of Maryland, School of Pharmacy.

Susan McClanahan, RN, BSN, is a director in the Clinical Services Group for Hospital Corporation of America (HCA). She joined the company in 1995. Through her work providing consultative and educational assistance to each of the HCA affiliates, she promotes foundational quality of care and compliance with accreditation, legislative, and regulatory standards. A graduate of the University of Tennessee at Knoxville, Ms. McClanahan specialized in emergency department nursing for eight years. After obtaining her certification as a paralegal in 1990, she worked as a claims investigator in the risk management department at Vanderbilt University Medical Center.

Nir Menachemi, PhD, MPH, is an associate professor of health care organization and policy at the University of Alabama at Birmingham (UAB). His research focuses on health information technologies, patient safety, medical malpractice, and health care quality issues. At UAB, Dr. Menachemi teaches courses in strategic management, health information management, and directs the doctoral program in public health.

John C. Morey, PhD, CHFP, is a board-certified human factors professional and the senior research psychologist at Dynamics Research Corporation. He has more than thirty years of experience in training evaluation and conducts research in teamwork training programs for aviation, combat systems, and health care. Dr. Morey was a member of the original development team for the MedTeams® project, a joint civilian and military program to transition lessons learned from aviation crew resource management to health care. He holds a doctorate in experimental psychology from the University of Georgia.

Jonathan B. Perlin, MD, PhD, MSHA, FACP, FACMI, is president of clinical services and chief medical officer for Hospital Corporation of America (HCA). He holds adjunct appointments as professor of medicine and biomedical informatics at Vanderbilt University and professor of health administration at Virginia Commonwealth University. Dr. Perlin previously served as the chief executive officer of the Veterans Health Administration, where his work helped propel the nation's largest integrated health system to international recognition for achievements in quality, safety, and use of electronic health records.

Matthew M. Rice, MD, JD, FACEP, is an ABEM-certified practicing emergency medicine physician who works clinically at more than 26 hospitals in the Pacific Northwest. Dr. Rice spent 22 years in the U.S. Army in various positions, retiring as a colonel in 2000 from Madigan Army Medical Center where he was department chair and program director of the Emergency Medicine Residency. He is a senior member of the American College of Emergency Physicians (ACEP), the national organization representing emergency medicine and chairs and is a member of various committees including the ACEP standards of care committee. He is on the board of directors of the National Patient Safety

Foundation. He has special professional interests in legal medicine, quality of medicine, local and national politics, and future issues in health care.

Douglas W. Roblin, PhD, is Senior Research Scientist with the Center for Health Research/Southeast at Kaiser Permanente Georgia (KPG) and adjunct assistant professor of health policy and management at the Rollins School of Public Health at Emory University. He is a social anthropologist with research interests in chronic disease management, health care access, social epidemiology, and association of patient-level outcomes with organizational and financial characteristics of delivery systems. Dr. Roblin has more than twenty years of experience with management and analysis of Kaiser Permanente (KP) databases and has directed a number of surveys of KP enrollees. He is KPG's site principal investigator for three large multisite research consortia of the HMO Research Network: the HMO Center for Research and Education on Therapeutics, the HMO Cancer Research Network (CRN), and the HMO Cancer Communication Research Center.

Daniel T. Risser, PhD, is an experimental social psychologist with thirty years of research experience examining teams and organizations. He is a senior scientist in the Concepts and Analysis Division of VT Aepco in Gaithersburg, Maryland. He has been a member of the American Society for Healthcare Risk Management (ASHRM), a member of the ASHRM Claim Data Gathering Task Force, and an assistant professor of organizational behavior in a business school. Dr. Risser was the lead researcher examining clinical errors in a large, 10-hospital project (the MedTeams Project) designed to improve teamwork and reduce errors in emergency departments. He has also conducted teamwork research on obstetrical delivery units and Army helicopter aircrews, conducted research on human links in weapon systems design, military command and control systems, and unmanned aerial systems (UAS), and helped to develop Human Systems Integration (HSI) policy for weapon design for the Office of Secretary of Defense.

Mary Salisbury RN, MSN, is a nurse commanding forty years of continuous service in operative, critical care, and emergency medicine with a current focus on safety research. A member of the original MedTeams® research team working to translate the principles of crew resource management into health care, Ms. Salisbury remains a participating author and designer of the TeamSTEPPS™ training and evaluation methodologies. As founder and president of the Cedar Institute, Inc., Ms. Salisbury provides services to both military and civilian health care organizations to translate research into practice—leader and team training, implementation, sustainment and performance coaching, and to focus work on the facilitating elements of team-driven safety to include simulation, evaluation, and managing disrupting behaviors.

Paul M. Schyve, MD, is the senior vice president of The Joint Commission. Before joining the Commission in 1986, he held a variety of professional and academic appointments in the areas of mental health and hospital and health system administration. A Distinguished Life Fellow of the American Psychiatric Association, he has served on numerous advisory panels for the Centers for Medicare and Medicaid Services, the Agency for Healthcare Research and Quality, and the Institute of Medicine, and published in the areas of psychiatric treatment and research, psychopharmacology, quality assurance, continuous quality improvement, health care accreditation, patient safety, health care ethics, and cultural and linguistic competence.

Robert Simon, PhD, has a doctorate in education from the University of Massachusetts. He is a human factors specialist and educator with more than thirty years experience. For the last twenty years he has specialized in research, development, and training for high-performance, high-stress teams in aviation and medicine. He was the principal investigator for the U.S. Army's Aircrew Coordination Training Program, the U.S. Air Force's Crew Resource Management Program, and the MedTeams® program. He joined the Center for Medical Simulation in Cambridge, Massachusetts, as education director in December 2002. He is the director of the Institute for Medical Simulation, a jointly sponsored endeavor of the Center for Medical Simulation and the Harvard-MIT Division of Health Science and Technology intended to foster high-quality simulation-based health care education.

Donna J. Slovensky, PhD, RHIA, FAHIMA, is a professor and associate dean for Academic and Student Affairs in the School of Health Professions at the University of Alabama at Birmingham (UAB). Her teaching and scholarship interests include health information management, strategic management, and health care quality issues.

Sven Ternov, MD, is a PhD student at Lund Institute of Technology, studying risk management in complex socio-technical systems. He is a consultant for the Swedish air traffic navigation and a provider and consultant for the Danish Board of Health. He previously served as an inspector for the Swedish Board of Health and Welfare at the regional unit in Malmoe.

PART 1

THE BASICS OF PATIENT SAFETY

CHAPTER 1

A FORMULA FOR ERRORS: GOOD PEOPLE + BAD SYSTEMS

Susan McClanahan
Susan T. Goodwin
Jonathan B. Perlin

LEARNING OBJECTIVES

- Understand the prevalence of health care–associated **errors** and error consequences
- Describe the concepts of latent failures and human factors analysis
- Demonstrate how to apply mistake-proofing techniques to reduce the probability of errors
- Discuss the role of leaders in supporting patient safety initiatives

Since this book was published in 2000, there has been ongoing news media coverage of medical misadventures, increasing evidence of quality, safety, and efficiency gaps, and thus **patient safety** has continued to be a growing concern for the public, policymakers, and everyone involved in the delivery of health care services. Although the standard of medical practice is perfection (error-free patient care), most health care professionals recognize that some **mistakes** are inevitable.

In this book, readers discover how to examine medical mistakes and learn from them. This first chapter sets the stage for this learning by providing a general overview of the causes of medical mistakes and what can be done to eliminate or reduce the occurrence of such errors. The chapter starts with a description of a case involving surgery on the wrong patient. The case scenario is extrapolated from actual events, although the details of the case have been materially altered, including the use of fictitious names, to protect patient privacy and confidentiality.

Surgery on Wrong Patient

Mr. Murphy slipped on a wet floor in the locker room of the clubhouse at his favorite golf course. He fell heavily on his right hip and was in pain when he arrived by ambulance at the hospital's emergency department (ED). While Murphy was being examined, Mr. Jenkins was being admitted to the same ED. Jenkins was a resident of a local long-term care facility and he had also fallen on his right side that morning.

In addition to caring for Murphy and Jenkins, the ED staff members were very busy with other patients. As was typical when the department was crowded, the admissions registrar was behind in getting patients fully registered and putting identification bands on each patient. The registrar's time was also occupied by other duties. To prevent delays in patient care and to maintain patient flow in an already overcrowded ED, the physicians typically ordered needed diagnostic tests and pain medication in advance of conducting a physical examination of a patient. Staff members providing care relied on their memory of each patient's name, and verbal verification from the patient, but this was not done consistently. Mr. Jenkins, who had no attendant or family members with him, was not coherent enough to speak for himself and only his transfer documents accompanied him from the long-term care facility. Orders for right hip radiographs for both Murphy and Jenkins were entered into the computer by the nursing staff.

Murphy was transported to the radiology department first. A requisition for a radiograph of the right hip was printed out in the radiology department; however, his medical record did not accompany him. The radiology technologist took the requisition from the printer and, noting that it was for a right hip radiograph, verbally confirmed with Murphy that he was hurting in his right hip and was there for a hip radiograph. The technologist did not identify the patient using two patient identifiers (which for this department in this facility were name and date of birth). Unfortunately, the radiograph requisition was for Jenkins and it was Jenkins' name that was placed on Murphy's radiographs.

While radiographs were being taken of Murphy's hip, Jenkins was transported to the radiology department. A technologist who had just come back from her lunch break took the Murphy requisition from the department's printer and confirmed with the transporter that the patient on the stretcher was there for a right hip radiograph. She proceeded to perform the diagnostic study. The technologist did not know that there was another patient in the department for the same study, and she assumed she had the right requisition for the right patient (essentially repeating the error of the first technologist). Murphy's name was then placed on Jenkins' radiographs.

After both patients were transported back to the ED, the radiologist called the ED physician to report that the radiographs labeled with Murphy's name indicated a fracture. The radiographs labeled with Jenkins' name were negative for a fracture. Because metabolic diagnostic studies done on Jenkins indicated other medical problems, he was admitted to the hospital. Murphy was also admitted with a diagnosis of "fractured right hip." The radiologist had not been given any clinical information related to either patient. If he had, he may have noted that one of Murphy's diagnoses was obesity and his radiographs showed very little soft tissue. Jenkins, however, was very frail and thin and his radiographs showed a large amount of soft tissue.

Having been diagnosed with a fractured hip, Murphy was referred to an orthopedist. The orthopedist employed a physician assistant (PA) who performed a preoperative history and physical examination, noting in the medical record that there was shortening and internal rotation of the right leg. The orthopedic surgeon did not personally confirm these findings prior to authenticating the history and physical examination, even though he had had to admonish the PA in the past for doing less than thorough exams. The orthopedic surgeon had not communicated the performance issues related to the PA to anyone at the hospital. Likewise, the hospital's quality management department did not collect or report performance measurement data or conduct ongoing professional practice evaluations for any allied health professionals.

Surgery for Murphy was scheduled for the next day. Meanwhile, Jenkins continued to complain of severe pain in his right hip and refused to bear weight on that side. A repeat radiograph of his right hip was performed late that evening. The radiologist read the radiograph the next morning and a fracture was noted. Although the staff recognized the discrepancy in diagnoses between the first and second radiographs, no immediate investigation of the reason for this was done. The case was merely flagged for retrospective peer review.

Although Murphy's diagnostic images were digitally available through the Picture Archiving and Communication System (PACS) at this facility, they were not appropriately displayed in the operating room in accordance with the hospital policy addressing the Universal Protocol and procedures for avoiding surgical errors involving the wrong patient, wrong site, or wrong procedure. Once again, the discrepancy between the patient's physique and the soft tissue evident in the radiographs was not detected. Surgery proceeded until after the incision was made and the surgeon found no fracture. While waiting for the patient to recover from anesthesia, the surgeon made a quick call to the hospital risk manager to discuss how he should deliver the news of the unnecessary surgery to Murphy and his family.

Prevalence of Incidents

Fortunately, incidents like the one described in the case scenario are not usual occurrences, but they happen more often than they should. As of March 31, 2010, wrong site/wrong patient surgery continues to be the most prevalent **sentinel event** reported to The Joint Commission (TJC) constituting 13.4% of the 6,782 sentinel events reviewed by TJC since 1995 (The Joint Commission, 2010).

How often do incidents involving patient **harm** actually occur? A study prepared by Healthgrades (2008) estimates that patient safety incidents resulted in 238,337 potentially **preventable** deaths during 2004 through 2006. It is estimated that each year 100,000 patients die of health care–associated infections (Klevens et al., 2002). Medication errors are among the most common medical errors, harming at least 1.5 million people every year (Institute of Medicine, 2006). Although the exact number of injurious **patient incidents** is not clearly known, what we do know is that medical errors can have serious consequences and may result in patient death, disability, or other physical or psychological harm, additional or prolonged treatment, and increased public dissatisfaction with the health care system. Health care can be made safer and making it safer is a national imperative.

Incident Contributors

The causes of wrong site/wrong patient surgery generally involve more than one factor and the case described at the start of the chapter illustrates some of the common causes: incomplete patient assessment, staffing issues, unavailability of pertinent information in the operating room, and organizational cultural issues.

Mr. Murphy was the unlucky victim of less than ideal circumstances that led to a series of human errors that were not caught and corrected. Emergency department staff members were busy caring for patients and, not surprisingly, as annual ED visits throughout the United States increased by 31% between 1995 and 2005 (Nawar, Niska, & Xu, 2007). High patient loads frequently caused overcrowding in this facility's ED (a contributing factor to this case, related in part to staffing challenges). Staff did not follow procedures for properly identifying patients and surgical site verification (an organizational cultural factor). The radiologist had not been given any clinical information related to either patient (a contributing factor related to incomplete patient assessment). Conflicting diagnostic test findings did not arouse curiosity and were not investigated immediately. The PA who performed a preoperative history and physical examination noted in the medical record that there was shortening and internal rotation of the right leg; however, the orthopedic surgeon did not personally confirm these findings prior to authenticating the history and physical examination (resulting in an incomplete patient assessment).

Although Mr. Murphy's radiographs were available for viewing electronically, they were not appropriately displayed in the operating room (a factor related to availability of pertinent information in the operating room). The end result, as James Reason observed, is that the greatest **risk** of **accident** in a **complex system** such as health care is "not so much from the breakdown of a major component or from isolated **operator** errors, as from the insidious accumulation of delayed human errors" (1990, p. 476). In this instance, each contributing factor or cultural issue—which alone would not necessarily lead to the untoward outcome—align like the holes in Reason's famous **Swiss cheese model**, allowing a **system failure** to penetrate each potential **barrier** and occur (Reason, 2000).

Why Mistakes Occur

Mistakes are unintended human acts (either of omission or commission) or acts that do not achieve their intended goal. No one likes to make mistakes, but everyone is quick to point them out. In the minds of society and medical professionals alike, health care mistakes are unacceptable. Why are health care professionals so quick to find fault and place blame? Psychologists call it "the illusion of free will." "People, especially in Western cultures, place great value in the belief that they are free agents, the captains of their own fate" (Reason, 1997). Because people are seen as free agents, their actions are viewed as voluntary and within their control. Therefore, medical mistakes have traditionally been blamed on clinicians who were characterized as careless, incompetent, or thoughtless.

However, because human action is always limited by local circumstances and the environment of action, free will is an illusion, not a certainty (Reason, 1997). Investigations of incidents such as the Three Mile Island and the Challenger disasters indicate that "accidents are generally the outcome of a chain of events set in motion by faulty system design that either induces errors or makes them difficult to detect" (Leape et al., 1995). Mr. Murphy's unnecessary surgery illustrates the relationship between human errors and faulty systems. Several erroneous decisions and actions occurred that had an immediate impact on the chain of events. These types of errors, known as **active failures**, are often conspicuous and recognized as slips, mistakes, and **violations** of rules or accepted standards of practice. Active errors are usually committed by the persons who appeared to be in control of the system at the time the incident evolved. Examples of active errors that led to Mr. Murphy's unnecessary surgery are summarized in Figure 1.1.

Errors by the "frontline operators" created the local immediate conditions that allowed the **latent failures** in the system to become manifest. Latent failures are contributory factors in the system that may have lain dormant for a long time (days, weeks, or months) until they finally contributed to the incident. delayed impact on the function of the system (Reason, 1997). Many times these latent failures are only recognized after an incident occurs. Listed below are some of the latent failures that created conditions which made possible the occurrence of an unnecessary surgery:

- Staffing for the admissions registration area was not adequate for the volume of patients experienced during the busier times in the ED. There was no contingency plan to increase staffing during these times. Instead, the staff prioritized their workload and improperly prioritized patient registration and placing of ID bands as a task that could wait. There were no policies and procedures set forth to guide staff more properly in what to do in a busy situation. Nor was there a "safety culture" that facilitated identifying the environment as potentially unsafe and encouraged resolution of concerns.

- The facility's policy regarding patient identification did not address safety measures to be taken in the event that the patient was uncommunicative or disoriented and therefore unable to verbally confirm his or her identity.

- There was a lack of standardized "hand-off" communication of important information. Patient identification was not appropriately communicated between caregivers.

- The quality management activities of the hospital did not cover an entire category of care providers. There was no performance measurement data or systematic ongoing professional practice evaluation for allied health professionals; in this case, the PA. Traditionally, the quality management activities of the hospital most frequently resulted in peer review letters of sanction, and fear of this had prevented the orthopedic surgeon from communicating performance information about the PA for whom he was responsible. The surgeon also did not provide adequate supervision of the PA.

FIGURE 1.1   Active Errors Leading to Mr. Murphy's
Unnecessary Surgery

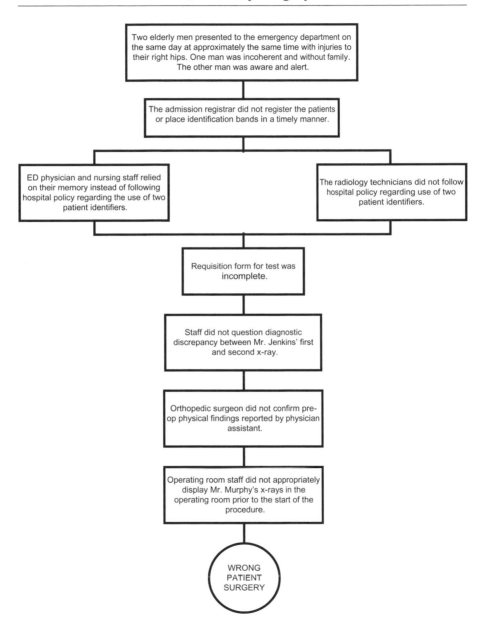

Combination of Factors

As shown by the accident scenario, adverse patient incidents rarely result from a single mistake. System safeguards and the abilities of caregivers to identify and correct errors before an accident occurs make single-error accidents highly unlikely. Rather, accidents typically result from a combination of latent failures, active errors, and breach of defenses (Leape, 1994). System defenses, often called barriers, function to protect potential victims and assets from potential **hazards**. Defenses include engineered mechanisms (for example: alarms, physical barriers, automatic shutdowns), people (surgeons, anesthesiologists, nurses), procedural or administrative controls (time-out procedures, patient identification verifications). The breach of a defense occurs when latent failures and active errors momentarily line up to permit a trajectory of accident opportunity, bringing hazards into contact with victims, as demonstrated by James Reason's Swiss cheese model (2000).

Evidence from a large number of accident inquiries indicates that bad events are more often the result of error-prone situations and error-prone activities than they are of error-prone people (Reason, 2004). The balance of scientific opinion clearly favors system improvements rather than individual discipline as the desired error management approach for the following reasons:

- Human fallibility can be moderated to a point, but it can never be eliminated entirely. It is a fixed part of the human condition partly because, in many contexts, it serves a useful function (for example, trial-and-error learning in knowledge-based situations).

- Different types of errors have different psychological mechanisms, occur in different parts of the organization, and require different methods of management.

- Safety-critical errors happen at all levels of the system; they are not just made by those directly involved in patient care.

- Corrective actions involving sanctions, threats, fear, appeals, and the like have only limited effectiveness, and in many cases these actions can harm morale, self-respect, and a sense of justice.

- Errors are the product of a chain of causes in which the precipitating psychological factors—momentary inattention, misjudgment, forgetfulness, preoccupation—are often the last and least manageable links in the causal chain.

Health safety researchers have come to realize that individuals are not the primary cause of occasional sporadic accidents. Individuals can, however, be dynamic agents of patient safety by identifying and eliminating factors that undermine people's ability to do their jobs successfully (Smith, Boult, Woods, & Johnson, 2010). In the next section readers are introduced to the science of **human factors analysis** and what health care organizations can learn from the error-reduction efforts in other complex, yet highly reliable, safe industries.

How to Error-Proof Processes

Systems that rely on error-free human performance are destined to fail. Traditionally, however, individuals have been expected to not make errors. The time has come for health care professionals to universally acknowledge that mistakes happen and to aim improvement activities at the underlying system failures rather than at the people who, though predominantly well intentioned, are working in systems that are not robust in protecting against mistakes or critically harmful outcomes. For example, if a nurse gives the wrong medication to a patient, typically two things occur. First, an incident report is completed and sent to the nurse's department manager and **risk management**. Next, the nurse is "counseled" by management to pay closer attention next time. She is possibly told to read educational materials on the type of medication that was given in error. She may be warned that a second incident will result in a letter of reprimand being placed in her personnel file.

These individual-focused actions, however, will not fix the latent failures (for example: look-alike or sound-alike medication names, confusing product packaging, similar patient names) that continue to smolder behind the scenes and will invariably manifest themselves when another medication error is made by a different nurse. There may be the rare case of purposeful malevolence, malfeasance, or negligence, which is appropriately dealt with by sanction, but it is inappropriate to react with disciplinary actions for every error.

Human Factors Engineering

The discipline of **human factors engineering (HFE)** has been dealing with the causes and effects of human error since the 1940s. Originally applied to the design of military aircraft cockpits, HFE has since been effectively applied to the problem of human error in nuclear power plants, NASA spacecraft, and computer software (Welch, 1997). The science of HFE has more recently been applied to health care systems to identify the causes of significant errors and develop ways to eliminate or ameliorate them. Two particular concepts from the science of HFE have been introduced to health care systems to proactively improve safety. One is the use of a **risk assessment** technique—**failure mode and effect analysis**—to anticipate failures that may occur in **high-risk processes**. The process is then redesigned to reduce the severity and frequency of failures (Burgmeier, 2002). A second very promising proactive concept is the identification and examination of **close call** events (where a mistake almost reached a patient but was caught just in time). Information derived from close call events provides an understanding of latent failures that need to be resolved to prevent an actual harmful event from occurring (Cohoon, 2003).

By adopting the error-reduction strategies that have been successfully applied in other industries, many health care delivery systems can be redesigned to significantly lessen the likelihood of errors. Some of the tactics that have been summarized in health care literature are illustrated in Figure 1.2 and described in the following paragraphs (Leape, 1994; Cook & Woods, 1994; Grout, 2007; Clancy, 2007; Zwicker & Fulmer, 2008).

FIGURE 1.2   Error-Reduction Strategies

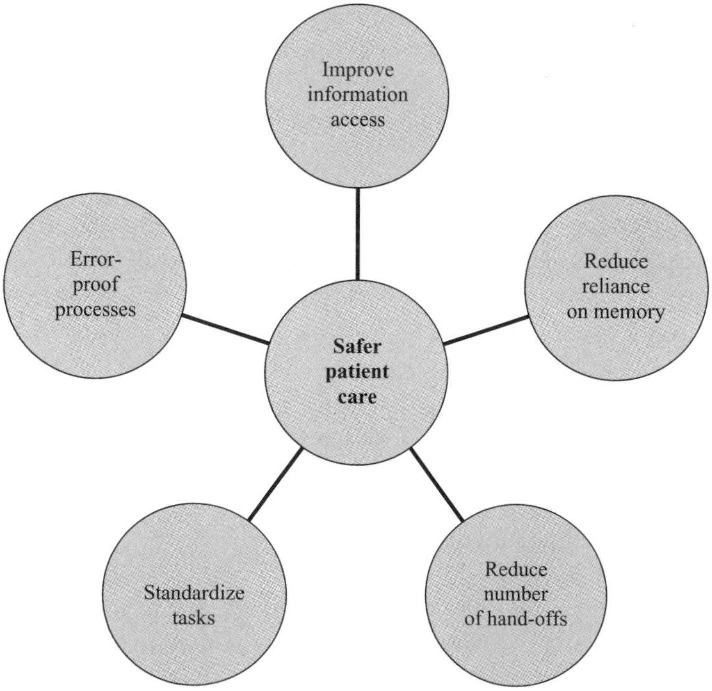

Reduce reliance on memory. Work should be designed to minimize the need for human tasks that are known to be particularly fallible, such as short-term memory and vigilance (prolonged attention). **Checklists**, protocols, and computerized decision aids are examples of tools that can be incorporated into health care processes to reduce mistakes. In a recent study related to clinical information technologies and patient outcomes, researchers found that hospitals with automated notes and records, order entry, and clinical decision support had fewer complications, lower mortality rates, and lower costs (Amarasingham, Plantinga, Diener-West, Gaskin, & Powe, 2009).

Improve information access. Creative ways must be developed to make information more readily available to caregivers. Information must be displayed where it is needed, when it is needed, and in a form that permits easy access by those who need it. For example, placing printed resuscitation protocols on "crash carts" gives caregivers a ready reference during cardiopulmonary resuscitation.

Mistake-proof processes. Where possible, critical tasks should be structured so that errors cannot be made. The use of **forcing functions** is helpful. For example, computerized systems can be designed in such a way as to prevent entry of an order for a lethal drug or to require weight-based dosing calculations for pediatric patients.

Standardize tasks. An effective means of reducing error is by standardizing processes wherever possible. If a task is done the same way every time—by everyone—there is less chance for error.

Reduce the number of hand-offs. Many errors come from slips in the transfer of materials, information, people, instructions, or supplies. Processes with fewer hand-offs reduce the chances for such mistakes.

The system and task redesigns suggested here could serve as the basis for improving processes that led to the unnecessary surgery described at the beginning of this chapter. The following specific corrective actions would likely be effective in decreasing the possibility of future adverse patient occurrences caused by latent failures in the system that cared for patients Murphy and Jenkins:

Reduce reliance on memory. In reverting to alternative procedures when patients were not wearing identification bands, the staff needed to remember to ask patients their identity. Strictly applied protocols for patient care treatment and diagnostic testing would incorporate the step of checking two patient identifiers and would not allow informal variations from this requirement.

Improve information access. The case illustrates many gaps in information communication (for example, patient identity, clinical information, and practitioner performance data). Health information technologies designed to permit access to clinical information by all appropriate practitioners may have helped the radiologist identify the error. Appropriate methods for collecting and trending practitioner performance data that can foster an improvement and safety culture are also needed to change the punitive culture generally associated with the peer review process.

Error-proof processes. Systems have been created that force the critical task of verifying patient identification before care can proceed. For example, by requiring patient identifier information to be entered into the system before the PACS allowed the radiology technologist to proceed with a diagnostic imaging study, the process would be more error-proof. A point-of-care bar-coding system that matches the identifying information in the system to the bar code on a patient's ID band would also greatly reduce mistakes.

Standardize tasks. Safety-critical tasks should be standardized and processes created to ensure that all steps are followed. An example is the use of a standardized checklist to ensure consistency and compliance with all measures of the Universal Protocol developed by TJC to prevent surgery on the wrong patient (The Joint Commission, 2009). Another example is the Surgical Safety Checklist developed by the World Health Organization (WHO) that helps ensure that OR teams consistently follow critical safety steps in the surgical process, with a goal of minimizing the most common and avoidable risks that may endanger surgical patients. Pilot testing of the WHO Surgical Safety Checklist in eight hospitals demonstrated the rate of death decreased from 1.5% to 0.8%, and the rate of complications decreased from 11% to 7% when the checklist was used (World Health Organization, 2008).

Reduce the number of hand-offs. If the steps of the ED admission process and related patient care activities were flowcharted, it would likely reveal unnecessarily complex steps and transfers of information. It is important to eliminate as many hand-offs as possible to prevent errors while at the same time recognizing the need to standardize the communication of important information during hand-offs.

Health care professionals also need to be indoctrinated with an understanding similar to aircraft pilots that safe practice is as important as effective practice (Helmreich, 2000). The staff involved in this unnecessary surgery should have been made aware of the process steps that are essential to safe practice, which would have made them less likely to circumvent these safety-critical steps.

Role of Senior Leaders

Efforts to successfully implement comprehensive patient safety improvement strategies require strong and sustained support, commitment, and actions by board members. administrators, medical staff leaders, and clinical leaders. These leaders must be committed to patient safety. Leaders must work together to ask what happened (not who should be blamed), establish values that place patient safety as a top priority, ensure adequate resources for patient safety, and require adherence to reliable, evidence-based practices. Several studies have substantiated the relationship between active senior leadership involvement and subsequent patient safety improvements (Leape et al., 2000; Lanier, 2006; Keroack et al., 2007; Ginsburg et al., 2010).

Senior leaders have a unique role in championing patient safety. The eight key steps for leaders to follow, as recommended by the Institute for Healthcare Improvement (IHI), are shown in the following list (Botwinick, Bisognano, & Haraden, 2006). By completing these steps, leaders can promote ever better patient safety in their organization.

Step One: Address strategic priorities, culture, and infrastructure

Step Two: Engage key stakeholders

Step Three: Communicate and build awareness

Step Four: Establish, oversee, and communicate system-level aims

Step Five: Track/measure performance over time, strengthen analysis

Step Six: Support staff and patients/families impacted by medical errors

Step Seven: Align systemwide activities and incentives

Step Eight: Redesign systems and improve reliability

Addressing the organization's culture of safety is a first step for leaders. There are various tools for conducting a safety culture assessment to determine factors needing improvement. (Nieva & Sorra, 2003) Borrowing from the Advisory Committee on the Safety of Nuclear Installations is a definition of a safety culture:

> "The safety culture of an organization is the product of individual and group values, attitudes, perceptions, competencies, and patterns of behavior that determine the commitment to, and the style and proficiency of, an organization's health and safety

management. Organizations with a positive safety culture are characterized by communications founded on mutual trust, by shared perceptions of the importance of safety and by confidence in the efficacy of preventive measures" (ACSNI, 1993).

As important as culture is to safety, there are indications that more work is needed in health care organizations. In a recent comparative study of **patient safety cultures** at 633 hospitals submitting data to the Agency for Healthcare Research and Quality (AHRQ), only 44% responded positively to having a nonpunitive response to errors (Sorra, Famolaro, Dyer, Khanna, & Nelson, 2009).

To change the safety culture and build trust, leaders must be visibly committed and supportive. This can be accomplished in several ways (Botwinick, Bisognano, & Haraden, 2006):

- Place patient safety issues at the top of the agenda at meetings of senior leaders, medical staff, and board meetings and educate board members and other leaders about patient safety.

- Engage the board in discussions of patient safety and share performance of the organization as compared with national best practices.

- Make patient safety a priority in hiring practices and spend time with new staff by providing information about patient safety at orientation.

- Provide existing staff with patient safety education and conduct unit walk-arounds focusing on patient safety—listen and respond to staff members' safety concerns.

- Promote and support reporting and analysis of **adverse events** to proactively identify and correct potential system failures.

- Provide support for those involved in a medical error.

- Implement evidence-based processes to increase safety and reliability and reduce errors (for example, rapid response teams, electronic health records with clinical decision support, physician order entry, and other automated error-reducing features).

- Improve, enhance, and reward teamwork.

- Align incentives with patient safety.

- Celebrate successes.

Conclusion

Health care professionals are entrusted with people's lives, and when they make a mistake, someone may suffer indeterminate harm or even death. This is a great burden that no true professional takes lightly. Health professionals have been traditionally socialized toward the unobtainable and unrealistic goal of being infallible. Thus, when they fail or make a mistake, their self-worth is diminished and they may face emotional devastation.

How does the same system that has placed professionals on this pedestal respond to an individual's mistake? It often accuses, ostracizes, sanctions, and even sues the person involved. After all, how can an error have occurred without negligence? Regulators and accrediting agencies ask health care organizations to report adverse events, yet when they do self-report, they are often punished with fines, probation, or even worse consequences. Is it really surprising that in a punitive (as opposed to a learning-oriented) safety culture that practitioners seek to conceal their mistakes or try to shift blame?

Patient safety improvements will only come about when leaders in health care organizations and the professionals providing care accept the notion that error is "an inevitable accompaniment of the human condition, even among conscientious professionals with high standards" (Leape, 1994). The very institutions that educate and regulate these clinicians must be the primary change agents for creating a learning-oriented safety culture. Only with acknowledgment that complete elimination of errors is beyond human control can we direct necessary focus on changing the systems in which humans work.

Changes in attitudes and practices—in short, culture change—will not occur overnight. People do not easily amend well-worn habits of thoughts and deeds. The physicist Max Planck wrote: "A new scientific truth does not triumph by convincing its opponents and making them see the light, but rather because its opponents eventually die, and a new generation grows up that is familiar with it" (cited in Millenson, 1997). The medical profession was issued an unprecedented challenge in May 1996 by the American Medical Association when this group announced that "it's time to acknowledge that medical mistakes happen—are even common" (Prager, 1996).

There is compelling evidence from the work under way in other complex industries that many medical errors can be eliminated with systems redesign and improved teamwork and through the sheer willpower of people committed to making it happen. Unfortunately, there are no quick fixes or magic bullets. Rather, research reveals a broad set of factors involved in failures related to potential and actual adverse events. Consequently, multiple directions for improvements must be coordinated to make progress on patient safety (Aspden,

Corrigan, Wolcott, & Erickson, 2004). To uphold our professional commitment to "first do no harm," we are now pursuing each and every one of these new directions.

Discussion Questions

1. Describe how the expectation of perfection among health care practitioners can undermine patient safety efforts.

2. Describe three system or task redesigns that will decrease the possibility of mistakes caused by latent failures.

3. Explain why a culture that punishes people for mistakes contributes to an unsafe culture.

Key Terms

Accident

Active failure

Adverse event

Barrier

Checklist

Close call

Complex system

Error

Failure mode and effect
  analysis

Forcing function

Harm

Hazard

High-risk process

Human factors
  analysis

Human factors
  engineering

Latent failure

Mistake

Mistake-proof processes

Operator

Patient incident

Patient safety

Patient safety culture

Preventable

Risk

Risk assessment

Risk management

Sentinel event

Swiss cheese model

System failure

Violation

References

ACSNI. (1993). *Advisory committee on the safety of nuclear installations, study group on human factors. Third report: Organizing for safety*. HMSO, London.

Amarasingham, R., Plantinga, L., Diener-West, M., Gaskin, D., & Powe, N. (2009). Clinical information technologies and inpatient outcomes. *Archives of Internal Medicine, 169*(2), 108–114.

Aspden, P., Corrigan, J., Wolcott, J., & Erickson, S. (Eds). (2004). *Patient safety: Achieving a new standard for care.* Washington, DC: National Academies Press.

Botwinick, L., Bisognano, & Haraden, C. (2006). *Leadership guide to patient safety.* IHI Innovation Series white paper. Cambridge, MA: Institute for Healthcare Improvement.

Burgmeier, J. (2002). Failure mode and effect analysis: An application in reducing risk in blood transfusion. *Joint Commission Journal of Quality Improvement, 28*(6), 331–339.

Clancy, C. M. (2007). Mistake-proofing in health care: Lessons for ongoing patient safety improvements. *American Journal of Medical Quality, 22*(6), 463–465.

Cohoon, B. D. (2003). Learning from near misses through reflection: A new risk management strategy. *Journal of Healthcare Risk Management, 23*(2), 19–25.

Cook, R., & Woods, D. (1994). Operating at the sharp end: The complexity of human error. In M. S. Bogner (Ed.), *Human error in medicine.* Hillsdale, NJ: Erlbaum.

Ginsburg, L., Chuang, Y., Berta, W., Norton, P., Ng, P., Tregunno, D., & Richardson, J. (2010). The relationship between organizational leadership for safety and learning from patient safety events. *Health Services Research, 45*(3), 607–632.

Grout, J. R. (2007). *Mistake-proofing the design of health care processes.* Rockville, MD: Agency for Healthcare Research and Quality.

Healthgrades. (2008). *Fifth annual patient safety in American hospitals study.* Retrieved from http://www.healthgrades.com/media/dms/pdf/HealthGradesPatientSafety Release2008.pdf.

Helmreich, R. L. (2000). On error management: Lessons from aviation. *British Medical Journal, 320*(7237), 781–785.

Institute of Medicine. (2006). *Preventing medication errors: Quality chasm series.* Washington, DC: National Academies Press.

Keroack, M., Youngberg, B., Cerese, J., Krsek, C., Prellwitz, L., & Trevelyn, E. (2007). Organizational factors associated with high performance in quality and safety in academic medical centers. *Academic Medicine: Journal of the Association of American Medical Colleges, 82*(12), 1178–1186.

Klevens, R., Edwards, J., Richards, C., Horan, T., Gaynes, R., Pollock, D., & Cardo, D. (2002). Estimating health care–associated infections and deaths in U.S. hospitals, 2002. *Public Health Report, 122*(2), 160–166.

Lanier, W. (2006). A three-decade perspective on anesthesia safety. *American Surgeon, 72*(11), 985–989.

Leape, L. L. (1994). Error in medicine. *Journal of the American Medical Association, 272*(23), 1851–1857.

Leape, L. L., Bates, D., Cullen, D., Cooper, J., Demonaco, H., … Edmondson, A. (1995). Systems analysis of adverse drug events. *Journal of the American Medical Association, 274*(1), 35–43.

Leape, L. L., Kabcenell, A., Gandhi, T., Carver, P., Nolan, T., & Berwick, D. (2000). Reducing adverse drug events: Lessons from a breakthrough series collaborative. *Joint Commission Journal on Quality Improvement, 26*(6), 321–331.

Millenson, M. L. (1997). *Demanding medical excellence: Doctors and accountability in the information age.* Chicago: University of Chicago Press.

Nawar, E., Niska, R., & Xu, J. (2007, June 29). *National hospital ambulatory medical care survey: 2005 emergency department summary. Advance data from vital and health statistics. Number 386.* Hyattsville, MD: U.S. Department of Health and Human Services, Centers for Disease Control and Preventions, National Center for Health Statistics.

Nieva, V., & Sorra, J. (2003). Safety culture assessment: A tool for improving patient safety in healthcare organizations. *Quality and Safety in Health Care, 12* (Supplement II), ii7–ii23.

Prager, L. O. (1996). Safety-centered care. *American Medical News, 36*(6), 1.

Reason, J. (1990). The contribution of latent human failures in the breakdown of complex systems. *Philosophical Transactions of the Royal Society of London, 327*(1241), 475–484.

Reason, J. (1997). *Managing the risks of organizational accidents.* Brookfield, VT: Ashgate.

Reason, J. (2000). Human error: Models and management. *British Medical Journal, 320*(3237), 768–770.

Reason, J. (2004). Beyond the organizational accident: The need for "error wisdom" on the frontline. *Quality and Safety in Health Care, 13* (Supplement II), ii28–ii33.

Smith, A., Boult, M., Woods, I., & Johnson, S. (2010). Promoting patient safety through prospective risk identification: Example from peri-operative care. *Quality and Safety in Health Care, 19*(1), 69–73.

Sorra, J., Famolaro, T., Dyer, N., Khanna, K., & Nelson, D. (2009, March). *Hospital survey on patient safety culture: 2009 comparative database report.* Agency for Healthcare Research and Quality. Publication No. 09–0030. Retrieved from http://www .ahrq.gov/qual/hospsurvey09/hospsurv092.pdf.

The Joint Commission. (2009, January). *Universal protocol.* Retrieved from http://www .jointcommission.org/PatientSafety/UniversalProtocol/.

The Joint Commission. (2010, May). *Sentinel event statistics.* Retrieved from http://www .jointcommission.org/SentinelEvents/Statistics.

Welch, D. L. (1997). Human error and human factors engineering in health care. *Biomedical Instrumentation and Technology, 31*(6), 627–631.

World Health Organization. (2008, June). *Surgical safety checklist.* Retrieved from http:// www.who.int/patientsafety/safesurgery/tools_resources/SSSL_Checklist_ finalJun08.pdf.

Zwicker, D., & Fulmer, T. (2008). Reducing adverse drug events. In E. Capezuti, D. Zwicker, M. Mezey, & T. Fulmer (Eds.), *Evidence-based geriatric nursing protocols for best practice* (3rd ed.) (pp. 257–308). New York: Springer.

CHAPTER 2

THE HUMAN SIDE OF MEDICAL MISTAKES

Sven Ternov

LEARNING OBJECTIVES

- Understand how complex systems function and why accidents occur
- Recognize human factors that contribute to mistakes
- Identify how humans solve problems and why errors occur
- Describe the common error mechanisms

Whether it is an automobile assembly plant or a hospital, a production system consists of many organized activities whose aim is to add value to whatever is put into the system. A production system is made up of human operators and various equipment that cooperate in a structured way. The different activities in the system are often called processes. The processes take place inside an organization. The organization contains the framework of rules for how groups of humans and equipment will cooperate to achieve the production goals of the organization. When these interdependent activities reach a certain volume, the system is labeled a complex system.

Systems theory is a field of study designed to understand and describe the properties of complex systems such as biology (ecosystems), sociology, and organizations. The conceptual framework for modern risk management is derived from organizational systems theory. By using systems theory, tremendous advances have been made toward prevention of accidents in complex technical systems (for example, nuclear power, air and rail traffic, and shipping). Similar advances in the health care have been slow to materialize.

This chapter introduces a systems view of accidents and describes how accidents occur in complex systems such as health care delivery. A model from cognitive science on how people solve problems is presented together with accident prevention recommendations derived from systems theory.

Health Care: A Unique Socio-Technical System

A health care system consists of staff, equipment, buildings, and patients receiving services. These components are interdependent and interact in a complex, nonlinear way. Compared to technical complex systems, health care is much more people-intense and people-driven and is thus called a **socio-technical system** (Van Cott, 1994). People working in nuclear power and aviation, for instance, are largely supervisors of automated processes. Few health care processes are fully automated; people do much of the actual work.

The health care system is made up of numerous autonomous units or disciplines, each having its own rules, procedures, and cultures. Individuals in each discipline must cooperate toward the same goal, such as diagnosis and treatment of a patient. Informal oral communication within and between these units greatly affects performance of health care processes, whereas many technical systems rely heavily on large volumes of written instructions to guide processes. In health care, information about system changes is communicated horizontally among caregivers, often with little structure for implementation. Changes in a technical complex system are often mediated vertically in a strict hierarchical organization. Thus, revisions to health care processes can be slow and unreliable and thus add to risks.

In health care, the relationship between an action and the effect of the action is often less obvious than in a technical system. For instance, if an operator in a nuclear power plant wrongly closes a valve that depletes the core of its coolant, the effect is very certain—the core temperature will rise. If a radiologist gives the wrong diagnostic conclusion following an x-ray examination the effect is less certain. It might lead to an adverse patient incident. However, the recipient of the radiologist's report might question the conclusion or the exam result may not significantly influence future patient treatment decisions. Thus the health care system is considered *loosely coupled*, whereas technical systems often are *tightly coupled*.

Although socio-technical complex systems have some unique characteristics, many accident causation and prevention theories in technical complex systems are also applicable to health care. Commonalities are interdependency, self-organizing behavior, adaptation to external influences, and the emergence of new system properties. A consequence of these characteristics is that a complex system is difficult to manage top-down.

Accident Models

Accident models based on systems theory have emerged following investigations of several past disasters in complex systems such as the Challenger shuttle explosion, the nuclear accidents at Three Mile Island and Chernobyl, the Bhopal chemical plant disaster, King's Cross metro station fire, and the Exxon Valdez oil spill in Alaska. The work of James Reason has played a major role in introducing systemic accident models together with the concept of latent failure (Reason, 1990; Reason, 1997). These accident models, though not derived from adverse event investigations in socio-technical complex systems, are relevant to health care (Ternov & Akselsson, 2005).

Reason divides errors into two classes: *active failures* and *latent failures*. Errors made by the operators performing the processes fall into the category of active failures. Latent failures—sometimes called latent system failures or latent conditions—are risks built into the system. These risks can be at an organizational level (such as understaffed work areas, purchase of difficult-to-use equipment), at a supervisory level (such as application of unsafe procedures, rule bending, staff not adequately trained in equipment use), or local workplace factors (such as distraction or noise). Latent failures increase the likelihood of active failures (people perform poorly, commit mistakes, forget to do something, and so forth).

A single latent failure seldom causes an accident, because safeguards in the system often prevent an accident. However, latent failures can combine in unforeseen ways to create accidents and they are not specific to a particular event. For instance, a certain latent failure may contribute to several different accidents.

Latent failures may exist for a long time without causing an accident. It is usually so-called **situational factors** (unlucky circumstances) that trigger the risk presented by a latent failure. This causes the operator to commit an active failure. For example, when the midwife in the case study in Exhibit 2.1 is distracted by a colleague, a latent failure comes into play.

Not infrequently, it is difficult to distinguish between latent failures and other **contributing causes** for an accident. The following criteria can be used for distinguishing between other contributing causes and latent failures:

- Latent failures are independent of the individual. For example, lack of training, new on the job, unfamiliarity with procedures, and so on are *not* latent failures.

- It is beyond the power of frontline individuals (sometimes called "sharp end staff") to remedy latent failures. Latent failures typically relate to concerns

EXHIBIT 2.1

CASE 1. MIDWIFE TAKES WRONG DRUG VIAL OFF THE SHELF

A midwife intends to give a pregnant woman with premature labor an infusion of a drug that inhibits labor. At the moment when she is going to take the vial from the shelf, she is distracted by a question from a colleague. She continues her intended action but chooses instead a vial containing a drug that stimulates labor. Fortunately, she discovers her mistake when she does the last procedural check before coupling the infusion set to the patient's intravenous line.

Commentary: The procedure that allowed a drug that inhibits labor to be stored on the shelf close to a drug that stimulates labor had never before resulted in a medication error. When the midwife was distracted (situational factor) the latent failure (faulty drug vial storage procedure) contributed to the midwife's selecting the wrong drug from the shelf. Another latent failure might be the working procedures that allow a nurse to be interrupted during medication preparation.

such as staffing practices, procedures, and organizational climate. These are issues that can only be remedied by management.

Safety Barriers

A safety barrier is an administrative or technical constraint that can act in one of two ways to prevent accidents. The safety barrier can hinder the individual from committing an active failure or it can contain the effect of the active failure. An example of a technical barrier is the manner in which ECG-electrodes are designed to prevent them from being plugged into the main power supply. The computerized system for prescribing drugs, which requires that dosage, route, and frequency be entered for all medication orders, is another example of a technical barrier.

A procedure that requires double checks of information before action by an individual is taken is an example of an administrative barrier. Safety barriers can be weak or strong and might even be called absolute or relative, depending on the barrier's ability to contain the effect of, or to prevent, active failures. It is easier to make technical barriers absolute, whereas active failures may slip through the cracks of administrative barriers.

FIGURE 2.1   Typical Medical Accident Trajectory

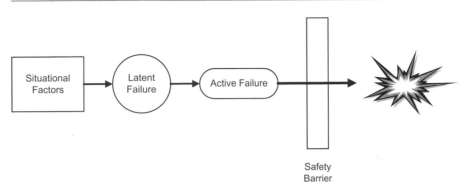

The Accident Trajectory

The relationship between situational factors, active and latent failures, and safety barriers in a medical accident is illustrated by the typical **accident trajectory** in Figure 2.1. A real accident situation is far more complex than suggested by this model. It is common to find that several latent failures were activated and these failures interacted with each other in a complicated manner before the **system defenses** (safety barriers) were breached to such an extent that an accident occurred.

Mechanisms that contribute to accidents in complex systems are summarized in the following list. Current concepts in modern risk management suggest that accidents in complex systems basically result from human-system interface problems. For example, poorly designed patient hospital rooms—inconvenient electrical outlets, hard-to-reach bed controls, inadequate supply storage, and the like—can cause human-system misfits that contribute to an accident.

- Several latent failures contribute to the accident.

- Latent failures can be found at different organizational levels: top management, supervision, and local workplace.

- Latent failures act as error traps for the operators, or create a messy problem-solving environment, or impede error detection.

- Safety barriers are insufficient or not in place.

- Situational factors trigger the risks in the system.

To prevent unexpected and undesirable patient outcomes that may result from human-system misfits, health care providers must have a better understanding of humans as problem solvers in a complex system, the interface between humans and the systems in which they function, and how humans exert influence on the system. In the next section readers learn more about how people make decisions and why social and system influences can cause human errors.

Humans as Problem Solvers

Certain models from the discipline of cognitive psychology help in understanding how humans solve problems and why errors occur. These models concern the concepts of long-term and working memory and the skill-rule-knowledge model for problem solving. The environment also affects the reliability of problem solving. Less than desirable work situations and stressful personal circumstances can greatly increase the chance of a mistake.

Long-Term and Working Memory

Long-term memory is a sort of knowledge database with seemingly unlimited capacity. Our long-term memory works quickly and without cognitive effort. It can process parallel bits of information and knowledge retrieval is mainly subconscious. Working memory, on the contrary, is slow and conscious. Working memory can only process one thing at a time (serial processing) and has a very limited capacity. Our working memory directs our attention to that part of a problem we are consciously dealing with. Due to the serial processing of the working memory we can only focus on one thing at a time. With training and experience, however, humans can learn to switch attention very fast.

According to one of several models in cognitive psychology, knowledge is stored in the long-term memory in chunks of information called schematas (or scripts or frames). Schematas contain knowledge structured in a functional way so that it is retrieved in a ready-to-use fashion and is made up of our previous experience of similar situations. The schematas are stored in a hierarchical system with main rules for solving a problem (for instance, a diagnostic problem) on the top, with side rules and exceptions from the rules further down in the hierarchy. The novice has only a limited number of schematas with main rules, but the expert problem solver has stored a lot of side rules and exceptions from the main rules.

Schematas have different strengths. A strong schema is more readily retrieved (and applied) than a weak one. What makes a schema strong is how recently and how frequently it has been used. That is, if a problem solver often uses solution A to a problem, the chances are high that he or she will use solution A instead of solution B even if solution B is the better choice or solution A downright wrong. The case study in Exhibit 2.2 illustrates how a physician's strong schema was unfortunately not the right choice.

EXHIBIT 2.2

CASE 2. WRONG METHOD USED FOR ANESTHESIA

A 42-year-old women undergoes a partial thyroidectomy. Shortly after the operation she shows signs of developing a hematoma in the wound area. The surgeon and the patient's nurse monitor this situation carefully for the next four hours. The surgeon finally decides to bring the patient back to the operating room for removal of the hematoma. He notifies the anesthesiologist by phone and later has a very short oral communication with him in a corridor outside the operating room. The surgeon then goes off to attend to some other matter and leaves the anesthesiologist in charge of the patient. The patient is doing fairly well and can talk to the anesthesiologist.

The anesthesiologist believes it best to intubate the patient right away. He starts an intravenous line, administers muscle relaxant, and then attempts to intubate the patient. The intubation is not successful and he tries to ventilate the patient with a mask, which also fails. He makes a new attempt to intubate the patient and initially believes the tube is in the patient's trachea, but after another minute finds the second intubation is also a failure. Now the surgeon has arrived and a lot of other staff as well. Some debate is going on between surgeon and anesthesiologist whether or not the patient is properly intubated. The situation is close to panic. After six minutes and more attempts, successful ventilation is finally established, but this is too late and the patient expires.

Skill-Based, Rule-Based, and Knowledge-Based Problem Solving

After studying operators who control complex technical systems (mainly nuclear power), Rasmussen and his associates (1986) suggested that human problem solving can be categorized into the following three levels:

1. Skill-based

2. Rule-based

3. Knowledge-based

Often referred to as the SRK model, this approach has been used in a large number of human factors studies.

Skill-based problem solving is used in highly automated work processes and involves stereotypical motor movements, like working on an assembly line, driving a car, or retrieving medication vials from a storage area. Rule-based problem solving is used in novel situations, in which we are able to recognize features from similar situations. The anesthesiologist in case #2 (Exhibit 2.2) was presented with a situation that he presumed was similar to other situations he had encountered. The anesthesiologist made a rule-based decision to intubate the patient right away, which later proved to be the wrong choice. The anesthesiologist performed the intubation the way he was used to doing it; that is, he gave the patient a muscle relaxant and then intubated. He used a rule that he very frequently used to solve this kind of problem and thus the rule was strong. But it was also a wrong rule. The anesthesiologist had a poor understanding of the situation, causing him to "read" the wrong cues. It might have helped if the surgeon had better conveyed to the anesthesiologist the patient's background and the dynamics of the problem. Lack of communication caused the problem to be cognitively underspecified for the anesthesiologist—a common cause for reading a problem wrong.

The use of a "strong-but-wrong" schema is not the whole explanation for the tragic outcome described in case #2. Often many things must go wrong before a patient is lost. This was also the situation in this case. Among other problems, the equipment for monitoring carbon dioxide in the patient's expiratory air was missing, thus delaying the detection of esophageal intubation.

According to one model (Reason, 1990) the schema or rules are "tagged" with certain "cues." When encountering a problem, the operator deciphers or "reads" the problem to identify relevant cues for solving the problem. These read cues are then matched against what is stored in the operator's working memory, and hopefully, a rule or solution that fits the problem is retrieved and applied to the situation. Supposedly, reading problem cues and retrieving a relevant solution occurs subconsciously, whereas application of the solution is a conscious act.

The operator uses knowledge-based problem solving in novel situations in which a ready solution to the problem cannot be retrieved from working memory. In knowledge-based problem solving it appears that we try to restructure the problem to give us hints as to which ready-made solutions from our long-term memory could be applied to the situation.

Error Mechanisms in the SRK Model

Mistakes caused by different error mechanisms can occur at each of the three problem-solving levels: **skill-based**, **rule-based**, and **knowledge-based errors**.

Skill-Based Errors

These errors are often labeled *slips* or *lapses*. The intention is right but the execution is wrong. These errors originate in the stereotype nature of the motor movements in this kind of "problem solving." The work is mainly done without conscious control, such as driving a car along a highway under favorable conditions or filling a syringe with medication. Now and then it is necessary to apply conscious control to ensure that the automatic actions proceed as intended. If this control is missed, you may find yourself speeding past the intended exit or administering the wrong medication. These conscious controls are very sensitive to distraction. As the operator is often not aware of committing a "slip of the mind" these errors are seldom detected in real-time. An example of a slip is found in case #1 (Exhibit 2.1). Thankfully, the midwife double-checked herself and was able to avert an adverse incident.

Rule-Based Errors

This type of error is often called a *mistake*. The intention is wrong because the operator applies a wrong rule. Misreading the problem is a common cause of retrieving the wrong rule. A problem can be misread because it is cognitively underspecified or because our attention is captured by salient but less important problem features. A cognitively underspecified problem is a problem where the important cues are difficult to read or detect. Several latent system failures contribute to this difficulty, such as inadequate presentation of necessary information or poor equipment design (for example, machine displays are difficult to read or understand).

Even if the problem is read correctly and the matching rule is retrieved, an error can still occur if the rule is wrong. Frequently and recently used rules are more easily retrieved. This is not a guarantee that they are correct. The rules may be strong but wrong. If an operator applies a not-so-good rule the circumstances will show this. The problem is not getting solved and things start to take a turn for the worse. At this point, the operator may be influenced by an error mechanism known as *confirmation bias*. This very powerful bias mechanism works like this: we subconsciously suppress new information signaling the problem is not getting solved and give undue attention only to information that reinforces the correctness of our course of action. Confirmation bias can cause people to continue with the wrong way of solving a problem for a much longer time than necessary. The information is there, but it is not noticed. Case #3 in Exhibit 2.3 illustrates the effect of confirmation bias on patient treatment decisions.

EXHIBIT 2.3

CASE 3. MISSED DIAGNOSIS OF DIABETIC KETOACIDOSIS

An elderly gentleman was brought to the emergency department complaining of breathing difficulties. He had a known asthmatic condition; however, the asthma medication he took at home had not brought relief to his symptoms. On physical examination the expected findings of wheezing were heard on the lungs, which disappeared with the usual infusion of asthma drugs. The patient's breathing difficulties, however, got only slightly better. The patient was admitted to an inpatient bed. X-ray studies of the patient's lungs did not show anything special and his condition remained a puzzle to several physicians.

After some hours a new doctor came on duty. Upon entering the patient's room, she immediately smelled acetone and located the laboratory test in the patient's chart, which revealed the patient's high blood glucose level and a very pathological acid-base balance. Within 30 seconds this physician made the correct diagnosis of diabetic ketoacidosis, a severe, life-threatening condition in diabetics, where the glucose regulation is utterly out of control. The physicians who had earlier treated the patient had their attention on the wrong condition. The asthma "label" followed the patient for hours before the real diagnosis was discovered.

Knowledge-Based Errors

Errors in knowledge-based problem solving are also considered mistakes. When presented with new situations, the individual makes an error due to lack of knowledge. Although knowledge deficits are more common with trainees or novices, experienced individuals can make knowledge-based errors. As mentioned before, the working memory is only able to process information serially (one thing at a time). This serial processing may cause us to wrongly focus on relatively unimportant parts of a problem. This serial processing can also cause

EXHIBIT 2.4

CASE 4. NURSE ADMINISTERS TEN TIMES THE PRESCRIBED AMOUNT OF INSULIN

The setting is a long-term care unit. An elderly patient with diabetes has stumbled and x-ray confirms a luxation of his hip prosthesis. During the evening the orthopedic surgeon makes an unsuccessful attempt under anesthesia to reduce the luxation. The surgeon orders the patient to be prepared for surgery for the next morning and the patient is transferred back to the long-term care unit.

The night nurse in the long-term care unit has very little experience in preparing patients for surgery. She tries to carry out the surgeon's orders, which are stated in very general terms and refer to numerous vaguely worded procedures. The nurse finds these procedures difficult to understand and they are apparently very outdated. She has to make several phone calls to physicians and staff to ask questions about what to do. Among other issues, she is very confused about the insulin infusion she has to prepare for the patient. When she finally calculates the dose of insulin, she commits an error and administers ten times too much insulin. The medication error was not detected until the caregivers in the post-anesthesia care unit had a difficult time awakening the patient. After checking the blood glucose level, which was very low, glucose was administered, the patient recovered, and the accident had a happy ending (for the patient, not the nurse).

knowledge-based errors. Time is often a limiting factor in medical problem solving and we may jump to conclusions or act before our working memory has processed all information. The case described in Exhibit 2.4 illustrates a knowledge-based error.

The nurse who made the medication error had very little experience with preoperative procedures. Thus her similarity matching for stored rules to solve the problem gave a meager result. She had to switch to knowledge-based problem solving and slowly, serially, and meticulously worked her way through the problem. During the hours of early morning when she finally was expected to prepare an insulin infusion, her working memory resources were depleted and she made the final miscalculation of insulin.

Conclusion

Risk management in areas where great disasters have occurred (nuclear power, air and rail traffic, shipping) has made tremendous advances during the past decade in understanding accident mechanisms in complex technical systems. Unfortunately, investigations of medical accidents are still largely a matter of finding and punishing the humans involved. This obsolete approach to medical accident investigations has serious negative effects:

- Staff members accused of having caused an accident feel guilt and shame during the rest of their professional career. This may have a negative effect on their future ability as problem solvers.

- The latent failures causing the accidents are not identified, thus there is no learning.

- Litigation is costly and the money could have been spent more productively on proper preventive actions.

Health care production takes place in what can be called a complex system. Risk management in complex technical systems has made tremendous advances during the past two decades but has thus far been applied only to a limited extent to health care, though health care also is a complex system, though a socio-technical system. The modern way of looking at accidents suggests that they basically result from interface problems between human and system.

The mechanisms contributing to human error can be understood from cognitive models concerning our problem-solving strategies. Our memory data-base is the long-term memory, which has seemingly unlimited capacity for storing information and works outside our conscious control. The working memory, on the contrary, is the conscious part of our thinking. It has a very limited capacity and quickly gets overloaded. Our working memory directs our attention toward important parts of a problem. By applying this knowledge concerning cognitive strategies, accident investigators can recognize how latent system failures exert negative influence on the caregiver's problem-solving capacity.

Discussion Questions

1. Describe the difference between a complex technical system and a complex socio-technical system. How do these differences affect safety improvement strategies?

2. What type of errors (skill-based, rule-based, and knowledge-based) contributed to the event described at the beginning of Chapter One?

3. Describe the difference between an active error and a latent failure. Give an example of each type of failure.

Key Terms

Accident trajectory	Rule-based error	Socio-technical system
Contributing cause	Situational factor	System defense
Knowledge-based error	Skill-based error	Systems theory

References

Rasmussen, J. (1986). Skills, rules and knowledge: Signals, signs and symbols, and other distinctions in human performance models. *IEEE Transaction on Systems, Man and Cybernetics, 13*(3), 257–266.

Reason, J. T. (1990). *Human error: Causes and consequences.* New York: Cambridge University Press.

Reason, J. T. (1997). *Managing the risks of organizational accidents.* Aldershot, UK: Ashgate.

Ternov, S., & Akselsson, R. (2005). System weaknesses as contributing causes for accidents in health care. *International Journal for Quality in Health Care, 17*(1), 1–9.

Van Cott, H. (1994). Human errors: Their causes and reductions. In S. Bogner (Ed.), *Human error in medicine.* Hillsdale, NJ: Erlbaum.

CHAPTER 3

HIGH RELIABILITY AND PATIENT SAFETY

Yosef D. Dlugacz
Patrice L. Spath

LEARNING OBJECTIVES

- Define the five basic principles of high-reliability organizations
- Understand how high-reliability principles can improve patient safety
- Recognize the relationship between patient safety culture characteristics and HRO principles
- Describe steps for improving the reliability of health care processes

High-reliability organizations (HROs) operate under difficult conditions with a great potential for errors. These organizations are considered high reliability because they experience fewer accidents than would be anticipated given the high-risk nature of the work. Some industries recognized as being highly reliable are naval and commercial aviation and nuclear power. The complex systems in these organizations consistently perform nearly error free, thereby avoiding potentially catastrophic failures.

Two factors contribute to the creation of HROs. First, senior leaders create an environment where everyone is keenly aware of the error potential in operations and safe behaviors and attitudes are rewarded. This culture of safety positively influences the reliability of systems and processes (Weick, 1987). In addition, work processes are designed to be reliable, which results in tasks being performed as expected a high proportion of the time. The combination of a supportive safety culture and **reliable processes** is essential to high reliability.

Health care organizations, especially hospitals caring for patients with serious conditions, are complex, high-risk systems. In contrast to HROs, the systems in health care organizations do not consistently perform nearly error free (Gaba, 2000). Patient safety is not always viewed as a strategic priority around which the entire efforts of the organization must be focused (Pronovost et al., 2003). Because processes are not well designed, people's vigilance and hard work are relied on to prevent accidents. System failures are often treated by local fixes rather than systematic reforms (Reason, Carthey, & de Leval, 2001).

The combination of supportive safety culture and process reliability found in HROs is lacking in most health care organizations. Resar (2006) posited four common themes to explain why health care delivery is not reliable:

- Improvements are dependent on caregivers' vigilance and hard work.

- Mediocre benchmarks give a false sense of reliability.

- Tolerance for clinical autonomy results in performance variation.

- Processes are not designed to meet specific reliability goals.

Often health care leaders understand what must be done to increase reliability, but struggle with how to accomplish it (Dixon & Shofer, 2006). In this chapter, readers learn what health care organizations can do to advance high-reliability principles and process improvement techniques that have proven to be successful in preventing accidents in other complex, high-risk industries.

High-Reliability Principles

HROs strive to avoid errors by stressing a commitment to consistently safe and reliable operations. This commitment is referred to as **collective mindfulness**. Weick and Sutcliffe, HRO theorists, describe this as a "clear and detailed comprehension of emerging threats and on factors that interfere with such comprehension" (2007, p. 33).

Readers may be more familiar with the concept of individual mindfulness. At the individual level, mindfulness represents "a heightened state of involvement and wakefulness or being in the present" (Langer & Moldoveanu, 2000, p. 2). Collective mindfulness also involves a heightened state of involvement or being, but at the organizational level. Mindful organizations are very sensitive to variations in their environment and continually update safety assumptions and perspectives (Fiol & O'Connor, 2003; Weick & Sutcliffe, 2007). Consistently safe and reliable operations rely on both individual and collective mindfulness.

Qualitative research in HROs suggest that collective mindfulness is created when organizations adopt five basic principles (Weick & Sutcliffe, 2007):

1. Sensitivity to operations

2. Preoccupation with failure

3. Deference to expertise

4. Commitment to **resilience**

5. Reluctance to simplify interpretations

Sensitivity to Operations

Being sensitive to operations is a belief that everyone—from senior leaders to frontline workers—must individually and collectively understand the big picture of current organizational operations. In an HRO, diverse information and viewpoints are shared at all levels throughout the organization. Sharing promotes systemwide knowledge of operations that facilitates error detection and prevention at the frontlines.

Preoccupation with Failure

Preoccupation with failure is a belief that the system is flawed and failure is always possible. Small mistakes are recognized as precursors of potentially catastrophic events. Therefore, HROs encourage individuals to monitor operations for even the smallest of mistakes. People are not fearful of retaliation when reporting unsafe situations and actual incidents. HROs actively evaluate operations to identify where errors might occur before they actually happen.

Deference to Expertise

Deference to expertise is a belief that decisions should be made by those with the greatest relevant expertise. HROs understand that rigid hierarchical decision making can lead to mistakes, especially during high-risk situations. People within the organization who have expertise in solving specific problems are consulted. In times of trouble or when the pace of operations change, decision-making authority can be easily shifted to individuals with the most expertise, regardless of their hierarchical position.

Commitment to Resilience

Being committed to resilience is a belief that all errors cannot be prevented. An HRO develops practices and procedures for quickly addressing and containing evitable mistakes to minimize the escalating consequences. In an HRO, workers are trained to anticipate errors and are not caught by surprise when mistakes occur.

Reluctance to Simplify Interpretations

Reluctance to simplify is a belief that the environment and the tasks of the organization are interactively complex. HROs are unwilling to accept the common tendency to provide simple answers to complex problems. Simplification runs the risk of covering up important information.

Principles of high reliability provide a way for organizations to *think* about safe processes and a safe environment. It is a cognitive, not a mechanistic, approach to improving safety. Adopting HRO principles involves deliberately embracing concepts that emphasize:

- Continuous vigilance to risk, where reports of flawed processes can be made without fear of censure or retribution.

- Efficient and respectful teamwork, where the contribution of every individual is equally valued.

- Effective communication that is democratic and respectful.

- Individual and organizational mindfulness of the potential dangers involved in various processes and functions.

- Ongoing education and training.

For health care organizations to become HROs, leadership must understand and overcome the unique challenges involved in changing long-entrenched organizational and individual habits.

Applying HRO Principles to Health Care

Since the publication of two Institute of Medicine (IOM) reports about deficits in patient safety (1999, 2001), the nation's attention has been focused on reducing medical errors and unsafe practices. Although health care organizations have made efforts to address safety issues, progress has been slow and preventable errors still occur (Wachter, 2010). The goal of ensuring that patients receive consistently safe and reliable care has not been reached.

A change is needed in the way health care professionals think about patient safety and the way things are done—and we must commit to sustaining these changes. By adopting HRO principles that have benefited other complex, high-risk industries, health care organizations can further reduce mistakes and prevent errors that can lead to catastrophic consequences.

The delivery of health care services is prone to errors for many reasons. Primary among them is its complexity and variability. Patients vary in their symptoms and responses to treatment. Patients often have multiple health issues; hospitalizations often involve multiple processes and tasks, with numerous professionals attending to a single patient. Coordination of services and communication among clinicians can be problematic. In high-risk areas, such as the operating room (OR) and intensive care unit (ICU), opportunities for errors are especially plentiful because of the many patient care steps that have to be correctly performed fairly quickly. Each step represents an opportunity for error.

Many health care organizations are structured with departments that function as independent, hierarchical silos. Caregivers become complacent; accepting errors as unavoidable treatment complications. Physician autonomy is often tolerated; leading to process variability and inevitably to process unreliability (Wennberg, 2002). Commitment to patient safety improvement among leadership may be weak and the resources needed for process changes are scarce. In a 2008 survey sponsored by American College of Healthcare Executives, 77% of hospital CEOs reported financial challenges as their top concern, with only 43% identifying patient safety and quality as a major concern (American College of Healthcare Executives, 2008).

High-reliability organizations encourage individuals and groups to observe, to inquire, and to make their conclusions known and, where observations concern important aspects of the system, to actively bring them to the attention of higher management (Westrum, 1992). For health care organizations to achieve collective mindfulness by fostering the five HRO principles, a culture change is needed. Organizational values must be transformed, roles redefined, expectations revised, and risk prevention made the highest priority. In the next section, the interrelated and somewhat abstract HRO principles are described within the context of health care delivery.

Sensitivity to Operations

Adopting the principle of sensitivity to operations requires that health care organizations have a better understanding of what is happening on the frontlines of patient care. Systems and processes must be measured and analyzed with both quantitative and qualitative information (Drain & Clark, 2004). Quantitative data are necessary for policy development and qualitative data are necessary to know what patients and frontline workers actually experience. Pronovost et al. (2006) recommend patient safety be measured at the institutional, task, and team levels. At the institution level, the organization needs to know how often patients are harmed and whether a culture of safety has permeated the organization. At the task and team levels, the organization needs to know how often patients receive appropriate interventions and whether people are learning from mistakes.

There must be a climate of open communication among all caregivers. A practice that can promote open communication is reporting of **near misses**— situations in which mistakes are caught and corrected before patient harm occurs. Reports of near miss events reveal operational trouble spots requiring further investigation. Organizational leaders must constantly emphasize the value of reporting these events for learning purposes. At the University of Louisville, for example, one near miss event is talked about each week at their morbidity and mortality conference (McCafferty & Polk, 2004). Regular discussion of near miss events heightens everyone's sensitivity to operations and reinforces the benefit of pointing out safety problems.

Preoccupation with Failure

In health care organizations preoccupied with failure, people are not complacent. Staff members are alert to the possibility of errors and concerned with doing tasks safety. For example, in a high-reliability health care organization the OR circulating nurse understands the importance of proper patient positioning and is careful to avoid mistakes. In an HRO, everyone that interacts with patients— food delivery staff, maintenance workers, clinicians, transport staff, and the like—is attentive to the potential danger of patient falls. People know how to keep patients from falling and they feel empowered to take action when they see a fall-risk situation. Health care delivery routine tasks do not become automatic and "mindless" in a highly reliable organization. To counter complacency, staff members continually and carefully monitor actions for even the smallest of errors or mistakes. Incidents and near misses are reported and dissected for cause and effect and work routines adjusted accordingly to improve process reliability.

Trinity Health System's Potential Error and Event Reporting System (PEERs) is an example of a successful error reporting initiative (Conlon, Havlisch, Kini, & Porter, 2008). Information reported into the PEERs Web-based system from 32 different hospitals and four home health agencies allows the organization, both at the local level and the system level, to identify and respond quickly to operational hazards. Approximately 90% of the 4,000 reports filed each month represent incidents and near misses that did not cause significant harm to patients. Analysis of these events reduces complacency and provides Trinity Health with the opportunity to identify and correct weaknesses proactively (Conlon et al., 2008).

Deference to Expertise

HROs make use of expertise within the organization and everyone's contribution is respected. This is not the norm in many health care organizations, where work often is conducted in "silos" with little understanding of the expertise of other disciplines, services, and staff. This is particularly problematic when the health care team is caring for patients at high risk for complications.

Research at the University of Pittsburgh Medical Center (UPMC) illustrates how deference to the relevant expertise of a care team member can ultimately improve patient safety and service efficiency. Harbrecht et al. (2009) report that UPMC respiratory therapist-driven protocols for assessment and management of non-ICU patients decreased hospital stays and overall hospital costs. Rather than viewing the therapists' involvement as "wrongly taking patient management out of my hands," UPMC physicians acknowledged (and ultimately validated) the value of the therapists' expertise.

Caregivers are interdependent, with effective and respectful collaboration necessary to ensure reliably safe patient care. Research shows that people working effectively together as a team make fewer errors than individuals acting on their own (Baker, Day, & Salas, 2006).

Commitment to Resilience

A resilient health care organization demonstrates two main capabilities: (1) the ability to learn, particularly from mistakes; and (2) the ability to quickly respond as events change over time and divert resources (knowledge, people, and equipment) to where the resources would be best used (Sutcliffe & Vogue, 2003).

In high-reliability health care organizations, a commitment to resilience is evident in a number of practices and procedures, such as the formation of prospective **risk assessment** teams (Bonnabry et al., 2006; Abujudeh & Kaewlai, 2006) and simulation-based training, that expose physicians and staff to new problems or unusual situations (Ziv, Small, & Wolpe, 2000; Henneman & Cunningham, 2005). Heightened error awareness and ongoing training are crucial components of HROs so that innovative safety solutions can be designed and implemented after a problem occurs.

Reluctance to Simplify Interpretations

Workers in high-reliability health care organizations are actively encouraged to question the way things are done and to question decisions made by others. Frequent interactions among care team members with diverse opinions are encouraged. For example, a patient safety specialist at Duke University Medical Center in Raleigh, North Carolina, regularly visits different clinical areas to learn about the patient safety concerns of frontline staff and gather their opinions on how risks can be reduced (Frush, Alton, & Frush, 2006).

Health care organizations must be unwilling to accept simple solutions to complex patient safety problems. An example of a complex problem is patient wandering behavior that can result in elopement. Of the 263 root cause analyses of missing patient events submitted by Veterans Administration (VA) facilities to the National Patient Safety Center, only 15% of the actions taken to prevent recurrence of a similar event were considered strong—an action that would eliminate vulnerabilities by making it impossible to do a task incorrectly (DeRosier, Taylor, Turner, & Bagian, 2007). The VA researchers found that when a strong action was developed and implemented, it was 2.5 times more likely to be effective as compared to intermediate and weak actions.

HRO Self-Assessment

Is your organization sufficiently sensitive to operations? Are caregivers preoccupied with failure? In high-risk situations, is expertise more important than hierarchical decision making? Do people hide from mistakes or seek to learn from them? When things go wrong, are quick-fix solutions too often the common response? Assess your organization's progress in adopting each HRO principle by determining your level of agreement with the statements listed in Exhibit 3.1.

EXHIBIT 3.1

ORGANIZATION SELF-ASSESSMENT OF HIGH-RELIABILITY PRINCIPLES

Score your organization from 1 to 5 for each statement.

1 = strongly disagree

2 = somewhat disagree

3 = neither agree nor disagree

4 = somewhat agree

5 = strongly agree

I. Sensitivity to Operations	**Score (1–5)**
1. Should problems occur during patient care delivery someone with the authority to act is always accessible and available to people on the front lines.	

2. Supervisors readily pitch in to assist with patient care whenever necessary.
3. During an average day we communicate sufficiently with one another to build a clear picture of the current situation with patients.
4. Managers and senior leaders are always looking for feedback from frontline workers about patient care activities that aren't going right.
5. People are familiar with tasks beyond their immediate jobs.
6. We have access to consultation or resources when unexpected patient care surprises crop up.
7. Senior leaders and managers frequently review information about safe practices and hazards at the front lines of patient care.
8. Managers constantly monitor workloads and are able to obtain additional resources or reduce workload if work becomes excessive.

Section I subtotal:

	Score (1–5)
II. Preoccupation with Failure	

1. We focus more on our patient care failures than on our successes.
2. We regard close calls and near misses as a kind of failure that reveals potential danger rather than evidence of our ability to avoid a harmful patient care event.
3. We treat near misses and errors as information about the safety of our patient care system and try to learn from them.
4. We often update our procedures after experiencing a close call or near miss to incorporate our learning and enriched understanding of hazards.
5. It is hard for people to hide patient care mistakes of any kind.
6. People are inclined to report patient care mistakes that have significant consequences even if nobody notices.
7. Managers seek out and report bad news about our patient care processes.
8. People are rewarded if they spot patient care problems, mistakes, errors or failures.

Section II subtotal:

	Score (1–5)
III. Deference to Expertise	

1. Everyone is committed to doing their job well.
2. People respect the nature and importance of one another's job activities.
3. If something out of the ordinary happens people know who has the expertise to respond.
4. People in this organization value expertise and experience over hierarchical rank.
5. In this organization the people most qualified to make decisions that affect patient care processes are the people who make the decisions.
6. If something unexpected occurs during patient care delivery the most highly qualified people, regardless of rank, make the decision in how to proceed.

7. People typically "own" a problem until it is resolved.
8. It is generally easy to obtain expert assistance when something comes up that the frontline staff members don't know how to handle.

Section III subtotal:

IV. Commitment to Resilience	Score (1–5)

1. Resources are continually devoted to training and retraining people on safe patient care practices.
2. People have more than enough training and experience for the kind of patient care they are assigned to do.
3. This organization is actively concerned with developing everyone's patient care skills and knowledge.
4. People around here are known for their ability to be innovative in designing safer patient care processes.
5. Building people's competence and repertoire of responses to unexpected patient care situations is a priority.
6. People have a number of informal contacts that they sometimes use to solve patient care problems.
7. People always learn from their mistakes.
8. People are always able to rely on one another for assistance.

Section IV subtotal:

V. Reluctance to Simplify Interpretations	Score (1–5)

1. People around here take nothing for granted when it comes to the provision of patient care; we strive to challenge—not maintain—the status quo.
2. Questioning about patient care is openly encouraged.
3. People in this organization feel free to bring up problems and tough issues relating to patient safety.
4. People generally prolong their analysis of patient care problems to better grasp the nature and cause of the problems.
5. People are encouraged to express differing viewpoints regarding patient care activities.
6. When differing viewpoints are expressed, people listen carefully; it is rare that someone's view is dismissed.
7. People are not shot down for surfacing information that could interrupt patient care operations.
8. When an adverse event occurs, people are more concerned with listening and conducting a complete analysis of the situation rather than advocating their point of view or jumping to conclusions.

Section V subtotal:

HRO Self-Assessment Total (sum of all five sections)

Source: Spath, P. L. (2010, March). Advancing innovation and sustainable improvements in patient safety. Conference sponsored by the Maryland Patient Safety Center, Elkridge, MD. Used with permission. Adapted from: Weick, K. E. & Sutcliffe. K. M. (2007). *Managing the unexpected: Resilient performance in an age of uncertainty* (2nd ed.). San Francisco: Jossey-Bass, 2007.

Safety Culture Versus High-Reliability Principles

Patient safety experts are urging health care facilities to adopt a culture of safety that permeates the organization. Organizations with a positive safety culture are characterized by communications founded on mutual trust, by shared perceptions of the importance of safety, and by confidence in the efficacy of preventative measures (Pizzi, Goldfarb, & Nash, 2001). Various researchers have substantiated the relationship between a positive safety culture and fewer mistakes (see, for example, Hickam et al., 2003; McFadden, Stock, & Gowen, 2006; Angermeier, Dunford, Boss, Boss, & Miller, 2009). Why should health care organizations adopt HRO principles if a positive safety culture is sufficient?

Many of the statements corresponding to the five HRO principles (Exhibit 3.1) also describe an organization with a positive safety culture, however there are some subtle but important differences. Only a portion of the behaviors documented in case studies of HROs are measured by most patient safety culture survey instruments (Vogus & Sutcliffe, 2007). Drawing on their own research on HROs and their fieldwork in health care, Vogus and Sutcliffe translated the five HRO principles into nine corresponding survey items with which to evaluate the actions and interactions of hospital nurses. Instead of asking whether, for example, nurses feel like their mistakes are held against them (U.S. Department of Health and Human Services, 2009), the HRO-based survey asks if nurses spend time discussing what patient safety risks to look out for (preoccupation with failure). Instead of asking whether other people help out when the unit gets busy (U.S. Department of Health and Human Services, 2009), the HRO-based survey asks if collective expertise is rapidly pooled to respond to patient crises (deference to expertise). The HRO-based survey asks if nurses are aware of the talents and skills of other people on the unit (sensitivity to operations), whether they talk about how errors can be prevented (commitment to resilience), and whether alternatives to normal work activities are discussed (reluctance to simplify).

Creating a positive patient safety culture involves factors that promote safety, such as leadership involvement, creation of safer processes and procedures, and encouragement of open communication and reporting of errors. The five interrelated HRO principles focus on the behavioral aspects of patient safety that create collective mindfulness among frontline employees. Collective mindfulness allows HROs such as aircraft carrier flight desks and nuclear power plants to operate in a nearly error-free environment. Collective mindfulness can also reduce errors in the complex environment of health care delivery where work is highly interdependent and time pressures are common. Survey instruments such as the nine-item Safety Organizing Scale developed by Vogus and Sutcliffe (2007) measure concrete behaviors positively associated with patient safety that are not commonly measured by many patient safety culture surveys (Colla, Bracken, Kinney, & Weeks, 2005).

Highly Reliable Processes

One aspect of achieving high reliability in a health care organization is creation of a positive safety culture that includes adoption of HRO principles. However, culture change alone is not sufficient; it must be coupled with creation of more reliable work processes. Reliability is the measurable capability of a process, procedure, or health service to perform its intended function in the required time under commonly occurring conditions (Berwick & Nolan, 2003). A reliable process is one that performs as expected a high proportion of the time. An **unreliable process** is one that performs as expected a low proportion of the time. Unfortunately, many health care processes fall into the unreliable category (Amalberti, Auroy, Berwick, & Barach, 2005).

In the next section, readers are introduced to **reliability science** concepts and steps for changing an unreliable process into one that performs as expected a high proportion of the time. Specific techniques for improving the reliability of health care processes are detailed in several of the later chapters.

Creating Reliable Processes

In Chapter Two Dr. Ternov describes how humans solve problems and why mistakes occur. These factors influence how health care professionals interact with the systems of patient care. The science of human factors engineering (sometimes called reliability science) involves creating a "good fit" between humans and work processes (Luria, Muething, Schoettker, & Kotagal, 2006). Since the 1940s, researchers have studied human-system interactions in various industries to determine the best way to minimize human "malfunctions" (Van Cott, 1994). The findings are now being used to improve human-system interactions in health care. Several researchers have applied the reliability improvement lessons learned in other industries to health care processes (see, for example, Nolan, 2000; Gosbee, 2002; Resar, 2006; Nemeth, Wears, Woods, Hollnagel, & Cook, 2008).

Though there are many ways of making a process more reliable, human factors research suggests that certain actions are more likely to result in sustained improvements. For instance, it is unlikely that staff retraining will result in fewer errors, especially considering that most mistakes are made by individuals already known to be competent at doing their jobs. Nolan's hierarchy of controls, based on reliability science, is presented in descending order of power to effect lasting change (2000):

1. Engineer the problem away

2. Reduce complexity of tasks

3. Optimize information processing

4. Automate wisely

5. Use procedural constraints

6. Use cultural constraints

The patient safety improvement action categories developed by the Department of Veterans Affairs' National Center for Patient Safety are also based on reliability science (Exhibit 3.2). Stronger actions are viewed as those that are more likely to be successful in accomplishing the desired results, resulting in greater utility for the effort expended (Department of Veterans Affairs, 2009). Some of the strong actions taken by Veterans Health Administration facilities to reduce patient wandering events have included (DeRosier et al., 2007):

- Installing new doors for fire escapes with alarms that cannot be disconnected by staff

- Placing black floor tiles in front of each door area, leaving a perception of a dark hole

- Not allowing committed patients to have off-ward privileges unless approved by the mental health unit chief of staff

The desired level of reliability for a particular process influences the choice of improvement actions. For instance, if it is acceptable for a process to perform as expected 80–90% of the time (1–2 failures out of 10 opportunities) it may be sufficient to use weaker actions, for example, standardizing, periodically measuring compliance. People's vigilance and hard work would then be relied on to catch and correct the evitable errors. For a **noncatastrophic process**—one that generally does not lead to patient death or severe injury within hours of a failure—good outcomes are dependent on having at least 95% process reliability. If at least 95% process reliability is the goal, improvement actions must be stronger. Actions should include more sophisticated failure prevention and basic failure identification and mitigation strategies (Resar, 2006).

EXHIBIT 3.2

NATIONAL CENTER FOR PATIENT SAFETY HIERARCHY OF IMPROVEMENT ACTIONS

Stronger Actions

- Architectural/physical plant changes
- New device with usability testing before purchasing
- Engineering control or interlock (forcing functions)
- Simplify the process and remove unnecessary steps
- Standardize on equipment or process or caremaps
- Tangible involvement and action by leadership in support of patient safety

Intermediate Actions

- Increase in staffing/decrease in workload
- Software enhancements/modifications
- Eliminate/reduce distractions (sterile medical environment)
- Checklist/cognitive aid
- Eliminate look and sound alikes
- Read back
- Enhanced documentation/communication
- Redundancy

Weaker Actions

- Double checks
- Warnings and labels
- New procedure/memorandum/policy
- Training
- Additional study/analysis

Source: Department of Veterans Affairs, National Center for Patient Safety. (2009, December). *Root cause analysis tools.* Retrieved from http://www4.va.gov/NCPS/CogAids/ RCA/index.html#page=page-14

Some health care processes are considered catastrophic—that is, there is a high likelihood of patient death or severe injury immediately or within hours of a process failure. Examples of **catastrophic processes** include identification of correct surgery site and administering ABO compatible blood for a transfusion. Good outcomes for these processes are dependent on having 99.9% or better process reliability. Achieving this level of process reliability requires a thorough understanding of process failures—how often and why they occur. Information about failures is regularly examined and used to design intermediate or strong actions to prevent or identify and mitigate failures (Resar, 2006).

Summarized in Table 3.1 are examples of system and process redesign strategies necessary to achieve and sustain a specific level of process reliability. These strategies are similar to Nolan's hierarchy of controls (2000), with higher level controls more likely to achieve higher levels of process reliability.

Table 3.1 Process Reliability Levels and Related Improvement Strategies

Desired Level of Sustained Reliability	System and Process Reliability Improvement Strategies
80–90%	This is achieved through "intent, vigilance, and hard work" and beginning to standardize some process elements representing the agreed way of doing things. Interventions include: • Use common equipment • Implement standard order sheets—the doctor only needs to check a box to prescribe standard pain relief medication • Create personal reminder checklists • Feedback information to staff on the rates of success—daily, weekly • Conduct awareness and training about the "agreed way of doing things around here" and using the above interventions
95%	This is achieved with a more deliberate focus on systems and processes to improve reliability. Interventions include: • Build decision aids and reminders built into the system • Make the desired action the default choice • Have independent back-ups; for example, when patients know what to expect they can act as a reminder • Take advantage of people's habits and work patterns • Standardize processes; for example encourage use of protocols for elements of patient care that have strong scientific evidence.

Table 3.1 *Continued*

Desired Level of Sustained Reliability	System and Process Reliability Improvement Strategies
99.5%	Investigate the cause of failures and redesign systems and processes to improve reliability using a three level design: prevent, identify, and mitigate. <ul><li>Prevent—this is about designing the system to prevent failure. There is a lot of focus on making sure critical steps in the process act independently of each other, so failures can be easily recognized.</li><li>Identify—this is about designing procedures and relationships to make failures visible when they do occur so that they can be caught before causing harm.</li><li>Mitigate—this is about designing procedures and building capabilities for fixing failures when they are identified; or mitigating the harm caused by failures when they are not caught and corrected.</li></ul>
> 99.5%	To get beyond 99.5% reliability nearly always requires technology and advanced system design. This usually means making significant resource investments.

Adapted from: National Health Service, Institute for Innovation and Improvement. (2008). *Quality and service improvement tools: Reliable design.* Retrieved December 16, 2009 from http://www.institute.nhs.uk/quality_and_service_improvement_tools/ quality_and_service_improvement_tools/reliable_design.htmlQuality

Use the information in Table 3.1 to evaluate the potential impact of various patient safety improvement strategies detailed in later chapters. Reaching 95% or better process reliability involves four main steps:

1. Have a common agreement on how reliability is to be measured

2. Measure how often the common agreement happens (a baseline)

3. Establish reliability goals for the measures

4. Make stepwise improvements and measure success

Agree on Reliability Measure

Process reliability can be measured in several ways and people should agree on the method or methods to be used. The process output or outcome can be measured. For example, suppose the average patient fall rate on all medical/

surgical units in your hospital is 4.6 falls per 1000 patient days. This is a measure of outcome. Reliability is calculated using the following formula:

Reliability calculation: $(1{,}000 - 4.6)/1{,}000 = 0.995$, or 99.5%

A second method for measuring reliability is to determine the reliability of the independent elements. For example, suppose prevention of a patient fall requires satisfactory completion of five tasks:

- Conduct initial patient assessment using the Morse Fall Risk Assessment tool

- Record total fall risk score on the patient's interdisciplinary care plan

- Implement a high-risk fall prevention plan for patients with a Morse Fall Risk score of 50 or higher *or* if the nurse judges the patient to be at higher than normal risk for fall

- Communicate patient's fall risk to other disciplines

- Monitor high-risk patients according to policy/procedure and fall risk reassess as indicated

The reliability of each task is calculated by dividing the number of times the task is completed as expected by the total number of times the task should have been completed.

A third method for measuring reliability is to calculate system reliability. System reliability is calculated by multiplying the reliability of the independent elements. For example, suppose you find that each fall prevention task is completed successfully 90% of the time. Using the following formula, you discover that the fall prevention system reliability in your hospital is only 59%.

System reliability calculation: $0.9 \times 0.9 \times 0.9 \times 0.9 \times 0.9 = 0.5905$

Not all process steps affect patient safety. Measure only those elements of practice that people agree are most likely connected to improved patient outcomes.

Measure Baseline Performance

Gather the data necessary for judging current process reliability. The data required for this purpose depends on how process reliability is to be measured—a decision made in the previous step. The results of data collection create a baseline against which future process improvements will be compared.

Establish Reliability Goals

Express these goals in the same way that baseline reliability was measured. For instance, if the reliability of the current patient fall prevention system was measured by calculating the reliability of the independent elements, set a reliability goal for each element. If system reliability was also calculated, set a goal for system reliability.

For many health care processes, 95% reliability may be sufficient, especially if the organization supports HRO principles. Better patient safety can often be achieved by bringing several chaotic processes to consistent 95% reliability rather than concentrating on advancing just a few processes from 95 to 99% reliability.

Make Stepwise Improvements

After reliability goals have been established, actions are taken to achieve the goals. The Institute for Healthcare Improvement (IHI) recommends that these actions be done in three-step fashion, starting with the lower levels of Nolan's hierarchy of controls and proceeding up to the higher levels (IHI, 2007).

Once process reliability of 80% or more is achieved and maintained, the next level of improvement strategies are initiated. At this point, the reliability improvement model advanced by the IHI recommends that at least 25% of the interventions be intermediate or strong (actions listed in the 99.5% reliability category in Table 3.1). Test the impact of each intervention before implementing the next one. Evaluate failures and use this learning to design the next intervention. Repeatedly implement and test the success of interventions until 95% reliability has been reached and maintained.

If process reliability of better than 95% is the goal, the next step is to identify failures that occur after simplification, standardization and implementation of stronger actions. To achieve 99.5% or better reliability requires an understanding of which failures are occurring, how often they occur, and why they occur. Targeted interventions are then designed and tested until the desired level of reliability is achieved and maintained.

Conclusion

Complex, high-risk industries have long recognized the value of adopting HRO principles that contribute to collective mindfulness and fewer catastrophic events. Unfortunately, health care organization and practice diverge from many of the

HRO elements (Gaba, 2000). Of course, health care differs in many respects from industries considered to be highly reliable, yet many of the factors contributing to high reliability can be incorporated into health care delivery. Patient safety is not a matter of separate individual accomplishments, but of a multitude of attitudes, behaviors, practices, and processes that interact.

First and foremost, health care leaders must differentiate between HRO principles and the human factor considerations that go into designing safer processes. Much has been written about how to reduce human errors by creating more reliable processes. Thus, the term "reliability" has come to refer to something that improvement teams must consider when they redesign processes. However, a highly reliable health care organization is not just focused on **mistake-proofing** tasks at the front lines of patient care. Leaders in an HRO are also personally involved in advancing HRO principles—sensitivity to operations, preoccupation with failure, deference to expertise, commitment to resilience, and reluctance to simplify interpretations. The two building blocks of reliability—HRO principles and reliability science—are what contribute to the extremely low accident rate in some complex yet highly reliable industries. These same two building blocks are essential for improving patient safety in the complex environment of health care services.

Discussion Questions

1. How can the five HRO principles can help health care organizations improve patient safety?

2. What are the challenges that health care organizations face in adopting HRO principles and how can they overcome these challenges?

3. What tactics could be used to improve the reliability of a particular health care process?

Key Terms

Catastrophic process

Collective mindfulness

High-reliability organization

Near miss

Noncatastrophic process

Reliable process

Reliability

Reliability science

Resilience

Risk assessment

Unreliable process

References

Abujudeh, H. H., & Kaewlai, R. (2006). Radiology failure mode and effect analysis: What is it? *Radiology, 252*(2), 544–550.

Amalberti, R., Auroy, Y., Berwick, D., & Barach, P. (2005). Five system barriers to achieving ultrasafe health care. *Annuals of Internal Medicine, 142*(9), 756–764.

American College of Healthcare Executives. (2008). *Top issues confronting hospitals: 2008.* Retrieved from http://www.ache.org/PUBS/research/ceoissues.cfm.

Angermeier, I., Dunford, B., Boss, A., Boss, R., & Miller, J. A. (2009). The impact of participative management perceptions on customer service, medical errors, burnout, and turnover intentions. *Journal of Healthcare Management, 54*(2), 127–140.

Baker, D., Day, R., & Salas, E. (2006). Teamwork as an essential component of high-reliability organizations. *Health Services Research, 41*(4 Pt 2), 1576–1598.

Berwick, D., & Nolan, T. (2003, December). *High reliability health care.* Presentation at the Institute for Healthcare Improvement 15th Annual National Forum in Quality Improvement in Health Care, New Orleans, Louisiana.

Bonnabry, P., Cingria, L., Ackerman, M., Sadeghipour, F., Bigler, L., & Mach, N. (2006) Use of a prospective risk analysis method to improve the safety of the cancer chemotherapy process. *International Journal for Quality in Health Care, 18*(1), 9–16.

Colla, J. B., Bracken, A. C., Kinney, L. M., & Weeks, W. B. (2005). Measuring patient safety climate: A review of surveys. *Quality and Safety in Health Care, 14*(5), 364–366.

Conlon, P., Havlisch, R., Kini, N., & Porter, C. (2008). Using an anonymous Web-based incident reporting tool to embed the principles of a high reliability organization. In K. Henriksen, J. B. Battles, M. A. Keyes, & M. L. Grady (Eds.), *Advances in patient safety: New directions and alternative approaches. Vol. 2. Culture and redesign.* AHRQ Publication No. 08–0034–2. Rockville, MD: Agency for Healthcare Research and Quality. Retrieved from http://ftp.ahrq.gov/downloads/pub/advances2/vol1/Advances-Conlon_50.pdf.

Department of Veterans Affairs, National Center for Patient Safety. (2009, December). *Root cause analysis tools.* Retrieved from http://www4.va.gov/NCPS/CogAids/RCA/index.html#page=page-14.

DeRosier, J. M., Taylor, L., Turner, L., & Bagian, J. P. (2007). Root cause analysis of wandering adverse events in the Veterans Health Administration. In A. Nelson & D. L. Algase (Eds.), *Evidence-based protocols for managing wandering behaviors* (pp. 161–180). New York: Springer.

Dixon, N. M., & Shofer, M. (2006). Struggling to invent high-reliability organizations in health care settings: Insights from the field. *Health Services Research, 41*(4 Pt. 2), 1618–1632.

Drain, M., & Clark, P. (2004). Measuring experience from the patient's perspective: Implications for national initiatives. *Journal for Healthcare Quality, 26*, W4–W16. Retrieved from http://www.nahq.org/ce/pdf/nahqce_article214.pdf.

Fiol, C., & O'Connor, E. (2003). Waking up! Mindfulness in the face of bandwagons. *Academy of Management Review, 28*(1), 54–70.

Frush, K. S., Alton, M., & Frush, D. P. (2006). Development and implementation of a hospital-based patient safety program. *Pediatric Radiology 36*(4), 291–298.

Gaba, D. M. (2000). Structural and organizational issues in patient safety: A comparison of health care to other high hazard industries. *California Management Review, 43*(1), 83–102.

Gosbee, J. (2002). Human factors engineering and patient safety. *Quality and Safety in Health Care, 11*(4), 352–354.

Harbrecht, B., Delgado, E., Tuttle, R., Cohen-Melamed, M., Saul, M., & Valenta, C. (2009). Improved outcomes with routine respiratory therapist evaluation of non-intensive-care-unit surgery patients. *Respiratory Care, 54*(7), 861–867.

Henneman, E. A., & Cunningham, H. (2005). Using clinical simulation to teach patient safety in an acute/critical care nursing course. *Nurse Educator, 30*(4), 172–177.

Hickam, D., Severance, S., Feldstein, A., Ray, L., Gorman, P., Schuldheis, S., … Helfand, M. (2003). *The effect of health care working conditions on patient safety.* AHRQ Publication No. 03-E031. Rockville, MD: Agency for Healthcare Quality and Research.

Institute for Healthcare Improvement. (2007, January). *Designing reliability into healthcare processes.* Cambridge, MA: IHI. Retrieved from http://www.qhn.ca/pdfs/Symp2007IHIpaper.pdf.

Institute of Medicine, Committee on Quality of Heath Care in America. (1999) *To err is human: Building a safer health system.* Washington, DC: National Academy Press.

Institute of Medicine, Committee on Quality of Health Care in America. (2001). *Crossing the quality chasm: A new health system for the 21st century.* Washington, DC: National Academy Press.

Langer, E. J., & Moldoveanu, M. (2000). The construct of mindfulness. *Journal of Social Issues, 56*(1), 1–9.

Luria, J. W., Muething, S. E., Schoettker, P. J., & Kotagal, U. R. (2006). Reliability science and patient safety. *Pediatric Clinics of North America, 53*(6), 1121–1133.

McCafferty, M. H., & Polk, H. C., Jr. (2004). Addition of "near-miss" cases enhances a quality improvement conference. *Archives of Surgery, 139*(2), 216–217.

McFadden, K. L., Stock, G. N., & Gowen, C. R., III. (2006). Exploring strategies for reducing hospital errors. *Journal of Healthcare Management, 51*(2), 123–135.

Nemeth, C., Wears, R., Woods, D., Hollnagel, E., & Cook, R. (2008). Minding the gaps: Creating resilience in health care. In Henriksen, K., Battles, J. B., Keyes, M. A. & Grady, M. L. (Eds.), *Advances in patient safety: New directions and alternative approaches. Vol. 3. Performance and tools.* AHRQ Publication No. 08–0034–3. Rockville, MD: Agency for Healthcare Research and Quality.

Nolan, T. (2000). System changes to improve patient safety. *British Medical Journal, 320*(7237), 771–773.

Pizzi, L., Goldfarb, N., & Nash, D. (2001). Promoting a culture of safety. In Shojania, K. G., Duncan, B. W., McDonald, K. M., & Wachter, R. M. (Eds.). *Making health care safer: A critical analysis of patient safety practices.* AHRQ Publication No. 01-E058. Rockville, MD: Agency for Healthcare Research and Quality.

Pronovost, P., Weast, B., Holzmueller, C., Rosenstein, B., Kidwell, R., Haller, K., … Rubin, H. (2003). Evaluation of the culture of safety: Survey of clinicians and managers in an academic medical center. *Quality and Safety in Health Care, 12*(6), 405–410.

Pronovost, P., Holzmueller, C., Needham, D., Sexton, J. B., Miller, M., Berenholtz, S., … Morlock, L. (2006). How will we know patients are safer? An organization-wide approach to measuring and improving safety. *Critical Care Medicine, 34*(7), 1988–1995.

Reason, J. T., Carthey, J., & de Leval, M. R. (2001). Diagnosing "vulnerable system syndrome": An essential prerequisite to effective risk management. *Quality and Safety in Health Care, 10*(Suppl II), ii21–ii25.

Resar, T. (2006). Making noncatastrophic health care processes reliable: Learning to walk before running in creating high-reliability organizations. *Health Services Research, 41*(4), 1677–1689.

Sutcliffe, K., & Vogue, T. (2003). Organizing for resilience. In Cameron, K., Dutton, J., & Quinn, R. (Eds.). *Positive organizational scholarship: Foundations of a new discipline.* San Francisco: Berrett-Koehler.

U.S. Department of Health and Human Services, Agency for Healthcare Research and Quality. (2009, March). *Hospital survey on patient safety culture.* Retrieved from http:// www.ahrq.gov/qual/patientsafetyculture/hospsurvindex.htm.

Van Cott, H. (1994). Human errors: Their causes and reduction. In Bogner, S. (Ed.) *Human error in medicine.* Mahwah, NJ: Erlbaum.

Vogus, T. J., & Sutcliffe, K. M. (2007). The safety organizing scale: Development and validation of a behavioral measure of safety culture in hospital nursing units. *Medical Care, 45*(1), 46–54.

Wachter, R. M. (2010) Patient safety at ten: Unmistakable progress, troubling gaps. *Health Affairs, 29*(1), 1–9. Published online December 1, 2009. Retrieved from http:// content.healthaffairs.org/cgi/reprint/hlthaff.2009.0785v2.

Weick, K. E. (1987). Organizational culture as a source of high reliability. *California Management Review, 29*(2), 112–127.

Weick, K. E. & Sutcliffe. K. M. (2007). *Managing the unexpected: Resilient performance in an age of uncertainty* (2nd ed.). San Francisco: Jossey-Bass, 2007.

Wennberg, J. E. (2002). Unwarranted variations in healthcare delivery: Implications for academic medical centers. *British Medical Journal, 325*(7370), 961–965.

Westrum, R. (1992). Cultures with requisite imagination. In J. Wise, V. Hopkin, & P. Stager (Eds.). *Verification and validation of complex systems: human factors issues* (pp. 401–416). Berlin: Springer-Verlag.

Ziv, A., Small, S. D., & Wolpe, P. R. (2000). Patient safety and simulation-based medical education. *Medical Teacher, 22*(5), 489–495.

PART 2

MEASURE AND EVALUATE PATIENT SAFETY

CHAPTER 4

MEASURING PATIENT SAFETY PERFORMANCE

Karen Ferraco
Patrice L. Spath

LEARNING OBJECTIVES

- Identify methods for measuring the safety of health care services
- Recognize safety critical tasks that should be regularly evaluated
- Describe common sources of patient safety measurement data
- Be aware of challenges associated with gathering valid and reliable measurement data

Management of errors in complex organizations has two components: **error containment** and **error reduction** (Reason, 1997). Error containment consists of actions taken to limit adverse consequences once an incident happens, whereas error reduction consists of actions taken to limit the occurrence of errors. This chapter describes an important component of error reduction: performance measurement of high-risk processes. Such evaluations provide an organization with vital information about the incidence of mistakes as well as insight into the **error-producing factors** that may ultimately lead to a harmful incident.

Health care performance measures can be used to evaluate many aspects of quality (for example, appropriateness of resource use, financial viability, clinical outcomes, effectiveness of treatment, patient satisfaction, and so on). This chapter focuses primarily on measures related to patient safety, although many quality measures serve a dual purpose. For example, hospital cancer programs annually report the number of new cancer cases and stage at time of diagnosis. A common quality of care measure is "Percent of new breast cancer cases diagnosed as Stage 0 (in situ) or Stage 1 (localized) at time of diagnosis" (Legorreta, Chernicoff,

Trinh, & Parker, 2004). This performance measure helps the organization identify access and patient management improvement opportunities. However, failure to identify suspicious breast lesions is a significant risk management concern for primary care physicians as well as radiologists. Failure to correctly and rapidly arrive at the right diagnosis can lead to an adverse patient outcome and may increase the chance of patient injury and subsequent legal action.

The purpose of patient safety measurement is to discover, assess, and correct problem areas before a significant untoward patient incident occurs. Evaluation of individual adverse events is often the primary source of information about patient safety. By evaluating the circumstances surrounding an event, clinicians identify sources and causes of the undesirable event, which may in turn result in immediate behavioral or process changes. However, health care organizations cannot rely solely on case-by-case analysis to ensure the safety of high-risk processes. Common patient safety problems will not be identified and corrected if the review focus is only on disastrous events that largely occur randomly and can only be examined after the fact. Case-by-case review must be supplemented by ongoing monitoring of safety-critical steps in high-risk processes. Regular analysis of high-risk process performance gives the organization a snapshot view of patient safety and an understanding of the potential for process failures that may lead to grievous consequences. The data are used to identify and change undesirable practices that increase the chance of an adverse patient event.

Measuring patient safety is a multidimensional endeavor. This chapter explores various patient safety measurement approaches. The reader is provided examples of different types of measures and sources of information that can be used to evaluate the safety of high-risk processes.

Monitor High-Risk Processes

The safety of all patient care processes should be subjected to some type of evaluation. However, there are so many disciplines, technical procedures, and individual decisions made in health care that it is economically impossible to measure all aspects. Therefore, measures must be focused on high-risk processes. In the context of this chapter, a high-risk process is defined as one that, if not planned or implemented correctly, has a significant potential for having an adverse impact on patient safety (The Joint Commission, 2005). From a risk management perspective, a high-risk process is one that could negatively affect important organizational dimensions if a failure occurs (National Institutes of Health, 2008):

- Mission: failure to achieve strategic goals and objectives

- Public trust: decrease in the level of confidence of individuals or groups outside of the organization

- Financial: increased cost to the organization

Analysis of malpractice claims data has shown certain activities to be associated with a greater risk of patient injury. These include the following (Physician Insurers Association of America, 1997; Weeks, Foster, Wallace, & Stalhandske, 2001; Phillips et al., 2004):

- Diagnostic and therapeutic decision making

- Patient assessment and observation (by physicians, nurses, and other caregivers)

- Transfer of patient care responsibilities between caregivers and facilities

- Communication (among caregivers and between caregivers and patients)

- Monitoring of patients during and immediately following high-risk interventions (for example, procedures performed under anesthesia or restraint/seclusion)

- Medication administration (prescribing, preparing, and dispensing medications) and monitoring their effects

Most people would agree that malpractice claims are merely the tip of the iceberg. However, data derived from claims analysis serve as one more piece of evidence that organizations can use in selecting the risk-prone activities that should be constantly monitored for performance problems.

High-Risk Patients

The patient population being cared for in the organization or by the individual clinician can have an impact on the riskiness of health care activities. For example:

- Hospitalized patients with longer lengths of stay, a diagnosis of diabetes mellitus, and more medications prescribed at discharge have been found to be at greater risk of post-discharge **medication errors** (Forster, Murff, Peterson, Gandhi, & Bates, 2005).

- Patient falls are generally associated with host factors long known to promote falls: increasing age, debility or decreased functioning, and central nervous system depressant medication (Ganz, Bao, Shekelle, & Rubenstein, 2007).

- Patients under treatment for depression or other psychiatric conditions may be at higher risk of an untoward incident as evidenced by the sentinel event database of The Joint Commission. Between January 1995 and September 2009, 770 patient suicides were reported to The Joint Commission by accredited facilities (The Joint Commission, 2009a).

- Patients with autoimmune deficiencies or those who cannot easily recover from the physical assault of a clinical error or mishap (for example, neonatal patients, patients receiving chemotherapy, severely ill or frail elderly patients) are at high risk for adverse events (Giraud et al., 1993).

Once an organization identifies the high-risk processes and patient groups that should be regularly evaluated, the next step is to define measurements to be used in this evaluation. Some measures may already be in place within the organization's risk management or performance improvement program. In other instances it will be necessary to identify additional measures to strengthen patient safety monitoring activities.

Measure Performance

Good health care performance requires providing services that are appropriate for each patient's condition; providing them safely, competently, and in an appropriate time frame; and achieving desired outcomes (Institute of Medicine, 2001). Performance measurement is an activity that has long been required by government regulators of the health care industry as well as by voluntary accreditation organizations (Spath, 2007).

A measure of patient safety performance is some form of a rate, ratio, or proportion that can be used as a tool to evaluate one or more aspects of health care services. Safety performance measures can also be single numeric values, for example, *number of attempted inpatient suicides.* Knowing how many attempted suicides have occurred tells the organization something important about the safety of health care services. It is not always necessary to create a rate, ratio, or proportion.

A common method of creating a patient safety measurement is to identify a group of patients who received care during a given "time window" and then to determine how many of those patients experienced an adverse event. Patients who experienced an adverse event are counted in the numerator of the performance rate or score.

Performance measures can also be used to evaluate the safety of specific health care processes. For example, the number of medications prescribed during a given time window can be compared with the number of prescription errors during that same time period. The population under study by this performance measure is prescriptions, not patients.

The ultimate purpose of patient safety performance measures is to reduce the number of avoidable patient injuries and deaths. To achieve this purpose, safety-related performance measures must be like the canary in the coal mine, providing a reliable early warning of safety-related problems.

The incidence of actual significant injury to patients, clients, or residents is easily identified after the fact. The difficulty lies in the identification of patterns of near-miss behavior—those actions that did not result in a patient's death or serious physical or psychological injury but which, under different conditions or with additional failures, could have caused such an outcome. At this time there is no industry-wide consensus about what near-miss behaviors should be measured or how to measure them (Chang, Schyve, Croteau, O'Leary, & Loeb, 2005). Therefore, health care entities are left to themselves to determine which performance measures will be used to identify unsafe acts that need further investigation.

Two types of performance measures can be used to identify failures in high-risk processes. These are **process measures** and **outcome measures**. Process measures provide information about whether or not caregivers are "doing the right things." Outcome measures provide information about whether or not caregivers are "doing the right things well."

Process Measures

Provision of health care services, whether in an inpatient or outpatient environment, involves a multitude of activities. The performance of any number of these activities can be measured. When selecting patient safety-related measures, be sure to concentrate evaluation efforts on those elements most likely to affect the safe delivery of health care services.

Process measures can be used to evaluate what Donabedian called the structure or characteristics of the care setting (1980). Measures of the safety-related structural components would be used to evaluate performance in areas such as the following:

- Compliance with safety regulations and codes

- Adequacy of equipment maintenance

- Physician and staff certification, training, and continuing education
- Oversight of physician and staff competency
- Workplace ergonomics
- Staff scheduling
- Telecommunications and information systems

Other safety-related process measures would be used to monitor the incidence of variations from accepted policies, regulations, and standards of practice that could potentially result in patient harm. The number of medication errors that occur in a facility is a common process measure. A medication error is any variation from an expected process that may cause or lead to inappropriate medication use or patient harm. For example, when a physician orders an incorrect dose of a medication, this is a variation from the "right" process (appropriate drug ordering). Though the error may be caught and corrected before patient harm occurs, a process variance has still occurred.

Researchers have used the term adverse event to describe a situation in which an inappropriate decision (action or inaction) was made when, at the time, an appropriate alternative could have been chosen (Andrews et al., 1997). Data about the number of adverse events (using this definition) would tell caregivers how well the clinical decision-making process is working. Recently, Newman-Toker and Pronovost (2009) suggested that diagnostic errors resulting in an adverse event be more closely monitored. These authors define **misdiagnosis-related harm** as "preventable harm that results from the delay or failure to treat a condition actually present (when the working diagnosis was wrong or unknown) or from treatment provided for a condition not actually present" (Newman-Toker & Pronovost, 2009, p. 1060). This definition incorporates both process (clinical decision making) and outcome (harm).

Process measures have been found to be more sensitive than outcome measures when differentiating quality across providers or time, or both; in addition, they are often easier to interpret (Mant, 2001). Accountability is clearer when measuring process—either the right thing was done or it was not done (Pronovost, Nolan, Zeger, Miller, & Rubin, 2004).

Outcome Measures

Outcomes represent the cumulative effect of health care processes on patients. An example of an outcome measure of patient safety is the number of patient falls. Although caregivers may have followed the right process, something caused the patient to experience a fall. An outcome measure reflects the whole system of care processes that produced the outcome (Mant, 2001).

Counts of serious events would also be considered outcome measures. For example, an event involving a medical product is defined as serious by the Food and Drug Administration (FDA) MedWatch Program if any of the following outcomes occurred as a result of using a medical product (FDA, 2009):

- Patient's death is suspected as being a direct outcome of the adverse event.

- Patient was at substantial risk of dying or it was suspected that the use or continued use of the product would result in the patient's death.

- Patient required admission to the hospital or hospitalization was prolonged because of the adverse event.

- Patient experienced a significant, persistent, or permanent change, impairment, damage, or disruption in his or her body function or structure, physical activities, or quality of life.

- Patient was exposed to a medical product prior to conception or during pregnancy that resulted in an adverse outcome in the child.

- Patient developed a condition that required medical or surgical intervention to preclude permanent impairment or damage.

The **Patient Safety Indicators (PSIs)**, developed by the Agency for Healthcare Research and Quality (AHRQ) and the UCSF–Stanford Evidence-Based Practice Center are examples of outcome measures (AHRQ, 2007). The PSIs use administrative data (hospital discharge records), including ICD-9 diagnosis and procedure codes, to identify potential in-hospital patient safety events. The PSIs are expressed as rates: the numerator is the number of occurrences of the outcome of interest and the denominator is the total population at risk (AHRQ, 2007). Examples of PSIs are listed in Table 4.1. The PSIs are considered *indicators*, not *measures*, because they point to events that are considered potentially preventable (Rivard, Rosen, & Carroll, 2006). To learn whether an event was in fact preventable, clinicians must "drill down" into the circumstances surrounding the event.

The Joint Commission uses the phrase sentinel event to describe a serious event. A sentinel event is considered an unexpected occurrence involving death or serious physical or psychological injury or the risk thereof. The phrase risk thereof includes any process variation for which a recurrence would carry a significant chance of a serious adverse outcome (The Joint Commission, 2007).

Table 4.1   Examples of Patient Safety Indicators

Indicator	Definition
Complications of Anesthesia	Cases of anesthetic overdose, reaction, or endotrachial tube misplacement per 1,000 surgery discharges. Excludes codes for drug use and self-inflicted injury.
Death in Low Mortality DRGs	In-hospital deaths per 1,000 patients in DRGs with less than 0.5% mortality. Excludes trauma, immunocompromised, and cancer patients.
Decubitus Ulcer	Cases of decubitus ulcer per 1,000 discharges with a length of stay of five or more days. Excludes patients with paralysis or in MDC 9, obstetrical patients in MDC 14, and patients admitted from a long-term care facility.
Failure to Rescue	Deaths per 1,000 patients having developed specified complications of care during hospitalization. Excludes patients age 75 and older, neonates in MDC 15, patients admitted from long-term care facility, and patients transferred to or from other acute care facility.
Foreign Body Left During Procedure	Discharges with foreign body accidentally left in during procedure per 1,000 discharges.
Iatrogenic Pneumothorax	Cases of iatrogenic pneumothorax per 1,000 discharges. Excludes trauma, thoracic surgery, lung, or pleural biopsy, or cardiac surgery patients, and obstetrical patients in MDC 14.
Selected Infections Due to Medical Care	Cases of secondary ICD-9-CM codes 9993 or 00662 per 1,000 discharges. Excludes patients with immunocompromised state or cancer.
Postoperative Hip Fracture	Cases of in-hospital hip fracture per 1,000 surgical discharges. Excludes patients in MDC 8, with conditions suggesting fracture present on admission and obstetrical patients in MDC 14.
Postoperative Hemorrhage or Hematoma	Cases of hematoma or hemorrhage requiring a procedure per 1,000 surgical discharges. Excludes obstetrical patients in MDC 14.
Postoperative Physiologic and Metabolic Derangement	Cases of specified physiological or metabolic derangement per 1,000 elective surgical discharges. Excludes patients with principal diagnosis of diabetes and with diagnoses suggesting increased susceptibility to derangement. Excludes obstetric admissions.
Postoperative Respiratory Failure	Cases of acute respiratory failure per 1,000 elective surgical discharges. Excludes MDC 4 and 5 and obstetric admissions.
Postoperative PE or DVT	Cases of deep vein thrombosis or pulmonary embolism per 1,000 surgical discharges. Excludes obstetric patients.

Table 4.1 *Continued*

Indicator	Definition
Postoperative Sepsis	Cases of sepsis per 1,000 elective surgery patients, with length of stay more than three days. Excludes principal diagnosis of infection, or any diagnosis of immunocompromised state or cancer, and obstetric admissions.
Postoperative Wound Dehiscence	Cases of reclosure of postoperative disruption of abdominal wall per 1,000 cases of abdominopelvic surgery. Excludes obstetric admissions.
Accidental Puncture or Laceration	Cases of technical difficulty (such as accidental cut or laceration during procedure) per 1,000 discharges. Excludes obstetric admissions.
Transfusion Reaction	Cases of transfusion reaction per 1,000 discharges.
Birth Trauma— Injury to Neonate	Cases of birth trauma, injury to neonate, per 1,000 liveborn births. Excludes some preterm infants and infants with osteogenic imperfecta.
Obstetric Trauma— Vaginal Delivery with Instrument	Cases of obstetric trauma (4th degree lacerations, other obstetric lacerations) per 1,000 instrument-assisted vaginal deliveries.
Obstetric Trauma— Vaginal Delivery without Instrument	Cases of obstetric trauma (4th degree lacerations, other obstetric lacerations) per 1,000 vaginal deliveries without instrument assistance.
Obstetric Trauma— Cesarean Delivery	Cases of obstetric trauma (4th degree lacerations, other obstetric lacerations) per 1,000 Cesarean deliveries.
Obstetric Trauma with 3rd Degree—Vaginal Delivery with Instrument	Cases of obstetric trauma (3rd and 4th degree lacerations, other obstetric lacerations) per 1,000 instrument-assisted vaginal deliveries.
Obstetric Trauma with 3rd Degree—Vaginal Delivery without Instrument	Cases of obstetric trauma (3rd and 4th degree lacerations, other obstetric lacerations) per 1,000 vaginal deliveries without instrument assistance.
Obstetric Trauma with 3rd Degree— Cesarean Delivery	Cases of obstetric trauma (3rd and 4th degree lacerations, other obstetric lacerations) per 1,000 Cesarean deliveries.

Source: AHRQ. (2007, March). Guide to patient safety indicators, version 3.1. Retrieved from http://www.qualityindicators.ahrq.gov/psi_download.htm.

A measure of the number of sentinel events is an outcome measure. These data do not necessarily tell caregivers how well they are doing at following the right processes; however, it does provide information about how often serious events actually occur.

Organizations should have a mix of process and outcome measures to evaluate patient safety. Listed in Exhibit 4.1 are examples of common process and outcome measures that would be useful for identifying error-related problems in various types of facilities. Data from these measures could be reported for the organization as a whole and could also be stratified by individual departments or services. Additional examples of process and outcome measures related to patient safety are available on the National Quality Measures Clearinghouse Web site (www.qualitymeasures.ahrq.gov) sponsored by the Agency for Healthcare Research and Quality.

EXHIBIT 4.1

GENERAL RISK-RELATED PERFORMANCE MEASURES

Inpatient and Long-Term Care

- Percentage of patients who are unexpectedly admitted or retained following a complication of outpatient surgery or anesthesia event

- Number of unplanned readmissions within 48 hours

- Number of delayed diagnoses (organization to define "delayed")

- Number of missed diagnoses (organization to define "missed")

- Number of cases in which a significant change in the patient's condition or diagnosis did not result in a reassessment (organization to define "significant")

- Number of adverse events occurring during anesthesia use (including conscious sedation)

- Percentage of cases in which attending physician was promptly notified about out-of-range or unusual diagnostic test results (organization to define "prompt notification")

- Rate of nosocomial infections, stratified by type of infection

- Percentage of live births entering intermediate or intensive care nurseries

- In-hospital mortality rate for low birthweight babies

- Perinatal mortality rate

- Number of patient suicides (attempted/successful)

- Patients admitted following attempted suicide for whom there is no documented suicide prevention plan

- Percentage of patients at suicide risk who receive appropriate consultation prior to a leave of absence (organization to define "appropriate")

- Percentage of patients who are adequately searched after returning from leave of absence (organization to define "adequate")

- Percentage of locked units with adequate security (organization to define "adequate")

- Percentage of patients in restraint/seclusion who are adequately monitored (organization to define "adequate")

- Ratio of patient restraint/seclusion hours to patient days

- Ratio of medication errors to medications dispensed or administered

- Ratio of potential adverse drug events to number of medications ordered (a potential adverse drug event is a serious medication error that had the potential to harm the patient but, either by luck or interception, did not)

- Percentage of patients who develop an adverse drug reaction

- Percentage of patients undergoing procedure requiring isotope injection who develop an adverse reaction to the isotope agent

- Ratio of transfusion reactions to total units transfused

- Percentage of patient falls resulting in patient injury

- Number of patients falls per 1,000 patient bed days

- Percentage of fire alarms/protection equipment tested as required

- Percentage of new devices/equipment added to inventory only after relevant physicians/staff have received in-service training

- Percentage of equipment maintenance checks completed within required time frame (organization to define requirements)

- Percentage of significant hazards identified through surveillance that are resolved within acceptable time frame (organization to define "significant hazard" and "acceptable time frame")

- Number of open and pending liability claims

- Percentage of long-stay patients who experience an unplanned weight loss problem (5% change in 30 days or 10% change in 180 days)

- Percentage of patients who develop a pressure ulcer at Stage II or higher, when no ulcers were previously present at Stage II or higher

- Number of serious resident injuries/deaths that may have been related to the use of a medical device

Home Health Services

- Percentage of clients on home IV therapy who require hospital admission

- Percentage of clients on ventilators who develop respiratory infection

- Percentage of cases with documentation of adequate patient education regarding home safety (organization to define "adequate")

- Percentage of cases with documented evidence that the physician remains involved in the care of the patient (organization to define "documented evidence")

- Percentage of clients failing to meet functional health status goals without evidence of care plan assessment and revision

- Ratio of medication errors to medications administered

- Number of adverse drug reactions

- Number of serious client injuries/deaths that may have been related to the use of a medical device

- Percentage of clients developing complications following venipuncture (hemolyzed specimens, hematoma, infection, and so on)

- Number of mislabeled or misplaced specimens obtained by caregiver during home visit

- Number of times that client records are missing or unavailable at time of scheduled home visit

- Percentage of abnormal diagnostic results or physical findings not communicated to physician within established time frames

- Percentage of clients developing new contractures or pressure sores while receiving rehabilitation therapy

- Percentage of clients referred to the appropriate treatment program (organization to define treatment appropriateness criteria for different conditions)

Clinic/Outpatient Services

- Number of patients who return to clinic within 72 hours due to failure to improve

- Number of missed appointments for high-risk patients (organization to define "high-risk")

- Number of patients who are noncompliant with medications without evidence of caregiver intervention

- Percentage of patients on more than five prescribed medications without evidence of medication counseling

- Number of medication prescription errors

- Percentage of patient records lacking notation of allergies (or "no known allergies")

- Number of outdated medications in medication supply area

- Number of misplaced/misfiled/misidentified laboratory or radiographic findings

- Number of instances in which laboratory results fell outside established quality control limits and no verification of findings was done

- Number of mislabeled/misplaced laboratory specimens

- Percentage of scheduled appointments at which patient's record was missing or unavailable at the time of the clinic visit

- Number of patient encounters (visit or telephone) not documented in record

---

The measures in Exhibit 4.1 are broad measures that offer a "snapshot" of the organization's patient safety performance. Although global measures of process and outcome such as these provide an overview of the incidence of errors or bad outcomes, these measures may not be sufficiently sensitive to provide early warnings of impending disasters. It is recommended that global measures be supplemented with measures that evaluate compliance with **safety-critical tasks**.

Measuring Safety-Critical Tasks

It is cost prohibitive to measure every aspect of a high-risk process. Therefore, it is important to identify the tasks most critical in keeping patients safe. It is these tasks that should be regularly examined for compliance. A safety-critical task is one that must be done properly all of the time (Dekker, 2009). For

instance, the National Center for Missing and Exploited Children (http://www
.ncmec.org) has identified several safety-critical actions that are important in
preventing infant abductions in hospitals:

- Confirm identification of people given access to the nursery
- Respond immediately when alarms sound (exit doors, electronic tracking systems, and so on)
- Promptly report people exhibiting unusual behavior to security
- Confirm identifications when releasing infant from facility
- Enforce visitor regulations

If a safety-critical task is performed incorrectly, the error could lead to catastrophic results. Though not all such errors will cause patient injury or death,
serious mistakes in high-risk processes can start an accident chain of events that
may be difficult to stop in certain circumstances. The criticality of a task in a
high-risk process can be expressed as:

$$\text{Level of risk} \times \text{likelihood of occurrence} = \textbf{task criticality}$$

The level of risk refers to the amount of damage expected when a failure
occurs at this step in the process. In this instance, damage refers to the severity
of patient injury. For example, an incorrect overdose prescription of a chemotherapy agent that is not caught before the drug is administered is more likely
to cause patient harm than the same error occurring in the prescription of a less
toxic drug. The likelihood of occurrence refers to the estimated frequency of
such errors happening. This prediction can be based on past performance measurement results or it may represent an educated guess by those intimately
involved in the process.

The matrix in Table 4.2 illustrates how this criticality scoring system can be
used to choose the tasks that should be regularly monitored for the process of
procuring, preparing and administering enteral feeding products to hospital or
nursing home patients. The tasks involved in the process are listed in stepwise
fashion in the first column. A numeric risk score and frequency score are assigned
to each task. The criticality score for each task is calculated by multiplying the
risk score times the frequency score. The highest possible criticality score for a
task is 16. Organizations should consider regularly monitoring the performance

Table 4.2   Task Criticality Scoring System for the Process of Enteral Feeding Product Procurement, Preparation, and Administration

Process Tasks	Risk Level[a]	Likelihood of Failure[b]	Task Criticality Score (risk level × likelihood of failure)
Purchase product			
Receive product			
Store product			
Thaw product			
Prepare product for delivery to nursing unit			
Deliver product to nursing unit			
Hold cold product on nursing unit			
Administer product			

a. Risk-Level Scoring Key:
   4 = Catastrophic (failure of this task could cause loss of patient life or permanent harm)
   3 = Serious (failure could cause severe patient harm or temporary disability)
   2 = Minor (failure could cause minor patient harm)
   1 = Negligible (failure is unlikely to cause patient harm)
b. Likelihood of Occurrence Scoring Key:
   4 = Probable (failure of this task occurs frequently)
   3 = Occasional (failure occurs sporadically)
   2 = Rare (failure is very uncommon, but it does happen)
   1 = Improbable (failure has never been known to occur)

of any process task that has a criticality score of 8 or higher to ensure that problems in this safety-critical step are quickly identified and resolved.

Examples of performance measures that can be used to evaluate various safety-critical steps are listed in Exhibit 4.2. These measures are sorted into major patient care functions and relevant sites of care.

It is not necessary or desirable for organizations to use all of the global measures listed in Exhibit 4.1 or gather measurement data for every safety-critical task. Collecting as much information as possible about patient safety can result in paralysis. It is much better to work with only a few measures that you understand and know how to use. It is also important to periodically evaluate your choice of safety-related measures to determine if changes or additions are needed.

EXHIBIT 4.2

EXAMPLES OF PERFORMANCE MEASURES FOR SAFETY-CRITICAL TASKS IN MAJOR PATIENT CARE FUNCTIONS

Operative and Other Procedures

Acute and Ambulatory Surgery

- Percentage of cases in which correct patient/surgical site was confirmed prior to start of operation (as required by policies/procedures)

- Percentage of cases requiring sponge/needle counts in which full count sheet is completed correctly

- Percentage of cases requiring sponge/needle counts with reported discrepancy

- Percentage of patients experiencing hypotension when receiving IV sedation

- Percentage of patients experiencing loss of sensation due to position during anesthesia

- Percentage of patients experiencing cardiac-related problems during withdrawal from general anesthesia

- Percentage of surgeries performed without history and physical examination present in patient's record

- Percentage of patients who experience a cardiac arrest within two post-procedure days of procedures involving anesthesia administration

- Percentage of surgeries delayed or cancelled due to unavailable or incomplete equipment or supplies

- Percentage of procedures in which there is a break in sterile techniques

- Percentage of total pathological specimens removed in the operating room that are lost or mislabeled

Behavioral Health Care

- Percentage of patients undergoing electroshock therapy (ECT) without pre-ECT workup, which includes: dental consultation, skull and spinal column x-ray studies, and electrocardiogram

Medication Management

Acute, Emergent, and Ambulatory Care

- Percentage of patients who experience extravasation during administration of chemotherapy

- Percentage of inpatients on Heparin and Coumadin therapy whose prothrombin times are not monitored according to approved guidelines

- Percentage of patients on Warfarin whose prothrombin times are maintained at 1.5–2.0 times the control value

- Percentage of outpatients on anticoagulants who do not have at least one prothrombin time test done every 30 days

- Percentage of high-risk surgery patients for whom deep vein thrombosis prophylactic measures/treatment are not implemented

- Percentage of patients receiving Pitocin without adequate documentation of the indications for use

- Percentage of medication prescriptions requiring clarification because of illegibility

- Percentage of medication prescriptions containing "nonapproved" abbreviations or acronyms

- Percentage of medication orders containing dosing that is incorrect for patient age or condition

- Percentage of patients on potassium whose plasma levels are greater than about 5 (exact level to be determined by organization)

- Percentage of diabetic patients whose glucose plasma levels are less than about 50 (exact level to be determined by organization)

- Percentage of patients receiving IV sedation in the emergency department (ED) who are released to appropriate family/significant other and instructed not to drive

- Percentage of cases in which information about patient's home medications is available to treating physician

- Percentage of patients admitted through the ED with a principal diagnosis of acute myocardial infarction who receive thrombolytic therapy

- Average time from patient admission to the ED to administration of thrombolytic for patients with a principal diagnosis of acute myocardial infarction

- Percentage of inpatients receiving Digoxin who have no corresponding measured drug level or whose highest measured level exceeds a specified limit

- Percentage of inpatients receiving Theophylline who have no corresponding measured drug level or whose highest measured level exceeds a specified limit

- Percentage of inpatients receiving Phenytoin who have no corresponding measured drug level or whose highest measured level exceeds a specified limit

- Percentage of outpatients receiving antihypertensives whose potassium levels are below normal

- Percentage of patients receiving antibiotics for surgical prophylaxis in which first dose was administered within one hour of surgical incision

- Number of medications administered but not documented

- Percentage of patients on Warfarin who have monthly INR monitoring

Behavioral Health Care

- Percentage of schizophrenic patients receiving doses of Haloperidol or Fluphenazine in excess of 20 mg per day

- Percentage of patients receiving MAO inhibitors without evidence of dietary monitoring

- Percentage of patients on Tegretol who have a complete blood count performed every two months

- Percentage of inpatients receiving lithium who have no corresponding measured drug level or whose highest measured level exceeds a specified limit

Skilled/Residential Care

- Percentage of patients regularly receiving more than five medications

- Percentage of patients who have a history of falls and are receiving tricyclic antidepressants, antipsychotics, or sleep agents

Home Care

- Percentage of clients receiving infusion therapy for whom therapy is discontinued before prescribed completion

- Number of interruptions in infusion therapy

Use of Blood and Blood Products

Acute and Ambulatory Care

- Percentage of contaminated units appropriately discarded (according to procedures)

- Number of outdated units in active blood supply

- Percentage of patients developing complications from too rapid administration of blood transfusion

Patient Rights/Organizational Ethics

Acute, Long-Term, Home, and Ambulatory Care

- Percentage of patients (or their families/significant others) queried about advance directives on admission

- Percentage of patients with advance directives who have a copy of the directive in their medical record

- Percentage of patients who refuse evaluation and treatment

- Percentage of patients seen in the ED who refuse transport to another facility for treatment

- Percentage of patients who change their primary care physician within a specified period

- Percentage of patients requiring foreign language or sign language interpretation who are provided such assistance within specified time frame (as defined by organization's policies)

Patient Assessment

Acute Care

- Average order-to-report times for critical diagnostic tests (organization to define "critical")

- Percentage of cases with abnormal diagnostic test results on admission without corresponding documentation in the patient assessment

- Percentage of inpatients with congestive heart failure for whom a weight is obtained on admission and thereafter at least daily

- Percentage of orthopedic procedures involving extremities in which descriptive CMS checks are not adequately documented by nursing staff the first 12 hours postop

- Percentage of newborn deliveries involving fetal distress in which the response time is 30 minutes or greater from the first sign of distress

- Percentage of radiology studies in which pathology identified later was not found on initial study

- Percentage of cases in which ED physician's interpretation of x-ray studies differs from radiologist's interpretation

- Percentage of patients admitted with a diagnosis of depressive disorder who are not assessed for the potential for harm to both self and others

- Number of patients that develop fluid overload due to inattention to the patient's intravenous line or rate of infusion

Ambulatory

- Number of patients with a breast mass that does not disappear or become smaller within six weeks of initial discovery (regardless of the mammogram findings) who do not undergo additional diagnostic tests

- Percentage of patients with an initial diagnosis of depressive disorder who are not assessed for the potential for harm to both self and others

- Percentage of patients with verified hypertension (for example, blood pressure > 140/90 taken on three occasions during a two-month period) who do not receive hypertensive workup/assessment and follow-up

Home Care

- Number of clients who develop aspiration pneumonia who did not have appropriate assessment and referral (organization to define "appropriate")

- Percentage of clients who have a home situation that puts them at risk of readmission to the hospital who are not evaluated by a clinical nurse specialist

Care of Patients

Acute and Emergency Care

- Percentage of patients identified as having functional needs who have an assessment/intervention by the appropriate therapist (organization to define "functional needs" requiring therapist consultation and "appropriate" therapist)

- Percentage of unsuccessful first attempts at orotracheal intubation

- Percentage of unsuccessful first attempts at intravenous line insertion

- Percentage of patients who develop latex anaphylaxis who have a known history of latex allergy

- Percentage of newborn deliveries in which physician or midwife is not in attendance

- Percentage of diagnostic tests requiring repeat due to technical error on first examination

- Percentage of patients undergoing fracture repair procedure who develop postop dislocation/displacement due to improper positioning

- Percentage of vascular grafts/cannulas that become occluded, requiring replacement

- Percentage of patients with suspected pulmonary edema who are positioned in high Fowler's position with lower extremities dependent

- Intraoperative mortality of trauma patients with a systolic blood pressure of less than 70 mmHg within two hours of ED or inpatient admission who did not undergo a laparotomy or thoracotomy

- Percentage of patients with endotracheal tube that develop complications related to cuff overinflation

- Percentage of patients that aspirate during a tube feeding

Ambulatory Care

- Percentage of patients with a diagnosis of intentional drug overdose or other suicidal gesture who are not referred for mental health counseling

- Percentage of patients followed through the full term of their pregnancy who have a minimum of five visits or a satisfactory reason for fewer than five visits is documented

- Percentage of known diabetic patients who undergo hemoglobin A1c measurement, ophthalmologic exam, and total cholesterol measurement at least annually

- Number of medication or treatment modalities that are not given because the stock is out of date, not available, damaged, or lost

- Percentage of indwelling vascular grafts/cannulas that become occluded, requiring replacement

Home Care

- Percentage of clients with diet-controlled diabetes who receive nutritional counseling

- Percentage of clients with two acute episodes of congestive heart failure in a six-month period who are not referred to the cardiopulmonary team

Patient Education

Acute, Ambulatory, and Home Care

- Number of readmissions due to insufficient/inadequate patient education on a prior admission

- Percentage of cases in which there is documentation that patient/family demonstrated an understanding of postdischarge precautions

- Inpatients with a diagnosis of insulin-dependent diabetes mellitus who demonstrate self-blood glucose monitoring and self-administration of insulin before discharge, or are referred for postdischarge follow-up for diabetes management

Continuum of Care

Acute, Emergency, Ambulatory, and Home Care

- Percentage of patients transferred to another facility from the ED without documentation of stable condition prior to transfer

- Percentage of cases in which ED physician's interpretation of x-ray studies differs from radiologist's interpretation and attending physician is not notified of discrepancy

- Percentage of home health care cases requiring physician contact (according to agency policy) in which physician was contacted within required time frame

- Percentage of patients given IV/IM Demerol, Valium, or other sedatives with no evidence that family or friend drove them home

Behavioral Health

- Percentage of cases in which a written relapse prevention plan is documented prior to the patient's discharge from inpatient care

- Percentage of patients for whom a follow-up appointment is scheduled within two weeks of inpatient discharge

---

Measuring the Safety Culture

Attributes of a supportive organizational culture of patient safety were described in Chapters One and Three. This culture becomes reality through what senior leaders and management do—its practices, procedures, and processes. To determine the success of these actions, the organization must periodically evaluate the culture by asking, how well have we created a culture of safety? (Pronovost et al., 2006).

Measures of safety culture evaluate the beliefs and attitudes of people working in the organization. For instance, do staff members believe they can report errors and near-misses without fear of recrimination? Do staff members

Table 4.3 Commonly Used Patient Safety Culture Assessment Tools

Survey Instrument	Developer/Sponsor
Hospital Survey on Patient Safety Culture	Agency for Healthcare Research and Quality (www.ahrq.gov/qual/patientsafetyculture)
Medical Office Survey on Patient Safety Culture	Agency for Healthcare Research and Quality (www.ahrq.gov/qual/patientsafetyculture)
Nursing Home Survey on Patient Safety Culture	Agency for Healthcare Research and Quality (www.ahrq.gov/qual/patientsafetyculture)
Physician Practice Patient Safety Assessment	Health Research and Educational Trust (HRET), the Institute for Safe Medication Practices (ISMP) and the Medical Group Management Association (MGMA) (http://www.mgma.com/PatientSafety/)
Safety Attitudes and Safety Climate Questionnaires	University of Texas, Center for Healthcare Quality and Safety (http://www.uth.tmc.edu/schools/med/imed/patient_safety/)

feel that their safety improvement suggestions will be acted upon by management? A number of researchers have created patient safety culture surveys that can be used to measure people's beliefs and attitudes. Commonly used culture assessment tools are listed in Table 4.3. Health care organizations can use these survey assessment tools to:

- Assess their patient safety culture

- Track changes in patient safety over time

- Evaluate the impact of patient safety interventions

Collect Measurement Data

A challenge in any performance measurement effort is the data collection process. To ensure that valid information is gathered it is important to identify reliable data sources. Various handwritten documents and computerized databases can be used to collect data for the numerator, denominator, and other data elements necessary to calculate the measure. Many factors affect the choice of a data source for a particular performance measure. The considerations include the following:

- What information is contained in the data source

- The accuracy and reliability of the data

- Which patients and processes are covered by the data

- The costs involved in capturing the data

- Whether the data are computerized or manually recorded

- The timeliness of the data

Primary sources of patient safety data include:

1. Direct observation

2. Patient records

3. Administrative data

4. Patient incident reports

5. Patient/family feedback

The accuracy and completeness of the information in the data source will determine the level of confidence one can have about the measurement results.

Direct Observation

Direct observation of patient care practices is considered to be the "gold standard" for gathering data for patient safety measures. Although observations can be more costly due to the staff resources required, such reviews can provide detailed and useful information on processes of care (Rivard, Rosen, & Carroll, 2006). For example, observing whether people are washing their hands before caring for patients provides specific information on who is performing hand hygiene and what factors may contribute to noncompliance (Haas & Larson, 2007).

Observation requires someone directly watch and record the behaviors or actions of health care workers. The form in Exhibit 4.3 is used by an observer to document whether housekeeping staff are in compliance with the department's infection control practices.

The observation method of data collection has some limitations and potential biases. Not only is it labor intensive, it is also subject to the Hawthorne effect (people change behavior because they know they are being observed). Sampling bias can occur if observations are done only during one shift or on certain units or days of the week.

EXHIBIT 4.3

FORM USED TO GATHER OBSERVATION DATA TO MEASURE HOUSEKEEPING STAFF COMPLIANCE WITH INFECTION CONTROL PRACTICES

Employee ID:	Date:		Date:		Date:		Date:	
	Met	Not Met	Met	Not Met	Met	Not Met	Met	Not Met
Employee wears clean, neat, un-torn, and appropriate clothing								
Closed shoes in good repair with safety soles are worn								
Personal hygiene (including hair and body cleanliness) is practiced								
Fingernails are trimmed and clean								
Hair is worn in a neat fashion								
Strict hand washing procedures (ex: between patient areas) are followed								
Employee refrains from direct patient contact except in emergency situations								
Utility gloves are worn to protect hands from harsh chemical cleansers/germicides								
Employee avoids touching, or clothing touching, patient belongings or equipment								
Gowns, gloves and masks are worn, as appropriate								
Bagging, double-bagged and labeling procedures are followed, as appropriate								

Source: Spath, P. L. (2005). *Fundamentals of health care quality management* (2nd ed.). Forest Grove, OR: Brown-Spath & Associates. Used with permission.

If you choose to gather data for patient safety measures using an observation method several factors must be considered (The Joint Commission, 2009b):

- What behavior or action do you want to observe?

- Whom do you want to observe?

- Who will conduct the observations?

- When and where will observations be conducted?

- How many observations will be conducted?

To gather reliable observation data, the data collector must be adequately trained in differentiating between safe and unsafe actions or compliant and noncompliant behaviors. The success of observation reviews depends on accurate calculation of adherence rates, careful training of data collectors, and the data collectors' use of clear, easy-to-understand forms (The Joint Commission, 2009b).

Patient Records

Patient records are common sources of data for patient safety measures. However, paper-based records are costly to review. In a study of the burden of collecting data from patient records for four quality measurements, researchers estimated that gathering data from 80 records took approximately 8.5 days, broken down as follows: 0.5 days to sample the medical records, 2 days to retrieve the medical records from archives, 4 days to abstract the sample, 1 day to enter the data on computer, and 1 day to check data quality (Corriol, Daucourt, Grenier, & Minvielle, 2008).

Rather than manually review records after patients have completed the episode of care (for example, after hospital discharge), many health care organizations have initiated concurrent record reviews. Gathering data concurrently while patients are still receiving care provides an opportunity to catch and correct safety concerns before patient harm occurs. For instance, using a 36-item patient safety checklist nurse reviewers in the neonatal intensive care unit at Children's Hospital Boston (MA) identified and facilitated correction of errors associated with delays in care, equipment failure, diagnostic studies, information transfer and noncompliance with hospital policy (Ursprung et al., 2005).

In recent years, progress has been made toward creation of electronic health records (EHRs) that contain much of the same information traditionally found in paper-based records. Although having an automated alternative to manual chart review has obvious advantages, it is also not without its challenges. For instance, many EHR systems do not routinely incorporate common process and outcome measures used by health care organizations to monitor patient safety (Kilbridge & Classen, 2008). Adding the functionality of automated extraction of measurement data from EHRs, using query templates, can reduce the cost of data collection. When combined with administrative data, the EHR provides an even richer source of information for assessment of patient safety factors.

A pitfall of using patient records, whether paper-based or electronic, is the lack of detail. For example, if a hospitalized patient receives the wrong dose of a medication, the record entry may read something like, "Patient received 10 mg instead of the 5 mg that was ordered by the physician." Information about the patient's response to the medication will also be recorded. What is likely to be missing from the record is the cause of the event. Perhaps the doctor's handwriting was unclear, and because of the urgency of the situation, the staff did not clarify the order with the physician. Information documented in the patient's records can be used to count the incidence of medication errors, but the record is not likely to contain answers to such questions as the following:

- How often does illegible handwriting result in a medication error?

- How frequently does staff fail to question puzzling orders?

- Do lower staffing levels in the nursing unit correlate with higher medication error rates?

Unless the cause of the event is documented in another location, answers to these questions will be unavailable.

Administrative Data

Administrative data are another source of performance measurement information, particularly malpractice claims and billing data. Malpractice claims can provide facts about potentially preventable clinical and system errors that lead to undesirable patient outcomes (Phillips et al., 2004). However, claims data are not without pitfalls and weaknesses. Many claims are filed in the absence of actual clinical errors. Plus (thankfully) the number of actual claims filed is small, making aggregate analyses suspect. Regardless, many people suggest that claims data can be useful in determining types of mistakes made in patient care and for suggesting changes that need to be made (Carroll & Buddenbaum, 2007; Conklin, Bernstein, Bartholomew, Oliva-Hemker, 2008; Griffen et al., 2008; Griffen & Turnage, 2009). In addition, detailed claims investigation reports prepared by the risk management department can stimulate further inquiry and suggest solutions to some types of safety problems.

The organization's billing database, which typically contains information such as patient demographics, codes that identify diagnoses and procedures performed, and charges billed to payers, is another data source. Electronic billing records use International Classification of Diseases, 9th Revision, Clinical Modification (otherwise known as ICD-9-CM) and procedures in the Current Procedure Terminology, Version 4 (known as CPT-4). The advantage of using billing data as a source of information for patient safety measures is its availability—almost every health care organization has this database.

The billing claims database can provide the data elements necessary for the denominators of some patient safety-related performance measurements (such as number of discharges, number of deaths, and so on). The coded diagnosis and procedure data can also be useful in identifying instances of iatrogenic events. For example, the E-codes and some of the diagnosis codes contained in the ICD-9-CM represent complications or comorbidities. Listed in Table 4.4 are examples of diagnosis codes for maternal and fetal complications of in utero procedures (ICD9Data.com, n.d.).

Table 4.4   ICD-9-CM Diagnosis Codes for Maternal and Fetal Complications of in Utero Procedures

Code	Description
679.00	Maternal complications from in utero procedure, unspecified as to episode of care or not applicable
679.01	Maternal complications from in utero procedure, delivered, with or without mention of antepartum condition
679.02	Maternal complications from in utero procedure, delivered, with mention of postpartum complication
679.03	Maternal complications from in utero procedure, antepartum condition or complication
679.04	Maternal complications from in utero procedure, postpartum condition or complication
679.10	Fetal complications from in utero procedures, unspecified as to episode of care or not applicable
679.11	Fetal complications from in utero procedures, delivered, with or without mention of antepartum condition
679.12	Fetal complications from in utero procedures, delivered, with mention of postpartum complication
679.13	Fetal complications from in utero procedures, antepartum condition or complication
679.14	Fetal complications from in utero procedures, postpartum condition or complication

A simple count of these ICD-9-CM codes is not an absolute measure of adverse events; however, the codes could be used for screening purposes (Hougland et al., 2008). Further analysis of the cases to which these codes apply would be necessary to determine if inappropriate caregiver actions contributed to these conditions.

Another problem with the use of many diagnosis and procedure codes is that the data do not typically indicate when the event occurred. For hospitalized Medicare patients, this data collection problem has been partially resolved with present on admission (POA) indicators now required for diagnoses reported on claim forms (Centers for Medicare and Medicaid Services, 2009). However, lack of documentation or insufficient clinical information can make it difficult to judge whether the patient had a particular diagnosis prior to admission. A recent study by the Office of Inspector General (2010) found that POA diagnosis codes were inaccurate or absent for seven of the 11 Medicare hospital-acquired conditions identified by physician reviewers. At this time billing data may not be a reliable source of information for determining whether Medicare patients developed potentially preventable conditions or complications *after* being admitted to the hospital.

Administrative databases that contain primarily billing information are of limited value in providing risk-related performance measurement data. Gaps in clinical information and the billing context may compromise the facility's ability to derive valid patient incident and outcome data from administrative data. The data provide insufficient clinical information, especially with regard to errors of omission and commission. However, the growing availability of electronic clinical information is changing the nature of administrative data and strengthening its usefulness as a source for safety-related performance measures.

Patient Incident Reports

Incident reports, sometimes called variance or occurrence reports, have long been used as a source of risk management information. A patient incident or occurrence is a situation or provision of service which is not consistent with routine patient care and adversely affects or has the potential to adversely affect the life, health, comfort or safety of a patient. Any time a patient is harmed, it is usually considered reportable even if the injury is a known risk of the procedure or was caused unintentionally. Examples of incidents representing patient safety concerns include:

- Deviation in patient care (for example, blood drawn on wrong patient, wrong procedure done, delay in care)

- Allergic or untoward reaction to a procedure, treatment, medication, or transfusion (even if it is a known risk)

- Accidents with or without known injury that occur to patients (for example, falls)

- Acts of violence by or upon patients (for example, fighting, attempted suicide)

- Failure of patient equipment which does or could have caused an injury

- Medication error (whether or not there is any harm)

- Elopements and signing out against medical advice (AMA)

- Skin breakdowns

Most health care facilities require staff members to fill out a report when an incident has occurred. These reports are meant to be nonjudgmental, factual accounts of the event and its consequences, if any. An example of an incident report form is shown in Figure 4.1.

Obtaining accurate, valid, and reliable information from incident reports is not without its challenges. Following are the four primary problems found with most **incident reporting** programs:

1. All incidents may not be reported, depending on people's willingness to report.

2. Data items are not well defined or understood by the staff.

3. Reports lack sufficient detail for effective analysis.

4. Reports may not be completed for all near-miss situations or truly serious events.

Willingness to Report

The first problem—an individual's willingness to report an incident—is strongly linked to the organizational culture and how the information is used. If the involved staff member is blamed for the event and disciplined or dismissed by management because of the error, it's unlikely that people will voluntarily incriminate themselves or their colleagues by completing incident reports.

Experience has shown that when caregivers are provided protection from disciplinary actions, they are more willing to report incidents (Barach & Small, 2000; Evans et al., 2004). This phenomenon is consistent with what has been discovered by officials of the NASA Aviation Safety Reporting System and the

FIGURE 4.1   Patient Incident Report Form

INCIDENT REPORT

Complete immediately for every incident
and send to manager

—Confidential Report of Incident—
—Not a Part of the Medical Record—

(Addressograph or name and address)

Please Print

Patient _____ Age _____ Sex ___ Unit/room _____
       (Last name)   (First name)

Date of incident _____ Time _____ Physician notified? __ Yes __ No

Physician _____

Physician's response _____

Bed rails up? __ Yes __ No   Safety belt in place? __ Yes __ No

Bed position: __ High __ Low

Exact location of incident _____

Account of incident _____

_____

Signature_____ Date: _____

**Department
Manager's Action:**

List of persons involved or familiar with incident:

Name: _____

Name: _____

Classification of Incident
(Check one that most closely defines)

__ Fall without injury   __ Medication error
__ Fall with injury   __ Missed dose/order
__ Fracture/dislocation   __ Extra dose
__ Delayed test/   __ Wrong medication
   treatment   __ Wrong dose
__ Missed test/treatment __ Wrong time
__ Adverse reaction
__ Other:_____

British Airways Safety Information System. These groups have found that the following five factors are important in determining both the quantity and quality of incident reports (Reason, 1997):

1. Indemnity against disciplinary proceedings (as far as it is practical)

2. Confidentiality or de-identification

3. The separation of the agency or department collecting and analyzing the reports from those bodies with the authority to institute disciplinary proceedings and impose sanctions

4. Rapid, useful, accessible, and intelligible feedback to the reporting community

5. Ease of making the report

Creating a climate of trust is an essential component of an incident-reporting system. It must also be easy for people to file reports. The Institute for Healthcare Improvement's National Collaborative on Reducing Adverse Drug Events and Medical Errors (1997) recommended several ways of making reporting easy for caregivers. These recommendations include establishing dial-in hotlines and instituting simplified, anonymous error-reporting mechanisms.

Several studies have documented the value of electronic reporting of incident data. Organizations that have implemented user friendly, intranet-based reporting systems often find the number of reported incidents goes up (Bae et al., 2005; Nakajima, Kurata, & Takeda, 2005; Conlon, Havlisch, Kini, & Porter, 2008; Bilimoria et al., 2009). Ease of making the report seems to strongly correlate with higher levels of reported events, including near misses.

Data Definitions

The second challenge related to incident reporting is that the data items are not well defined or understood by the staff. For example, there must be a clear understanding of what constitutes a medication error to ensure that all such events are consistently reported. The National Coordinating Council for Medication Error Reporting and Prevention (NCC MERP) defines a medication error as any preventable event that may cause or lead to inappropriate medication use or patient harm while the medication is in the control of the health care professional, patient, or consumer. Such events may be related to professional practice, health care products, procedures, and systems, including prescribing; order communication; product labeling, packaging, and nomenclature; compounding; dispensing; distribution; administration; education; monitoring; and use (NCC MERP, 2010).

This definition suggests that any error involving medication usage should be reported. However, in actual practice it is common for caregivers to question aspects of this definition. For example: Does this mean that the patient actually had to receive the wrong medication? Does this mean I have to report someone else's error if I discover it? Does this mean I have to complete two incident reports if the pharmacy sent the wrong drug and I gave it to the patient? Questions such as these are an indication that the definition of a reportable medication error is still not clear.

The same definitional problems can be found for other types of incidents. For example, if a patient is found lying unharmed on the floor, is this situation considered a fall? Many hospitals use a definition of patient fall that is consistent with the taxonomy used in the National Database of Nursing Quality Indicators®, a program of the American Nurses Association's National Center for Nursing Quality (NDNQI®, 2010):

A patient fall is an unplanned descent to the floor (or extension of the floor, e.g., trash can or other equipment) with or without injury to the patient. All types of falls are to be included whether they result from physiological reasons (fainting) or environmental reasons (slippery floor). Include assisted falls—when a staff member attempts to minimize the impact of the fall.

Organizations should develop objective definitions of the types of incidents that must be reported by staff. Definitions originating from organizations such as the American Society of Health-System Pharmacists, the World Health Organization, the Joint Commission, and others should be considered when developing internal definitions. Of particular note are the patient incident definitions developed for use by **Patient Safety Organizations (PSOs)**. The Patient Safety and Quality Improvement Act of 2005 (Patient Safety Act) authorized the creation of PSOs to improve the quality and safety of U.S. health care delivery (AHRQ, n.d.). The PSOs provide a framework by which hospitals, doctors, and other health care providers may voluntarily report patient safety information to an outside entity without fear of legal discovery. A set of common definitions and reporting formats have been developed by AHRQ, with input from various stakeholders, to guide the process (AHRQ, 2009). Shown in Table 4.5 are examples of data definitions applicable to patient safety information reported to a PSO.

Table 4.5   Data Definitions Applicable to Reporting to a Patient Safety Organization

Word or phrase	Definition
Fall	A sudden, unintended, uncontrolled downward displacement of a patient's body to the ground or other object.
Healthcare-associated infection	A localized or systemic condition resulting from an adverse reaction to the presence of an infectious agent(s) or its toxin(s). It is acquired during the course of receiving treatment for other conditions within a health care setting, with no evidence that the infection was present or incubating at the time of admission.
Near miss	An event that did not reach a patient. For example: discovery of a dispensing error by a nurse as part of the process of administering the medication to a patient (which if not discovered would have become an incident); discovery of a mislabeled specimen in a laboratory (which if not discovered might subsequently have resulted in an incident).
Patient safety concern	Any circumstance involving patient safety; encompasses patient safety event (both incident and near miss) and unsafe condition.
Patient safety event	A patient safety event that reached a patient, and either resulted in no harm (no harm incident) or harm (harm incident). The concept "reached a patient" encompasses any action by a health care practitioner or worker or health care circumstance that exposes a patient to harm.
Side effect	An effect (usually an adverse outcome) caused by something (such as a drug or procedure) that was not the intended or indicated effect. The occurrence of a known side effect, even if an adverse outcome, by itself, is not a patient safety incident.
Severe permanent harm	Severe lifelong bodily or psychological injury or disfigurement that interferes significantly with functional ability or quality of life.
Temporary harm	Bodily or psychological injury, but likely not permanent.
Unexpected adverse outcome	Adverse outcome that was not expected to be a result of the patient's treatment plan; harm suffered as a result of an incident.
Unplanned intervention	An intervention that was not part of a patient's treatment plan prior to the event that necessitated the additional intervention.
Unsafe condition	Any circumstance that increases the probability of a patient safety event; includes a defective or deficient input to or environment of a care process that increases the risk of an unsafe act, care process failure or error, or patient safety event. An unsafe condition does not involve an identifiable patient.

Source: *AHRQ Common Formats Version 1.0, Users Guide*—August 2009 Release. Retrieved from https://www.psoppc.org/web/patientsafety/commonformats.

The Patient Safety Act also directs AHRQ to support the development of a network of patient safety databases. This data will be used to analyze national and regional patient safety trends with the findings to be made public in AHRQ's *National Healthcare Quality Report*, available in hard copy and electronically on the AHRQ Web site (www.ahrq.gov).

Level of Detail

Incident reports can also lack sufficient detail about the event that limits the value of aggregate data analysis. The goal of evaluating incident report data is to identify which safety-critical tasks are failing and how often these failures occur. Often, incident reports don't contain sufficient task-level information; that is, the activity that contributed to the occurrence. Without meaningful data there can be no meaningful analysis. Consider the patient incident summary report illustrated in Figure 4.2. The report provides a count of incidents in each category that occurred in units reporting to the vice president of nursing. Summary counts such as these are not focused or specific and do not reveal which safety-critical tasks are failing. At best, they provide a "snapshot" of the organization's patient safety performance.

Reports that communicate the causes of incidents will generally be more useful than simple counts of how many times an incident occurs (Wheeler, 2000). However, obtaining data about what happened to cause the event using incident reports as the sole source of information can be problematic. Staff would need to report a lot more detail about what may have led up to the event—problems involving communication, written procedures, workplace design, physical environment, working environment, task supervision, or training. If the incident reporter doesn't know the causes or doesn't take the time to document suspected problems, the information must be gathered later. Often this is done during a more in-depth analysis of the incident by a manager or another individual (perhaps the patient safety officer or risk manager). As with any data source consideration, there are trade-offs between what information is desirable for measuring patient safety versus what resources are available to support the data gathering effort.

Organizations voluntarily submitting patient incident data to PSOs will be providing fairly detailed descriptions of each event including the extent of patient harm and interventions attempted to reverse or halt the progression of harm. For near-miss events, the reporter must answer such questions as, what prevented the near miss from reaching the patient? (AHRQ, 2009).

Failure to Report

The fourth problem with using incident reports as a data source for **error management** purposes is that not all reportable events end up getting

FIGURE 4.2   Sample Summary Report of Incidents for One Month

Incident Report for the Vice President of Nursing
Reporting Period: **July**

UNIT NAME	Event	Number	Severity	Number
Medical Inpatient	IV/Blood	5	None	5
	Medication	3	Minor	5
	Falls	2	Moderate	1
	Misc.	3	Significant	2
	Equipment	1	Death	1
	Total:	**14**	**Total:**	**14**
Surgery Inpatient	IV/ Blood	1	None	2
	Medication	2	Minor	1
	Falls	3	Moderate	3
	Misc.	1	Significant	2
	Equipment	1		
	Total:	**8**	**Total:**	**8**
Pediatric Inpatient	Medication	1	None	2
	Misc.	1	Minor	1
	Equipment	1		
	Total:	**3**	**Total:**	**3**
Psych Inpatient	Misc.	1	None	1
	Self-Injury	1	Moderate	1
	Total:	**2**	**Total:**	**2**
Intensive Care Unit	Medical	2	Minor	1
	Misc.	1	Moderate	2
	Total:	**3**	**Total:**	**3**
Coronary Care Unit	Medical	1	None	1
	Falls	2	Minor	2
	Total:	**3**	**Total:**	**3**
Emergency Services	IV/Blood	1	Moderate	1
	Procedure	1	Death	1
	Total:	**2**	**Total:**	**2**
Operating Room	Misc.	2	None	1
			Moderate	1
	Total:	**2**	**Total:**	**2**
Post Anesthesia Recovery Unit	Procedure	1	Moderate	1
	Total:	**1**	**Total:**	**1**

documented. Institutions may have specific policies about what incidents to report, but studies have shown that when faced with real clinical situations, clinicians do not appear to consistently comply with such policies (Leape, 2002). For instance, in a study of adverse events occurring while children are sedated, researchers found that minor adverse events associated with procedural sedation were underreported, despite clear perianesthesia documentation in the medical record that an event had occurred (Lightdale et al., 2009). As a result, much important information about errors is lost. All errors and near misses should be reported regardless of the surrounding circumstances. With this is mind, it is important to promote an atmosphere that encourages honest and thorough reporting.

There is also a belief in the risk management community that incident reports are rarely completed for truly serious events. Many professional liability carriers report that of total claims filed, only one-third ever had incident reports generated. This underreporting of serious events may be caused by staff not perceiving a problem whereas the patient does. Consider this example: A patient with a history of heart disease has a cardiac arrest on the first postoperative day. The staff feels everything was handled without error if the resuscitation is successful. From the patient's perspective, however, something went very wrong. The patient believes that the physicians and staff knew about his predisposing cardiac problems and should have taken appropriate precautions. Such differences in perception can cause the patient to initiate legal action, and yet no incident report of the event is completed by the staff.

In addition, injuries that evolve over a period of time (for example, deterioration in condition, neurological impairment, vascular compromise, and so on) are generally not reported because there may not be one particular point in time when something actually happened to cause the injury. Therefore, an incident report is not completed.

Even in the best of situations and environments, it is unlikely incident reports will ever be the sole data source for patient safety measurement. The information gleaned from incident reports will need to be supplemented by data obtained from other sources.

Patient and Family Feedback

Feedback from patients and family members has traditionally been used to gather information about satisfaction with service amenities. Now health care organizations are using this feedback to identify patient safety concerns (Zimmerman & Amori, 2008). Feedback can be gathered through surveys administered over the telephone, electronically (over a computer network or via the Internet), on paper (on-site or via mail) or through in-person interviews and focus groups. A study in the medicine unit of a Boston teaching hospital found that after leaving the hospital, patients are able to identify adverse events that had affected their care. Many of these events had not been reported by the staff during the patient's hospital stay (Weingart et al., 2005).

Health care organizations should encourage patients and family members to report safety concerns directly to caregivers. Staff members at one neonatal intensive care unit routinely ask parents such questions as, "Are there aspects of your child's care that you find concerning?" or "What do you worry about when you leave your child?" (Alton, Mericle, & Brandon, 2006). To use this information as a data source for patient safety measures, the organization must have a mechanism for documenting these concerns. At University Children's Hospital, Zurich, Switzerland, safety issues reported by parents are integrated with the incident reporting system (Frey et al., 2009). Examples of safety concerns that parents brought to the attention of neonatal caregivers at the Zurich hospital include:

- Wrong prescription (Carvedilol 265 mg/d instead of 261 mg/d)

- Infant's swollen, bluish leg (thrombosis of the femoral vein)

- Infant's respiratory distress

- Wrong infant weight on the prescription chart

In addition to the data sources mentioned above, performance measurement information may also be obtained from other sources, including referral logs, staff surveys, medication records, appointment books, and minutes of relevant meetings. Collecting data for patient safety measures is complex and requires a thorough understanding of multiple data sources and how to construct measures from disparate data types.

When planning the data collection strategy, evaluate existing data sources to determine where the information necessary to create each performance measure can be found. First determine if the necessary data are accessible in an existing information system. If they are, then check to be sure the data definitions are consistent with what you need for the measure. Although it may seem as if every possible data element is now being gathered, there may be times when the data needed to calculate a particularly important measure are not readily available and new data sources will need to be developed.

Conclusion

This chapter describes the use of performance measurement data for monitoring patient safety in an organization along with important points regarding data collection. Although there is not a singular formula for selecting performance measures, the chapter raises several fundamental questions about how safety performance can be evaluated and how the information can be gathered. By addressing each of these questions, organizations will eventually discover the most effective measurement strategy for their environment. Remember, performance measures tend to be evolutionary rather than revolutionary. No one starts with the perfect set of measures; successful organizations evolve their set of measures.

Measuring performance of high-risk processes with the intention of reducing errors is a multifaceted undertaking. It is possible to use any number of performance measures. Currently there is no industry-wide consensus on what safety-critical tasks should be regularly evaluated and what constitutes a reportable incident—although with the formation of PSOs and development of a network of patient safety databases this may soon change. Health care entities should formulate a plan for identifying high-risk processes and safety-critical tasks for focused measurement activities. Then, with input from patient safety, risk management, and quality improvement departments, the organization's leaders must decide which performance measures will yield the more worthwhile data.

Discussion Questions

1. For high-risk patient care activities two types of measures can be used: process and outcome measures. Identify one process measure and one outcome measure that could be used to evaluate the safety of the patient care process described below. The process shown in Figure 4.3 illustrates what happens

FIGURE 4.3   Flowchart of Blood Transfusion Process

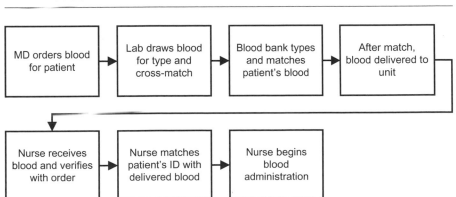

from the time the physician orders a blood transfusion for a hospitalized patient until the blood transfusion is administered to the patient.

2. Suppose the hospital's patient safety director wants to gather data to report performance results for the measures you've chosen. What data source could be used to gather information for the measures? Why would these data sources be best for gathering reliable data?

3. Query the National Quality Measures Clearinghouse (http://www.qualitymeasures.ahrq.gov) and identify two process and two outcome measures that could be used to evaluate patient safety in outpatient or ambulatory services. List each measure, the organization or group that developed the measure, and the date of publication.

Key Terms

Error containment

Error management

Error-producing factor

Error reduction

Incident reporting

Medication error

Misdiagnosis-related harm

Outcome measure

Patient safety indicator (PSI)

Patient safety organization (PSO)

Process measure

Safety-critical task

Task criticality

References

AHRQ. (n.d.). Patient safety organization information: Background. Retrieved from http://www.pso.ahrq.gov/psos/overview.htm.

AHRQ. (2007, March). *Guide to patient safety indicators, version 3.1* Retrieved from http://www.qualityindicators.ahrq.gov/psi_download.htm.

AHRQ. (2009, April). Common formats: Facilitating learning from patient safety data. Retrieved from http://www.pso.ahrq.gov/formats/brochurecmnfmt.pdf.

Alton, M., Mericle, J., & Brandon, D. (2006). One intensive care nursery's experience with enhancing patient safety. *Advances in Neonatal Care, 6*(3), 112–9.

Andrews, L. B., Stocking, C., Krizek, T., Gottlieb, L., Krizek, C., Vargish, T., & Siegler, M. (1997). An alternative strategy for studying adverse events in medical care. *Lancet, 349*(9048), 309–313.

Bae, S., Khouangsathiene, S., Morey, C., O'Connor, C., Rose, E., & Shakil, A. (2005). Implementation of a Web-based incident-reporting system at Legendary Health System (pp. 114–120). In L. Einbinder, N. Lorenzi, J. Ash, C. Gadd, & J. Einbinder (Eds.). *Transforming health care through information: Case studies.* New York: Springer.

Barach, P., & Small, S. (2000). Reporting and preventing medical mishaps: Lessons from non-medical near miss reporting systems. *British Medical Journal, 320*(7327), 759–763.

Bilimoria, K., Kmiecik, T., DaRose, D., Halverson, A., Eskandari, M., Bell, R., Soper, N., & Wayne, J. (2009). Development of an online morbidity, mortality, and near-miss reporting system to identify patterns of adverse events in surgical patients. *Archives of Surgery, 144*(4), 305–311.

Carroll, A. E., & Buddenbaum, J. L. (2007). Malpractice claims involving pediatricians: Epidemiology and etiology. *Pediatrics, 120*(1), 10–17.

Centers for Medicare and Medicaid Services. (2009, September 21) Hospital-acquired conditions (present on admission indicator). Retrieved from http://www.cms.hhs .gov/HospitalAcqCond/.

Chang, A., Schyve, P. M., Croteau, R. J., O'Leary, D. S., & Loeb, J. M. (2005). The JCAHO patient safety event taxonomy: a standardized terminology and classification schema for near misses and adverse events. *International Journal for Quality in Health Care, 17*(2), 95–105.

Conklin, L. S., Bernstein, C., Bartholomew, L., Oliva-Hemker, M. (2008). Medical malpractice in gastroenterology. *Clinical Gastroenterology and Hepatology, 6*(6), 677–681.

Conlon, P., Havlisch, R., Kini, N., & Porter, C. (2008). Using an anonymous Web-based incident reporting tool to embed the principles of a high reliability organization. In K. Henriksen, J. B. Battles, M. A. Keyes, & M. L. Grady, (Eds.), *Advances in patient safety: New directions and alternative approaches. Vol. 2. Culture and redesign.* AHRQ Publication No. 08–0034–2. Rockville, MD: Agency for Healthcare Research and Quality. Retrieved from http://ftp.ahrq.gov/downloads/pub/advances2/vol1/ Advances-Conlon_50.pdf.

Corriol, C., Daucourt, V., Grenier, C., & Minvielle, E. (2008). How to limit the burden of data collection for quality indicators based on medical records? The COMPAQH experience. BMC Health Services Research, 8, 215. Retrieved from http://www .biomedcentral.com/1472–6963/8/215.

Dekker, S. W. (2009). Just culture: who gets to draw the line? *Cognition Technology and Work, 11*(3), 177–185.

Donabedian, A. (1980). *Explorations in quality assessment and monitoring, volume I: The definition of quality and approaches to its assessment.* Ann Arbor, MI: Health Administration Press.

Evans, S. M., Berry, J. G., Smith, B. J., Esterman, A., Selim, P., O'Shaughnessy, & DeWit, M. (2004). Attitudes and barriers to incident reporting: A collaborative hospital study. *Quality and Safety in Health Care, 15*(1), 39–43.

Food and Drug Administration. (2009, August 17). *What is a serious adverse event?* Retrieved from http://www.fda.gov/Safety/MedWatch/HowToReport/ucm053087.htm.

Forster, A., Murff, H., Peterson, J., Gandhi, T., & Bates, D. (2005). Adverse drug events occurring following hospital discharge. *Journal of General Internal Medicine, 20*(4), 317–323.

Frey, B., Ersch, J., Bernet, V., Baenziger, O., Enderli, L., & Doell, C. (2009). Involvement of parents in critical incidents in a neonatal-paediatric intensive care unit. *Quality and Safety in Health Care, 18*(6), 446–449.

Ganz, D., Bao, Y., Shekelle, P., & Rubenstein, L. (2007). Will my patient fall? *Journal of the American Medical Association, 297*(1), 77–86.

Giraud, T., Dhainaut, J., Vaxelaire, J., Joseph, T., Journois, D., Bleichner, G., Sollet, J., Chevret, S., & Monsallier, J. (1993). Iatrogenic complications in adult intensive care units: A prospective two-center study. *Critical Care Medicine, 21*(1), 40–51.

Griffen, F. D., Stephens, L. S., Alexander, J. B., Bailey, H. R., Maizel, S. E., Sutton, B. H., & Posner, K. L. (2008). Violations of behavioral practices revealed in closed claims reviews. *Annals of Surgery, 248*(3), 468–474.

Griffen, F. D., & Turnage, R. H. (2009). Reviews of liability claims against surgeons: What have they revealed? *Advances in Surgery, 43*(1), 199–209.

Haas, J. P., & Larson, E. L. (2007). Methods of measuring compliance with hand hygiene with advantages and disadvantages. *Journal of Hospital Infection, 66*(1), 6–14.

Hougland, P., Nebeker, J., Pickard, S., Van Tuinen, M., Masheter, C., Elder, S., Williams, S., & Xu, W. (2008). Using ICD-9-CM codes in hospital claims data to detect adverse events in patient safety surveillance. Advances in patient safety: New directions and alternative approaches. Volumes 1–4, AHRQ Publication Nos. 08–0034 (1–4). Agency for Healthcare Research and Quality, Rockville, MD. http://www.ahrq.gov/qual/advances2/.

ICD9Data.com. (n.d.) Free 2010 medical coding data. Retrieved from http://www.icd-9data.com/.

Institute for Healthcare Improvement. (1997). The quest for error-proof medicine. *Drug Benefit Trends, 9*(6), 18, 23, 27–29.

Institute of Medicine, Committee on Quality of Health Care in America. (2001). *Crossing the quality chasm: A new health system for the 21st century.* Washington, DC: National Academy Press.

Kilbridge, P. M., & Classen, D. C. (2008). The informatics opportunities at the intersection of patient safety and clinical informatics. *Journal of the American Medical Informatics Association, 15*(4), 397–407.

Leape, L. (2002). Reporting of adverse events. *New England Journal of Medicine, 347*(20), 1633–1638.

Legorreta, A., Chernicoff, H., Trinh, J., & Parker, R.G. (2004). Diagnosis, clinical staging, and treatment of breast cancer: A retrospective multiyear study of a large controlled population. *American Journal of Clinical Oncology, 27*(2), 185–190.

Lightdale, J., Mahoney, L., Fredette, B., Valim, C., Wong, S., & DiNardo, J. (2009). Nurse reports of adverse events during sedation procedures at a pediatric hospital. *Journal of Perianesthesia Nursing, 24*(5), 300–306.

Mant, J. (2001). Process vs. outcome indicators in the assessment of quality of health care. *International Journal for Quality in Health Care, 13*(6), 475–480.

Nakajima, K., Kurata, Y., & Takeda, H. (2005). A Web-based incident reporting system and multidisciplinary collaborative projects for patient safety in a Japanese hospital. *Quality and Safety in Health Care, 14*(2), 123–129.

National Institutes of Health. (2008, June 17). *NIH risk management guidebook: A step-by-step guide.* Retrieved from http://omar.nih.gov/documentation/RM_Guidebook.pdf.

NCC MERP. (2010). About medication errors: What is a medication error? Retrieved from http://www.nccmerp.org/aboutMedErrors.html.

Newman-Toker, D. E., & Pronovost, P. J. (2009). Diagnostic errors—The next frontier for patient safety. *Journal of the American Medical Association, 301*(10), 1060–1062.

NDNQI® (2010, May). *Guidelines for data collection on the American Nurses Association's National Quality Forum endorsed measures.* Retrieved from https://www.nursingquality.org.

Office of Inspector General. (2010, March). *Adverse events in hospitals: Methods for identifying events.* Department of Health and Human Services. OEI-06–08–00221. Retrieved from http://www.oig.hhs.gov/oei/reports/oei-06–08–00221.pdf.

Phillips, R., Bartholomew, L., Dovey, S., Fryer, G., Miyoshi, T., & Green. (2004). Learning from malpractice claims about negligent, adverse events in primary care in the United States. *Quality and Safety in Health Care, 13*(2), 121–126.

Physician Insurers Association of America. (1997). *Radiology practice standards claims survey.* Reston, VA: American College of Radiology.

Pronovost, P., Nolan, T., Zeger, S., Miller, M., & Rubin, H. (2004). How can clinicians measure safety and quality in acute care? *Lancet, 363*(9414), 1061–1073.

Pronovost, P., Holzmueller, C., Needham, D., Sexton, J. B., Miller, M., Berenholtz, S., … Morlock, L. (2006). How will we know patients are safer? An organization-wide approach to measuring and improving safety. *Critical Care Medicine, 34*(7), 1988–1995.

Reason, J. (1997). *Managing the risks of organizational accidents.* Brookfield, VT: Ashgate.

Rivard, P. E., Rosen, A. K., & Carroll, J. S. (2006). Enhancing patient safety through organizational learning: Are patient safety indicators a step in the right direction? *Health Services Research, 41*(4, part II), 1633–1653.

Spath, P. L. (2007). Taming the measurement monster. *Frontiers of Health Services Administration, 23*(4), 3–14.

The Joint Commission. (2005). *How to meet the most challenging Joint Commission requirements for home care.* Oakbrook Terrace, IL: Joint Commission Resources.

The Joint Commission. (2007, July). Sentinel event policy and procedures. Retrieved from http://www.jointcommission.org/SentinelEvents/PolicyandProcedures/.

The Joint Commission. (2009a). Sentinel event statistics as of September 30, 2009. Retrieved from http://www.jointcommission.org/NR/rdonlyres/377FF7E7-F565 –4D61–9FD2–593CA688135B/0/SE_Stats_9_09.pdf

The Joint Commission. (2009b). Measuring hand hygiene adherence: Overcoming the challenges. Oakbrook Terrace, IL: The Joint Commission. Retrieved from http://www.jointcommission.org/NR/rdonlyres/68B9CB2F-789F-49DB-9E3F-2FB387666BCC/0/hh_monograph.pdf.

Ursprung, R., Gray, J., Edwards, W., Horbar, J., Nickerson, J., Plsek, P., Shiono, P., Suresh, G., & Goldmann, D. (2005). Real time patient safety audits: Improving safety every day. *Quality and Safety in Health Care,14*(4), 284–289.

Weeks, W. B., Foster, T., Wallace, A. E., & Stalhandske, E. (2001). Tort claims analysis in the Veterans Health Administration for quality improvement. *Journal of Law Medicine & Ethics, 29*(3–4), 335–345.

Weingart, S., Pagovich, O., Sands, D., Li, J., Aronson, M., Davis, R., Bates, D., & Russell, P. (2005). What can hospitalized patients tell us about adverse events? Learning from patient-reported incidents. *Journal of General Internal Medicine, 20*(9), 830–836.

Wheeler, D. J. (2000). *Understanding variation: The key to managing chaos* (2nd ed.). Knoxville, TN: SPC Press.

Zimmerman, T. M., & Amori, G. (2008). Patient involvement in system failure analysis: Engaging the overlooked partner (pp. 201–233). In P. L. Spath (Ed.). *Engaging patients as safety partners: A guide for reducing errors and improving satisfaction.* Chicago: Health Forum.

CHAPTER 5

ANALYZING PATIENT SAFETY PERFORMANCE

Karen Ferraco
Patrice L. Spath

LEARNING OBJECTIVES

- Identify techniques for reporting patient safety measurement data
- Recognize the strengths and weakness of measurement data
- Describe how measurement data are interpreted
- Identify situations requiring further investigation

Selecting patient safety measures and collecting data for these measures is merely the first step toward analyzing patient safety performance. An effective error management strategy requires that performance measurement results be processed and presented in meaningful ways to clinical and administrative staff. The collected measurement data must be synthesized so that people can make informed assumptions about what is happening, why safety performance might vary from what was expected, and what corrective action might be required. Put another way, the purpose of analyzing performance data is insight. The measurement results should provide people with a meaningful safety performance profile of the department or service to which the measures apply.

Before data can be used for monitoring the safety of patient care practices, they must be analyzed, interpreted, and assimilated. Although good data are collected, analysis will be difficult or the wrong conclusions reached if data are inadequately summarized or poorly displayed.

Reporting Measurement Data

Safety measurement data should be reported in a way that makes it easier to draw conclusions. Reporting can take many forms. Sometimes a single data grouping will suffice for the purposes of decision making. In complex situations, and especially when larger amounts of data must be dealt with, multiple groupings are necessary to create a clear picture of performance. Measurement data can be presented in many different formats. The most common are tabular reports and graphical representations.

Tabular Reports

To create a tabular report (sometimes called a *data table*) the raw data are translated into performance rates so that people can monitor **performance trends**. Illustrated in Figure 5.1 is an example of a tabular report showing patient safety measurement results in a hospital. The results are shown for four consecutive quarters.

Dashboards are a special type of tabular report that use symbols and/or colors to draw people's attention to performance concerns (Spath, 2005). Figure 5.2 shows an excerpt from dashboard-style format used to report organization-wide patient safety measurement results to a hospital governing board and senior leaders. Stars and colors are used to signify the hospital's actual performance. A key to understanding the meaning of the number of stars used to report results is provided at the bottom of the report. The actual report is printed in color with

FIGURE 5.1   Tabular Report of Inpatient Patient Safety Measures

	1st Qtr	2nd Qtr	3rd Qtr	4th Qtr
Measures				
Patient falls per 1,000 inpatient days	4.93	3.22	2.17	3.20
Patient falls with injury per 1,000 inpatient days	1.86	1.15	0.84	1.19
Percent of inpatients that developed pressure ulcers stage II +	0.92	1.70	1.43	1.01
Number of inpatients with a blood transfusion reaction	0	0	1	0
Medical-Surgical ICU: Number of catheter-associated urinary tract infections per 1,000 device days	0.3	0	1.1	1.6
Medical-Surgical ICU: Number of central line associated blood stream infections per 1,000 device days	0.2	1.2	0	0.3
Medical-Surgical ICU: Number of ventilator-associated pneumonias per 1,000 device days	0.6	0	0.8	1.5
Neonatal ICU: Percent of patients with coagulase negative staphylococcus infection	2.4	2.7	1.2	3.5
Neonatal ICU: Percent of patients with fungal infections	0.5	0	0	0.2

FIGURE 5.2   Dashboard Tabular Report of Inpatient Patient
Safety Measures

	Actual Year-to-Date Performance	Performance Goal
Infection Control		
Hospital-wide infection rate	★★★★	★★★★
Surgical site infection rate	★★★★	★★★★★
Rate of ventilator-assisted pneumonia	★★★★	★★★★★
Rate of infections possibly due to intravenous lines	★★★★★	★★★★★
Patient Incidents		
Falls	★★★★	★★★★
Falls with injury	★★★	★★★★
Pressure ulcers, Stage II+	★★★★	★★★★★
Blood transfusion error	★★★★★	★★★★★
Other/Miscellaneous	★★★★	★★★★★
Medication Errors		
Prescription errors	★★★	★★★★
Dispensing Errors	★★★★	★★★★★
Administration errors	★★	★★★★

Key   Exceptional =   ★★★★★ (Green)   Below Normal =   ★★ (Red)
      Above Normal = ★★★★ (Green)   Marginal =   ★ (Red)
      Normal =   ★★★ (Yellow)

the stars reported in different colors. Not only can board members and senior leaders quickly see how well the organization is doing by counting the stars they can also judge results by the color-coding.

Creating a safety performance dashboard that relies on symbols and/or color to denote results requires some behind-the-scenes decisions. People must decide on the numeric levels that equate to the performance ratings. For example, what is an "Exceptional" rate of patient falls versus one that is classified in the "Normal" category? This decision must be made on a measurement-by-measurement basis with input from all stakeholders. In addition, these definitions should be revisited periodically to ensure the organization is working toward ever-better patient safety.

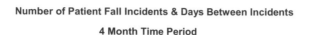

FIGURE 5.3   Bar and Line Graph of Patient Fall Incidents

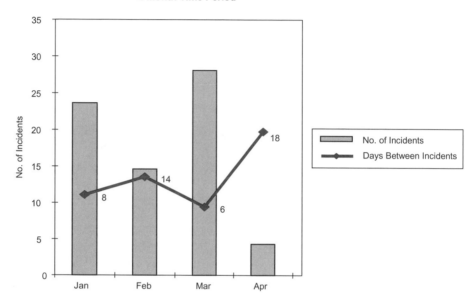

Graphical Representations

There are many ways to communicate measurement results through graphical means. The same set of data can often be graphed in different ways. The hard part is determining the best graph to emphasize the point you want to make and also accurately tell the story in the data. Two common graphical representations used to communicate patient safety measurement results from several time periods are line graphs and bar charts. Figure 5.3 shows a report that combines these two data displays. The graph shows the number of patient falls each month (bars) and the number of days between fall incidents each month (trend line).

Safety Measurement Results

Individual departments should receive reports of patient safety measurement data relevant to their area. In addition, leadership groups that oversee patient safety should receive aggregate safety-related performance measurement results for analysis. To create this aggregate report, start by gathering together all the measures that relate to patient safety so they can be merged into one report. Next use data analysis techniques to identify the early warning signs of safety-related problems that require immediate investigation and action.

Compile Safety-Related Measures

Health care organizations commonly create department- or service-specific performance reports, each of which include some safety-related measurement data. For example, hospital nursing units could be measuring compliance with medication administration protocols whereas the emergency department might be reporting the percentage of charts lacking information about patients' home medications. Although data for these measures are collected and included on separate, department-specific reports, there should be also at least one leadership group that has a comprehensive picture of how well the entire organization is doing.

To gain a thorough understanding of how well caregivers are performing high-risk processes, the safety-related performance measures from department-specific reports should be duplicated onto a patient safety summary. This summary report would include the results of every department's measures of performance for high-risk processes plus relevant outcome measures. Combining these data into one report can make it easier to identify relationships between process breakdowns and outcomes. For example, there may be a correlation between surgical site infections and missed or delayed doses of antibiotics. However, this correlation will be difficult (if not impossible) to see if the measurement data appear on separate reports.

Combining all safety-related measures into one organization-wide report can also help to ensure that small problems that are prevalent in more than one department are discovered and corrected. For example, nurses in the operating room may be experiencing periodic problems with broken equipment. Although this is an annoyance, the number of incidents may never reach the threshold for further investigation. Home health nurses may also be having the same problems, but they don't take any action either as the number of incidents is so small. Unless one central leadership group can see that the same equipment-related problems are occurring in several service areas, this circumstance will likely go uncorrected and could lead to serious patient injury.

Start the process of aggregating performance data about high-risk processes by listing each department's current patient safety-relevant process and outcome measures. Have the patient safety committee review the list to be sure all important functions are covered as well as all safety-critical tasks. It may be necessary to add some new measures. Once the inventory of measures is finalized, the next

Table 5.1 Organization-Wide Report of Safety Measures for the Function of Medication Administration

	1st Quarter	2nd Quarter	3rd Quarter	4th Quarter
Percent of records with patient's allergies noted prior to administration of antiarrhythmic medications	89%	90%	91%	88%
Percent of cases in which titration of IV Pitocin was done per hospital policy	85%	88%	98%	99%
Percent of patient medication profiles in pharmacy that correspond to physician's orders	97%	98%	100%	100%
Percent of benzodiazepine doses ordered correctly for patient age and/or condition	62%	84%	98%	100%
Number of restock errors involving automated medication dispensers	12	15	18	12
Percent of IV antibiotics administered within 1 hour of physician's order	83%	84%	78%	83%
Average thrombolytic therapy "Door to Needle" time (minutes) in the emergency department	25 min.	26 min.	19 min.	22 min.
Percent of patients reporting 5 or less on a pain scale of 1–10 on post-op day one	72%	80%	75%	78%

step is to capture the numbers from each departmental report and merge them into an organization-wide patient safety report. The measures can be sorted into categories for reporting purposes. For instance, the report shown in Table 5.1 is an excerpt from a larger hospital-wide report of safety measurement results. This excerpt shows results from measures related to medication administration that have been collected throughout the organization. Similar reports can be created for each major patient care function.

Understand Data Strengths and Weaknesses

Combining all measures into one report makes it easier for the patient safety committee to detect significant undesirable trends. Before taking action on these trends, it is important for the committee to consider the strengths and weaknesses of the data. This step allows for the identification of misinformation that might bias the analysis. Misinformation is information that is incorrect because of such factors as misinterpretation, improper recording, underreporting, and data collection mistakes.

The biggest problem with safety-related data is reporting inconsistencies. If people are punished when they report high error rates, they will start reporting lower rates regardless of the actual number of errors. Gross underreporting of patient incidents has been widely documented (Lawton & Parker, 2002). Discrepancies between actual number and reported incidents make it difficult to know how to react to performance measure results. High error rates may be an indicator of good detection and reporting by health care professionals, whereas low rates may be due to either lack of reporting or highly successful error prevention tactics (Leeuwen, 1994).

Not all risk-related performance measures will be affected by reporting inconsistencies. Generally, measures that rely on data that are voluntarily reported tend to be less reliable than data obtained through standardized patient record reviews, database queries, or observational studies. Therefore, accuracy may be judged differently for different types of information and can involve cross-checking information between reports; verifying numbers with knowledgeable respondents; or assessing the plausibility, detail, documentation, consistency, and overall "ring of truth" (Bauer, 2009). If the data are not considered to be reasonably accurate, the patient safety committee should concentrate organizational efforts on improving the quality of the information. In some organizations, getting good numbers is the most important first step in the error management initiative.

Analyze Results

Data analysis techniques should be used to identify the early warning signs of safety-related problems that require immediate investigation and action. It is not the intent of this chapter to address each and every analysis method that can be used to evaluate performance data. Methods range from fairly simple to fairly complicated. What is presented in this section is a very brief discussion of how to evaluate the fluctuations in performance data that will naturally occur from month to month. What the patient safety committee must determine is whether or not changes in the data represent random fluctuations in the process or if the changes represent an important signal that must be acted on.

The simplest tool that allows for identifying trends in performance measurement data is the line graph (sometimes called a run chart). This chart displays the data in the time order that they were collected. The run chart is constructed so that time is displayed on the horizontal axis and increases as you move to the right. The measurement data are plotted on the vertical axis. Figure 5.4. provides an example of a run chart showing the percentage of reported patient incidents that did not result in discomfort, infection, pain, or harm to the patient.

FIGURE 5.4   Percentage of Patient Incidents That Did Not Result in Discomfort, Infection, Pain, or Harm to the Patient

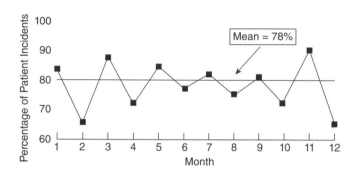

The mean of the values is plotted as a horizontal line across the graph. This mean line helps the patient safety committee detect patterns and trends. A pattern is formed when points on the run chart consistently "move" around the mean line in the same repetitive fashion (as shown in the graph). A trend is present when successive points on the run chart show either a consistent increase in value or decrease in value. Generally seven or more points all going up or all going down are considered a trend (Kelley, 1999).

Measurement data can also be analyzed using **statistical process control** by plotting the data on a **control chart** such as the example illustrated in Figure 5.5. A control chart includes the following:

- The performance measurement data

- An average (or center) line set at the mean (arithmetic average) of the data

- An upper control limit

- A lower control limit

A control chart is useful for determining if measurement results are attributable to **common cause variation** (random fluctuations in the process) or if the results indicate that **special cause variation** (something unusual in the process) is happening (Kelley, 1999). Wheeler (2000) provides an excellent reference for determining the correct approach for handling variation in most types of control charts. In general, he suggests that an estimate of the standard deviation be computed and then **control limits** established at three standard deviations above (the upper control limit) and below (the lower control limit) the mean. Common causes of variation produce data points on a control chart that over

FIGURE 5.5 Control Chart of Number of Patient Falls

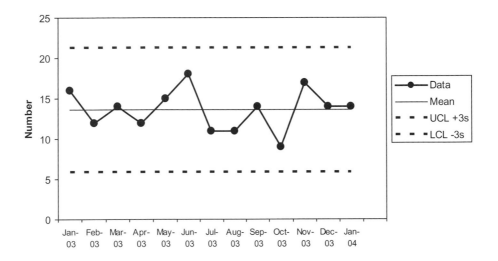

Number of Patient Falls
(All units)

time all fall inside the control limits. In this situation, no statistically significant trend is said to exist. The performance data do vary from point to point, but the fluctuations are due to random variation in the process.

The rate of patients falls shown on the control chart in Figure 5.5 shows no statistically significant trends. The number of falls does vary from point to point, but the fluctuations are due to random variation in the process. If a data point were to fall outside of a control limit (set at 3+ and 3− standard deviations from the mean), this signifies that a special cause variation has occurred. Special causes are specific issues acting on the process, such as personnel and equipment changes, weather delays, malfunctions, and other "unique" events. If the performance measurement data exceeds a control limit (upper or lower), this situation needs to be investigated or resolved. By using control charts instead of numeric reports or simple trend lines, the patient safety committee will be less likely to react to expected (and normal) data fluctuations.

If the performance data remain within control limits for 25 data points, the process is said to be "in control." To improve an "in control" process, the patient safety committee must examine all of the process information over the time period that the process has been stable. Improvement will hinge on determining the error-producing factors that have been acting on the process over this time and changing the process to remove or mitigate the sources of common cause variation (Kelley, 1999). In searching for common causes, it is important to perform the analysis over the entire time period that the process has been in control. The time interval chosen for the analysis population should correspond to an interval where no significant trends exist on the control chart.

A data point that falls outside of the control limit signifies that a special cause variation has occurred. Special causes are created by specific issues acting on the process, such as personnel and equipment changes, weather delays, malfunctions, and other unusual events. If the performance measurement data exceed a control limit (upper or lower), this situation needs to be investigated or resolved. The patient safety committee should also watch for significant trends that are evident from nonrandom patterns in the data, such as the following (Wheeler, 2000):

- Two out of three points in a row outside of two standard deviations above the average or two out of three points in a row outside of two standard deviations below the average

- Four out of five points in a row outside of one standard deviation above the average or four out of five points in a row outside of one standard deviation below the average

If one of these patterns is evident in the data over at least four complete reporting cycles, the process should be investigated for special causes. When a significant sentinel event has occurred, a formal root cause analysis should be initiated. Such a detailed analysis is not only important for understanding the specific event but is also required by the standards of the Joint Commission.

By using control charts instead of run charts to plot performance measurement data, the patient safety committee is less likely to view data fluctuations as coming from special causes. Considerable harm will be done (and certainly no improvement will be achieved) if endless hours are expended trying to explain why the most recent datum point occurred. Only if the most recent datum point was a statistically significant change on the control chart should there be an investigation into why the datum point came in at the value it did.

Regardless of the format used to report patient safety measures the information is only useful if it is analyzed. When safety concerns are identified, further investigation should be done. Consider the high rate of medication dispenser stocking errors in the report shown in Table 5.1. Questions such as the following can help the patient safety committee, as well as the pharmacy department, dig deeper into the problem:

- Are there any patterns or trends that are immediately obvious (for example, time of day, similar or identical errors)?

- Can you think of any reasons why errors might occur (for example, similar drug names, computer problems)?

- Do errors happen more frequently when the pharmacy is short-staffed?

- Does *all* staff involved in restocking medication dispensers receive training that enables them to detect errors (including staff who may provide cover)?

- Does any type of restocking error occur more frequently than the others (for example, wrong medication, wrong dose, wrong concentration)?

- Are there any obvious links or patterns between the type of medication involved in the stocking error and the restocking process?

- Do the contributing factors fall within one category more than others (for example, distraction, haste, inadequate double-checks, similar drug names)?

- Are there any patterns or trends associated with the circumstances (for example, they occur when the pharmacy is busier than usual, when regular technicians are not on duty)?

Compare Safety Performance

For some safety-related measures, comparative local, state, or national data from other organizations may be available. Some of these data are publicly available while other comparative databases are only accessible to project participants. Comparative data can help health care organizations answer the question, "Are we in the ballpark?" when it comes to the incidence of adverse patient events.

The *National Healthcare Quality Report* published annually by AHRQ includes a broad set of performance measures including data on patient safety (AHRQ, 2009a). The patient safety measures focus on **iatrogenic** conditions and postoperative complications such as accidental laceration during a procedure, blood clots in the lungs following surgery, fracture following surgery, and birth-related injuries. Rates of these occurrences have been calculated using hospital administrative data. Also included in the report are data from the National Nosocomial Infections Surveillance, a voluntary, hospital-based reporting system sponsored by the Centers for Disease Control and data on medication use derived from the Medical Expenditure Panel Survey. Eventually, patient safety data voluntarily submitted to Patient Safety Organizations (PSOs) will be included in the report.

Much of the information in this report could be used to compare your organization's patient safety experiences. The following patient safety topics are examples of data found in the 2008 *National Healthcare Quality Report* (AHRQ, 2009a):

- For the year 2006, the total percentage of surgical patients with postoperative catheter-associated UTIs was 5.4%.

- In 2005, the rate of iatrogenic pneumothorax was 0.65 per 1,000 hospital discharges of adults age 18 and over.

- In 2005, the rate of postoperative abdominal wound separation was 2.8 per 1,000 abdominopelvic surgery discharges in adults age 18 and over.

Health care organizations also have access to comparative data for safety culture surveys. One reason why so many hospital providers are using the safety culture survey available from AHRQ is that aggregate results are available for comparison purposes. AHRQ has established the Hospital Survey on Patient Safety Culture Comparative Database as a central repository for survey data from hospitals that have administered the AHRQ patient safety culture survey instrument (AHRQ, 2009b). The database serves as a resource for hospitals wishing to compare their patient safety culture survey results to those of other hospitals in support of patient safety culture improvement.

It can be challenging to obtain reliable numbers about the incidence of adverse events. However, knowing what is causing events—even when the exact number is not available—can be very useful. Some organizations are sponsoring databases that provide facts about the common causes of adverse events. This information is gathered in addition to or instead of incident prevalence data. The following list includes examples of national initiatives. There is also a growing number of state-sponsored and proprietary initiatives.

- The American Society of Anesthesiologists sponsors the Closed Claims Project, which is an in-depth investigation of closed anesthesia malpractice claims, designed to identify major areas of loss, patterns of injury, and strategies for prevention. This group also sponsors the Pediatric Perioperative Cardiac Arrest, an investigation of cardiac arrests and deaths of pediatric patients during administration of or recovery from anesthesia designed to identify the possible relationship of anesthesia to these incidents. For more information see: http://depts.washington.edu/asaccp/.

- The Institute for Safe Medical Practices provides an independent review of medication errors that have been voluntarily submitted to the Medical Errors

Reporting Program sponsored by the United States Pharmacopoeia. Information about the common factors causing medication errors and how to reduce such errors is distributed to health care facilities by ISMP through their biweekly *Medication Safety Alert* newsletter and various other educational offerings. For more information see: http://www.ismp.org.

- The Joint Commission has been tracking the occurrence of sentinel events in health care facilities since 1996. The findings of these review activities are regularly summarized and shared with the health care community through their *Sentinel Event Alert* newsletter. For more information see: http://www .jointcommission.org.

- The Safe Medical Devices Act of 1990 and the Medical Device Amendments of 1992 require that any "device-user facility" report certain types of medical device-related events to the Food and Drug Administration. Besides hospitals, device-user facilities include ambulatory surgical facilities, nursing homes, or outpatient diagnostic or treatment facilities. The FDA reviews all reports it receives and regularly publishes alerts regarding the causes of device-related incidents on their Web site at: http://www.fda.gov/MedicalDevices/.

As of November 2009, 27 states plus the District of Columbia had passed legislation or regulation related to provider reporting of adverse events to a state agency. These agencies create and disseminate reports that include incident prevalence data as well as recommendations for safety improvements based on what was learned in the analysis of reported incidents. The National Association of Health Data Organizations maintains a list of state-sponsored quality reporting initiatives (www.nahdo.org) and the National Academy for State Health Policy maintains a list of state-sponsored patient safety initiatives (www.nashp.org).

These types of "mishap" databases provide important learning opportunities for all health care organizations. Solutions to known patient safety problems no longer have to be reinvented by every facility. Adopting "best practices" in common work activities can prevent many adverse incidents.

It may be difficult for a health care organization to ever answer the question, "Are we in the ballpark when it comes to the incidence of adverse patient events?" Although the number of comparative databases is growing, many still lack consistency and precision. The total numbers are suspect because of the nature of voluntary reporting. There may be inaccuracy problems related to differing definitions, lack of data-quality controls, and limited capacity to account for differences in patient populations.

Dr. Charles Billings, who was involved in the design and implementation of NASA's Aviation Safety Reporting System (ASRS), suggests that counting voluntarily reported incidents is a waste of time (Billings, 1998). The benefit of the ASRS has been in capturing and disseminating information about the sequence of events and error-producing factors surrounding airline incidents, not merely reporting prevalence data. In health care, is it really necessary to know the exact number of adverse events that occur? Billings suggests that it is more important to recognize there are repeated mishaps involving the same drugs (for example, potassium chloride and lidocaine) or the same tasks (such as care of restrained patients) and improvements are needed.

Determine Need for Action

The final step in measuring patient safety performance is deciding whether there is need for further action. Any of the following situations signals the need for more in-depth investigation:

- Performance does not meet expectations

- Performance rates show undesired variation

- Performance differs significantly from comparison groups

- A significant harmful adverse event occurred

If none of the above situations exist, no further action may be needed. Patient safety will continue to be measured to be sure things don't change in the future.

If further action is warranted, the next step is to discover the cause of undesirable performance. To find out the reason for this situation more investigation must be done. Searching for the cause of undesirable performance is the starting point of patient safety improvement. Once the underlying causes are well understood, effective improvement interventions can be designed and implemented. Methods for examining the causes of safety problems and techniques for mistake-proofing health care processes are covered in later chapters.

Conclusion

Evaluating the results of patient safety measurement involves reporting and analysis of the data. The purpose of this analysis is to determine where there are safety improvement opportunities. There are several ways to evaluate measurement results: determine if undesired variation exists, compare results to internally set **performance expectations**, and compare results to what other facilities are able to achieve. When there is a **performance gap** between the expected and actual performance, further investigation is done to determine the cause and what needs to be done to fix the problem.

What an organization does with its patient safety measurement data is the most important indicator of its commitment to safety. Performance data can prompt the decision maker to ask for more information (what happened here?), but the performance measure data do not tell the decision maker why the data are the way they are. Trend information will not make decisions for the leaders nor will the data alone cause problem areas to vanish. Dedication and commitment are needed from senior leaders, physicians, managers, and staff. Those people intimately involved in the process must also have ownership in the analysis of performance and any subsequent improvements. Everyone must be accountable for making data-driven patient safety improvements.

Discussion Questions

1. Identify the measures of patient safety in the most current edition of the AHRQ *National Healthcare Quality Report*. According to this report, are the aspects of patient safety being measured showing an improving trend? If not, suggest ways of improving patient safety performance in these areas.

2. Using the most current information available in the AHRQ Hospital Survey on Patient Safety Culture Comparative Database (www.ahrq.gov/qual/patientsafetyculture/hospsurvindex.htm) identify which aspects of hospital culture are most problematic and suggest ways of improving these aspects.

3. What challenges are associated with creating a national network of patient safety databases? How can the federal government and health care organizations assist in overcoming these challenges?

Key Terms

Common cause variation	Dashboard	Performance trend
Control chart	Iatrogenic	Special cause variation
Control limits	Performance expectation	Statistical process control
	Performance gap	

References

AHRQ. (2009a, March). *National healthcare quality report, 2008.* Washington, DC: U.S. Department of Health and Human Services. AHRQ Publication No. 09–0001. Retrieved from http://www.ahrq.gov/qual/qrdr08.htm.

AHRQ. (2009b, April). Patient safety culture surveys. Agency for Healthcare Research and Quality, Rockville, MD. Retrieved from http://www.ahrq.gov/qual/patientsafetyculture/.

Bauer, J. C. (2009). *Statistical analysis for decision makers in healthcare: Understanding and evaluating critical information in changing times* (2nd ed.). New York: Productivity Press.

Billings, C. (1998). Incident reporting systems in medicine and experience with the aviation safety reporting system. In: R. Cook, E. Woods, & C. Miller (Eds.). *A tale of two stories: Contrasting views of patient safety. Report from a workshop on assembling the scientific basis for progress on patient safety.* McLean, VA: National Patient Safety Foundation at the AMA.

Kelley, D. L. (1999). *How to use control charts for healthcare.* Milwaukee, WI: Quality Press.

Lawton, R., & Parker, D. (2002). Barriers to incident reporting in a healthcare system. *Quality and Safety in Health Care, 11*(1), 15–18.

Leeuwen, D. H. (1994). Are medication error rates useful as comparative measures of organizational performance? *Journal on Quality Improvement, 20*(4), 192–199.

Spath, P. L. (2005). *Leading your healthcare organization to excellence: A guide to using the Baldrige Criteria.* Chicago: Health Administration Press.

Wheeler, D. J. (2000). *Understanding variation: The key to managing chaos* (2nd ed.). Knoxville, TN: SPC Press.

CHAPTER 6

USING PERFORMANCE DATA TO PRIORITIZE SAFETY IMPROVEMENT PROJECTS

Robert Latino

LEARNING OBJECTIVES

- Describe how to make the business case for patient safety improvement projects
- Identify steps of an Opportunity Analysis
- Recognize techniques for quantifying the cost of failure
- Describe how to identify the significant few problems most in need of fixing

Health delivery is in constant flux. Baby boomers are inundating the system and skilled health care professionals are in short supply. Each day it seems there are more tasks on our plate and the situation is not likely to change in the foreseeable future. In today's environment it can be challenging to prioritize patient safety improvement initiatives. Time pressures can sway the organization toward seeking short-term successes to satisfy immediate needs rather than tackling projects that have a more lasting and long-term influence on patient safety. These same time pressures also create an environment in which shortcuts become commonplace. Process improvement shortcuts intended to save time, effort, expenses, and so on serve as system band-aids which in the long term can compromise quality and increase the risk of adverse outcomes.

Rather than pursue improvement projects only in response to the latest external mandate or most recent adverse patient event, organizations must also look toward achieving longer term results likely to yield the greatest benefits (Leatherman et al., 2003). In this chapter readers are introduced to a systematic process that involves the use of performance data to select high-value patient safety improvement projects. First, the need for this analysis (the "whys) are covered and then the steps for applying the process (the "hows") are described. To aid in understanding and applying the analysis, a single case is presented and described throughout the chapter.

Quantify Opportunity Priorities

Opportunity Analysis (OA) is a data-driven technique used to identify specific failures that have occurred in a particular system. The failures to be identified are defined by the analyst and vary according to the priorities of the analysis. Typically the analyst looks back over a 12-month period and finds the occurrences and then measures the impact of the failures in either dollars or some type of weighted outcome rating. The calculation for measuring impact, to be described later in this chapter, is:

The data used for this analysis is historical; thus, it is factual in the sense that the failures *have* occurred. However, the technique looks at both the reality of the past and the "here and now." As such it helps identify trends in chronic or repetitive failures and assesses the impact over a 12-month period. This allows the analyst to identify the annual impact of high frequency, low cost failures. When viewed on an individual basis, the impact of occurrences is often not noticeable. But when viewed in the aggregate the story is often quite different.

For example, the cost of redrawing a patient's blood sample might appear to be minimal. However, at one of our client hospitals the average cost per redraw was calculated to be approximately $300 once all factors were taken into consideration—extended time the patient must spend in a nursing unit or the emergency department, technician and nurse time, supply and overhead costs. What was also found to be surprising was that this 225-bed hospital had over 10,000 redraws during the analysis period of the previous 12 months. This equates to over $3,000,000 coming out of the current budget and going unnoticed. Aside from wasted costs, there is the potential for patient harm associated with delayed test results and repeat blood draws.

When a blood redraw happens as a single occurrence does anyone really question the impact? Few organizations are likely to pursue prevention of redraws as an improvement goal. Whereas, when OA is used to select improvement projects the organization can be proactive in fixing chronic failures that have significant annual impacts. This concept is elaborated in greater detail in the remainder of the chapter.

Opportunity Analysis Goals

The results of an OA directly affect patient safety and the financial bottom line in the current period. The failures have occurred and the dollar losses are real and coming out of today's budgetary expenses. An OA demonstrates the yearly trend of such expenditures with the results providing the business case for tackling seemingly low-value improvement opportunities.

It can often be difficult to convince people to take on problems that, on the surface, appear to have minimal impact on patient safety or resource use. Essentially the quality director is selling the invisible when trying to justify an improvement with promises of lives saved or expenses reduced at some point in the future. We intuitively know the improvement project is the right thing to do yet we lack the numbers to back up our opinion. Well-intentioned improvement ideas must ultimately be accompanied by facts to justify the need for action. The organization's resources will not be allocated to projects that fail to demonstrate a certain return on their investment within a specific payback period.

We may have goodwill in mind, and the patient's best interest at heart, but if the improvement project's value cannot be translated into dollars, the fight is much more difficult to win. Thus, both cost and quality data must be available when recommending improvement projects. The OA provides a solution. It is designed to develop the financial justification for patient safety projects.

OA is a tool that allows people to look backward at events that are eating away at the organization's current resources. These are failures that affect patients, staff members and the financial bottom line in real time. The goal of an OA is to stop current failure trends from continuing in the future. When making the business case for patient safety improvement, be realistic about expressing cost-benefit relationships. If the interventions greatly reduce the frequency of a specific failure but also create another expense, then that other expense should be included in the cost-benefit calculation. The big picture must be accurately represented. For instance, in the renal community there is a national push to increase the use of arteriovenous (AV) fistulas as the primary means of access for hemodialysis patients. Although this is viewed as the best long-term option for qualified patients and it saves a considerable amount of money, it has also increased the number of catheters used across the country. The overall AV fistula savings will still outweigh the costs associated with increased catheter use but the added costs of additional catheters must be represented in the overall cost-benefit calculation in order to reflect reality.

Opportunity Analysis Steps

An OA is a useful tool to add to your process improvement analytical tool kit. Many health care organizations are not familiar with OA as there are no regulatory or accreditation requirements that specify an OA be done. Other analytic tools, such as root cause analysis and failure mode and effect analysis, are more familiar to health care organizations because of external requirements. Don't overlook OA just because it is not a required methodology. The process helps senior leaders, managers, and quality specialists uncover opportunities that often are in plain view, but are so ingrained in daily routines that people cannot see or quantify them. As in the blood collection example, who would think to analyze why blood is being redrawn from the same patient so many times? Why would someone perform such an analysis if it were not required?

Anyone can initiate an OA. In the blood redraw case study, the analysis was triggered by the finance director who wanted to reduce costs associated with nurses drawing blood. This prompted the need to know current costs for the blood draw system. Ultimately, the analysis uncovered patient safety concerns as well as opportunities to reduce costs.

Before proceeding through the OA, a group of people to facilitate and assist must be identified. The OA process is guided by a lead analyst. This individual directs the team toward a common objective. The lead analyst typically serves as facilitator for the subject matter experts on the team. As facilitator, the lead analyst keeps the analytical process on track during team sessions and makes sure that necessary information is methodically gathered from the expert team members. The lead analyst should be skilled in getting necessary information from team members and able to validate data gathered from the team with data found in various information systems (for example, risk management, quality or performance improvement databases, billing and outcome databases, and so on). The manager initiating the project may serve as the lead analyst or this position may be assigned to someone from within the department or in another department, such as quality or patient safety.

The makeup of the team varies according to the nature and scope of the analysis itself. For instance, the expert team members involved in an OA of patient falls in a geriatric inpatient unit would be different from the team assembled for an OA of patient blood draws in an emergency department. Team members are subject matter experts. These are typically the people closest to the actual work in the system selected for analysis. These individuals have experienced firsthand events that occur in the system and know whether the events were documented or not. Sometimes chronic failures such as blood redraws are not formally recorded as such. Knowledge of these events resides only in the memory of people doing blood draws. These are the type of failures or losses that OA strives to identify—the events buried in the system and not likely to be brought to light without tools like OA.

Once people who will facilitate and assist with the OA have been identified, the OA proceeds through the following steps:

- Perform preparatory work

    1. Define system to be analyzed

    2. Define team charter

    3. Define system "loss"

    4. Create process flow diagram of the system

- Set up OA worksheet

- Collect data

    1. Gather information at team meetings

    2. Query information systems

    3. Conduct literature review

- Calculate the loss

- Determine the significant few

- Issue the report

Preparatory Work

Like any analytical process, groundwork for the OA is vitally important. The more prepared the lead analyst, the more efficient the analysis will be. Good preparation helps ensure the OA accomplishes as much as possible in a short period of time. Just as important, the analysis team members will appreciate their time not being wasted by dealing with uncertainties (for example defining terminology in the team session) and by following a very structured path forward. The lead analyst should be accountable for ensuring proper preparations for the OA. The following steps summarize the OA preparation phase. To demonstrate the steps of an OA, the blood redraw example described earlier in the chapter is used throughout this section.

Define System to Be Analyzed

Step one for preparation is to clearly define boundaries for the scope of the analysis. Essentially, the system to be analyzed must be identified—where does it begin, what are the steps in the process flow, and where does the system end? For this case study example, the system to be analyzed is the blood drawing process, looking specifically at specimen integrity.

Define Team Charter

The OA team charter is usually a single paragraph describing why the particular team was formed. This paragraph should be short and concise. It serves as the mission statement or objective that guides the team toward its goal. For the blood draw case study, the following team charter was created:

> **This OA team is chartered to conduct an unbiased analysis of the blood drawing process. The "significant few" events and their associated recommendations will be submitted to management for review and approval.**

Define System "Loss"

Once the boundaries of the system have been established, the next step is to define how losses will be measured in that process. Though this step may appear to be relatively simple, it does require some forethought as the definition of a loss influences the focus of the OA.

Typically the losses being sought are derived from the team charter. If the OA was put together to analyze patient falls in a particular hospital unit, then falls would serve as the definition of the loss for that analysis. How the impact of losses will be measured depends on the analysis objective. For instance, in an OA being done primarily to reduce patient falls, losses would likely be measured using an outcome rating scale (such as severity of patient injury on a scale of 1 to 5). If the OA goal is reduction of costs associated with patient falls, losses might be based on costs such as claims, labor, materials, rehabilitation, and so forth. In some instances, both costs and outcomes are considered in the OA.

The lead analyst should discuss with their superior (or the person/group that commissioned the OA team) how losses are to be measured. Once decided, the lead analyst reports to the team how the losses will be measured for the OA. The team members do not usually define how to measure the losses, but rather follow the criteria set by the lead analyst.

Following are examples of possible failure or loss definitions in some systems:

- Any event or condition resulting in a sentinel event
- Any event or condition resulting in a near miss
- Any event or condition resulting in a never event
- Any event or condition resulting in patient harm
- Any event or condition resulting in a medication order process error
- Any event or condition resulting in a patient fall
- Any event or condition resulting in a treatment delay in excess of 60 minutes
- Any event or condition resulting in a patient complaint
- Any event or condition resulting in a claim

For this case study example, the definition of a loss is: Any event or condition resulting in a blood redraw.

Create Process Flow Diagram of the System

To communicate effectively with the analysis team, the lead analyst creates a **process flow diagram**. Essentially the entire process is the system to be analyzed. Each step within the system is referred to as a subsystem. These terms will be important when setting up the worksheet for the analysis, described in the next section. In Figure 6.1 is the basic blood drawing process to be evaluated.

FIGURE 6.1   Basic Blood Drawing Process Flow Diagram

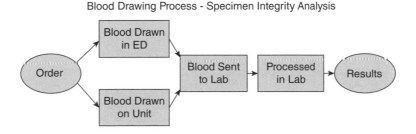

Blood Drawing Process - Specimen Integrity Analysis

Set up OA Worksheet

Now the process is defined both conceptually and graphically and the definition of loss or failure is established. At this point, the OA analysis is data-driven. Information is gathered from the subject experts on the team as well as other sources. A worksheet is used to organize the information. It is best to use an electronic spreadsheet program such as Excel to create the worksheet. There are also commercially available products that can be used to support the OA analysis (Latino, 2009).

The lead analyst prepares an electronic spreadsheet to facilitate evaluation of the data to be gathered. This is an important step because this document is used in team discussions. The OA spreadsheet contains terminology that may be unfamiliar to the OA team. A great deal of time can be wasted in team meetings explaining and debating the definitions. Avoid this problem by creating definitions for the various terms on the OA spreadsheet prior to the meeting and post the definitions on the wall during the meetings and within any handouts provided to the team members.

The OA spreadsheet contains fixed columns included in every analysis and some custom columns that are unique to the OA being conducted. Table 6.1 shows the spreadsheet column headings to be used for the blood draw process OA. The fixed columns that require inputs in the blood draw study case are:

1. Subsystem: Subsystems relate back to the process flow diagram and the major steps within the defined process

2. Event: The event is usually related to the definition of loss and is the last effect or consequence in a causal chain. In the case study example an event would be the occurrence of a redraw.

3. Modes: Modes are the high level reasons events occur. There is a direct cause-and-effect relationship between a mode occurring (cause) and the event (effect). In the blood drawing process, for example, a blood redraw can occur *because* the initial blood sample was contaminated. It is not the intent of an

Table 6.1   Blood Drawing Process Spreadsheet Headings

1	2	3	4	5	6	7	8
Subsystem	Event	Mode	Frequency/ Year	Labor	Lost Profit Opportunities	Materials	Total Annual Loss

OA to determine why the initial blood sample was contaminated. Modes are just the facts, not speculation of why the facts are happening.

4. Frequency/Year: This is a fixed column in an OA because in all analyses it is important to know how often the modes have occurred in the past. The usual time frame of looking back is 12 months but the time frame may be defined differently by the lead analyst and can go back as far as they would like.

There are also customizable columns on the OA spreadsheet that are dependent on the analysis at hand. For instance, the user defines the impacts per occurrence. There may any number of impact columns. Impacts can be dollars or non-dollar-weighted criteria. If the impact is to be defined in dollars, the analyst would look for expenditures incurred when the mode takes place. In most cases there is a labor component to the expenditures. Other financial impacts might be costs associated with:

- Extended length of patient stays (ELOS)

- Lost profit opportunities (LPO)

- Materials and supplies

- Liability claims paid

- Training

- Equipment

- Attorney fees

- Regulatory compliance

The costs to be considered in an OA are selected based on their suitability to the modes occurring in the process. When using dollars in an OA, it is imperative the lead analyst clearly define how costs will be calculated during the preparatory phase. For instance, for category of "labor," the dollar amount often reflects the average daily hourly rate of pay for the people involved (such as floor nurse, emergency nurse, physician, lab technician, and so on). If cost calculations are not defined upfront, valuable team meeting time may be spent debating the definitions. The same goes for ELOS and LPO definitions.

For the case study OA, blood redraws, dollars are used to measure the impact of failures. The three customized columns on the spreadsheet are Labor (column 5), Lost Profit Opportunities (column 6), and Materials (column 7).

In some situations it can be difficult to calculate the impact of failures using dollars. In these situations, it is acceptable to use criteria that are "weighted" based on their importance. Below are examples of criteria that might be used to measure impact:

- Customer satisfaction results
- Regulatory compliance
- Criticality of harm
- Loss of reputation
- Loss of market share
- Negative impact on quality
- Negative impact on patient safety

Each criterion is assigned a numeric "weight" relevant to its importance. You can either use an overall fixed weighting system (a total value for all criteria not to exceed 100, for example) or you can simply add as many criteria with their respective weightings as you wish.

The last column heading on the OA spreadsheet is **Total Annual Loss** (column 8). This is where the final OA calculations will be entered. As described earlier in the chapter, the equation for this calculation is simply:

$$\text{Frequency/Year} \times \text{Sum of Impact} = \text{Total Annual Loss.}$$

The preparatory phase of the OA is now complete. The system has been defined and the spreadsheet, with corresponding data definitions, has been created. Now it is time for the OA lead analyst to get ready for the first team meeting. Prepare a large easel pad with the following information:

- Definition of loss
- Process flow diagram
- Impact assumptions (for example, labor rate, costs per day for floor rooms and emergency department space)

This information should be written out with a bold-colored marker and taped to the wall or an easel in clear view of the team members.

The impact assumptions used in the blood redraw OA are found in Exhibit 6.1. These reflect the direct and indirect costs associated with a need to redraw blood due to an error on the first attempt for whatever reason.

EXHIBIT 6.1

IMPACT ASSUMPTIONS USED IN OA OF BLOOD REDRAW PROCESS

Additional Labor Costs

Average costs per redraw for:

1. RN = $2.62 (7 minutes @ $22.50 per hour),

2. Unit Secretary = $0.67 (5 minutes @ $8.00 per hour),

3. Lab Technician = $1.11 (5 minutes @ $13.30 per hour),

4. Medical Technician = $2.31 (7 minutes @ $19.84 per hour) and

5. Quality Assurance = $1.40 (3 minutes @ $28.00 per hour)

Additional Material Costs

Average costs for supplies associated with redraw:

Venipuncture Supplies

1. Tubes x 3 per SST, Lavender, Citrate = $0.28 each

2. Tourniquet = $0.11 each

3. Butterfly needle = $0.75 each

4. Luer adapters = $0.15 each

5. Gauze, alcohol, and band-aid = $0.10 each

Lab Testing Supplies

Reagents. = $1.00 per test ran. 33% ran

For the blood redraw OA, the Lost Profit Opportunity (LPO) costs were associated with using valuable emergency department time and space to redraw a blood sample after a failed attempt. It was estimated that the average redraw would cause the patient to remain in the ED an additional 30 minutes (7 minutes for the redraw, 20 minutes to test the sample and 3 minutes for routing the sample to and from the lab). Had this redraw not occurred, the space in the emergency department could have been used for other patients and this time would be billable. The average revenue per patient in the emergency department is $828 and the average length of stay (LOS) is 3 hours and 45 minutes, or 225 minutes. Therefore, the average lost profit per minute in the emergency department is $3.68. These costs do not reflect the impacts associated with additional safety risks or customer dissatisfaction. It is acknowledged that such esoteric parameters are difficult to measure in dollars but could easily outweigh the dollar values expressed.

Collect Data

Now it is time to populate the OA spreadsheet with data. Keep in mind throughout the OA process that the data will be used to build the case for process changes. People will be critical of the data sources. Knowing this, we must ask ourselves, "Where can we get the most credible numbers?" For dollar impact assumptions, accounting data in the finance department is often the best source. It may be more difficult to capture data on the frequency of modes. Some institutions have sophisticated electronic data systems that contain accurate, real time information about patient care activities. These health care organizations are in the minority. Many institutions rely on direct observation for gathering information that accurately reflects what is happening during the provision of patient care. This is why the OA team should consist of subject matter experts—the people who know the reality of what is happening. While data for completing the OA is a judgment call by the lead analyst, in the author's experience the most reliable data on mode frequency comes from the frontline workforce.

A cautionary note: don't inflate any numbers to make them look more impressive. When faced with a choice of using a higher or lower number, always go with the more conservative number. For instance, staff overtime costs may be a legitimate expense for some modes; however, critics can argue that overtime hours would be expended anyway because of staffing shortages. Though you may be able to make a solid case that extra labor was spent addressing a particular mode, arguing over this detail can erode the OA credibility.

There are several data collection strategies for filling in the blanks on the OA spreadsheet: gather facts at team meetings, query information systems, and review relevant literature sources.

Team Meetings

During OA team meetings, the facilitator leads the group through the analysis. Starting with the first block on the process flow diagram, team members are asked two questions:

1. In this subsystem, what modes have you experienced that have resulted in our definition of loss?

2. How often would you say this mode occurs?

The same questioning is repeated for each subsystem on the process flow diagram. As data is collected from team members it will likely be provided in non-uniform units. For example, some people may say a mode happens four times per year and another person may say it happens a week. Team members will also convey the amount of time they spend addressing a mode in minutes or hours. Take the information as it is provided and then later extrapolate it into common units for calculation purposes. The key to a successful analysis is to extract as much information as possible from the subject matter experts while they are together. The lead analyst can refine the data after the meeting.

At a minimum, the lead facilitator should ask team members to provide their impression of the "mode of failure" and the "frequency of occurrence." If labor hours expended is a measure of impact of the failure/loss, then team members should be asked to estimate how long it takes them, on average, to address the failure mode at hand. Other than these data, the lead analyst should already have in place supported assumptions such as cost per labor hour (nurse, tech, physician, and so on, and cost per hour for emergency department or nursing unit stay). Of course these assumptions will vary based on the impacts being measured but typically the team is not involved in addressing these issues. The goal of team discussions is to extract the raw information needed for the analysis and then later add the data to the spreadsheet.

In the blood draw case study, the people involved in the drawing process offered impressions on how often a day (frequency) they usually have to redraw blood and for what reason (mode). Since the labor impact was being measured, the lead analyst also asked how long, on average, it takes to do a blood redraw. The couple of minutes it takes a nurse to do a redraw are then added to the time of others in the blood processing cycle, such as the time of the lab technician or the person delivering the samples. If blood is redrawn because it hemolyzed during a delay in handling, the labor costs may be different than if it is redrawn because the first attempt was unsuccessful.

Query Information Systems

Once information has been gathered from the OA team members, use other information sources in the organization to substantiate the team's input. Although the data systems may not be as comprehensive as feedback from the experts, for credibility purposes it is helpful to demonstrate two reference points to support the results.

In the blood drawing example the material costs were validated by financial data analyst through a review of purchasing records for materials and supplies. The cost of labor was validated by human resource personnel. The cost of real estate for a floor room versus a room in the ED was also validated by the financial data analyst.

Literature Sources

Relevant journal articles can provide a third reference point, although the data from these sources should not be used independently for the OA. Use information from the literature to further support your data, not to populate the OA spreadsheet. Literature sources are merely benchmarking tools that demonstrate the experience of other organizations. For the OA, you want to report the unique experience at your institution.

For example, in the blood draw case study the team needed to validate the costs associated with blood culture contaminations due to improper collection practices. A second blood draw for a repeat culture must be done and this can delay the patient's treatment. It would have been nearly impossible to dig through the billing records of patients that had redraws to piece together an estimate of the direct and indirect costs associated with a blood culture contamination. The leader analyst sought out literature sources for average costs associated with handling blood culture contaminations. A credible source was found which identified the costs to be $5,000 per occurrence and that source was cited as the validation. At the end of the day the team must have confidence in the data and be able to defend their numbers. If the lead analyst and the team are comfortable with the data validations, they are usually ready to answer data credibility questions.

Calculate the Loss

After the blocks on the OA spreadsheet have been filled in, the OA advances to the computation step. In this step the lead analyst refines the data and calculates the loss. This step primarily involves data quality control.

First, data must be standardized. As mentioned earlier, information gleaned from team discussions should be reported in common units. Next, if data has been collected from different shifts there may be some redundancy in the reported modes because of handoffs between shifts. Evaluate the data to be sure the frequency numbers are not "double-dipping," which would inflate the actual results.

As much as possible, assess the credibility of the data. Start with what is likely the most reliable data source—the experience of the workforce. Combine this experience with data from the finance department. For example, suppose a nurse says she spends, on average, one hour correcting a situation caused by a mode and it happens once a week. The analyst then multiples 52 hours per year (1 hour per week time 52 weeks) times the average unit nurse loaded salary of $40 per hour. A loaded salary includes the cost of all benefits for the individual. This should be included as it is a cost not often seen by the workforce but nonetheless a real and significant cost to the organization. To calculate labor assumptions for the OA, multiply a loaded factor rate (usually available from the finance department) times the salary for that position. This calculation results in a figure for the loaded salary.

Continuing the example above, this equates to $2,080 per year for this one nurse to address this one mode. If each unit nurse reports the same experience and there are ten nurses, the total annual loss becomes $20,800 per year. Once the total annual losses for each mode have been calculated, look for other data that can be used to add credibility to the figures. Because each occurrence may not be documented, the frequency of modes may appear to be less than the actual number.

Do not be surprised if the frequency of occurrences reported by the team members varies from what is actually recorded in various information systems. This is especially true of chronic events that have not harmed a patient or are not recognized as a near miss. These events are not likely to be recorded in any fashion. This gap illustrates the benefit of an OA. The analysis makes obvious events that are "hidden" from view and have become accepted as just the cost of doing business. Defer to the experts—the OA team members. They should reach consensus on the number to be used for average frequency despite what numbers may be found in the information system. Note significant gaps in the OA report. If a root cause analysis of the problematic process is to be conducted, recommend the wide variations in actual versus reported event frequency be investigated.

Finally, it may be helpful to find literature sources of comparable data. For instance, what is the blood redraw rate at other hospitals? While the experience at other institutions is not the reality in your institution, it may be interesting to explore. In Table 6.2 is the completed OA spreadsheet for the blood redraw process.

Determine the Significant Few

The last step in the OA process is to identify the priorities for improvement. At this point all data has be refined, validated for accurate and readied for reporting. Now it is time to define the "significant few" modes or events that need to be eliminated. The significant few are the 20% or less that are costing 80% or

Table 6.2   Blood Redraw Process OA Spreadsheet

Subsystem	Event (effect)	Mode (cause)	Frequency/ Year	Labor	Lost Profit Opportunities	Materials	Total Annual Loss
Processed in Lab	Redraw	Blood Culture Contamination	480	0	5000.00	0	240000000.00
Blood drawn in ED	Redraw	Hemolyzed—ED	2597	8	110.40	1.39	311094.63
Blood drawn in ED	Redraw	Clotted—ED	409	8	110.40	1.39	49994.11
Blood drawn in ED	Redraw	QNS—ED	403	8	110.40	1.39	48275.37
Blood drawn in ED	Redraw	SUA—ED	211	8	110.40	1.39	25275.00
Blood drawn in unit	Redraw	QNS—Unit	1676	8	0	1.39	15737.64
Blood drawn in unit	Redraw	Hemolyzed—Unit	1557	8	0	1.39	14620.23
Blood drawn in unit	Redraw	Clotted—Unit	1540	8	0	1.39	14460.60
Blood drawn in ED	Redraw	Mislabeled—ED	67	8	110.40	1.39	8025.93
Blood drawn in Unit	Redraw	SUA—Unit	834	8	0	1.39	7831.26
Blood drawn in Unit	Redraw	Mislabeled—Unit	239	8	0	1.39	2244.21

QNS = Quantity not sufficient
SUA = Unsuitable for analysis

greater of our losses (dollars or weighted criteria). Apply the following steps to the OA spreadsheet to determine the significant few.

1. Sort the Total Annual Loss (TAL) column from highest to lowest

2. Take the TAL and multiply that number by 0.80. This is our significant few number.

3. Add up the highest modes TAL until we reach our significant few number or slightly greater.

Figure 6.2 shows a graphical depiction of the OA spreadsheet results. The first and most prominent bar shows that one mode (blood culture contamination) represents greater than 80% of all the losses associated with the blood redraws. In the ongoing blood redraw case study, blood culture contaminations were by far the most costly issue of the 10,013 annual redraws. The OA allows people to see, in a systematic and quantifiable manner, where the organization should focus its improvement efforts.

Issue the Report

As the OA steps progressed, the components were being constructed. At this point much is already done: losses calculated, process flow diagram created, data entered into the spreadsheet and validated, and significant few identified. Now it is time to step back, look at the information, and prepare conclusion and recommendation statements. The conclusion is basically a statement of what we learned from the analysis. What is the end result?

Recommendations are about the future. What is to be done with the analysis results? Should interim solutions be implemented now? Should longer term improvement projects be initiated to eliminate the significant few events? Will nothing be done? There are many options to consider. Exhibit 6.2 shows the conclusion and recommendation statements for the blood redraw OA.

The conclusions and recommendations are typically drafted by the OA team and finalized by the lead analyst. The subject matter experts on the team are the best source of ideas on how to overcome the identified modes, thus their input should be solicited. However, it is ultimately the decision of the lead analyst and their superiors if identified issues should proceed to a root cause analysis or another type of improvement project for further, in-depth investigation of why the significant few events are occurring.

When the OA report is complete it usually proceeds to a final presentation in front of those who commissioned the analysis. This group of stakeholders will

FIGURE 6.2 Blood Redraw Process Significant Few Events

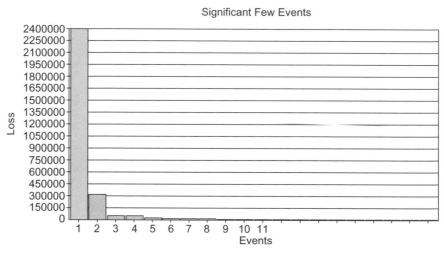

ID	Event	Mode	Frequency/Year	Total Annual Loss
1	Redraw	Blood Culture Contamination	480	240000000.00
2	Redraw	Hemolyzed – ED	2597	311094.63
3	Redraw	Clotted – ED	409	49994.11
4	Redraw	QNS – ED	403	48275.37
5	Redraw	SUA – ED	211	25275.00
6	Redraw	QNS – Unit	1676	15737.64
7	Redraw	Hemolyzed – Unit	1557	14620.23
8	Redraw	Clotted – Unit	1540	14460.60
9	Redraw	Mislabeled – ED	67	8025.93
10	Redraw	SUA – Unit	834	7831.26
11	Redraw	Mislabeled – Unit	239	2244.21

QNS = Quantity not sufficient

SUA = Unsuitable for analysis

EXHIBIT 6.2

CONCLUSIONS AND RECOMMENDATIONS FOR BLOOD REDRAW OA

Case Conclusion Statement

This analysis demonstrates that 4.8% of the occurrences (480/10013) are causing 82% of the annual dollar losses ($2,400,000/$2,896,560). Currently there are approximately 10,013 redraws per year (extrapolated for the period from 9/07 to 9/08) resulting in a consumption of man hours, material, and lost profit opportunities costing $2,896,560.

Recommendations

A literature search reveals that use of a well-trained phlebotomist staff will result in 98% successful draws on the first attempt. Given that statistic, this would indicate that a savings of $2,838, 629 ($2,896,560 × .98) would be realized under the current conditions. The cost of 25 full-time equivalent (FTE) phlebotomists is estimated at $697,400 per year. The cost/benefit then becomes:

Total Potential Returns: $2,838,629 per year

Total Initial Investment: $697,400 per year

Potential Return on Investment: 407%

Payback Period: ~3 months

Based on this empirical data, it is recommended that the institution establish an in-house phlebotomy team to bring consistency to the task of drawing blood, reduce the risk of errors, and increase overall patient safety.

In addition, it is recommended a root cause analysis be conducted to determine why there are 480 blood culture contaminations each year. Hiring a team of trained phlebotomists is unlikely to eliminate this problem. An in-depth investigation that results in corrective action is recommended.

---

approve, modify, delay, or reject the recommendations of the team. The team should provide a solid and well-grounded analysis to the decision makers, allowing them to make an informed decision on the next steps.

A considerable amount of time and effort are put into creating an OA. The team members will be watching to see what happens with the report. If no action is taken to eliminate the events and improve the process, staff members will be reluctant to participate in a future analysis. As time progresses, keep the team members informed about actions to be taken and successes. Eventually, when the organization establishes the collective efforts as being successful, celebrate in some fashion with the team members. Also, recognize the members for their efforts when the results are publicized. By following through on the OA recommendations and achieving sustaining improvements, the organization is demonstrating to its workforce what they are capable of achieving.

Conclusion

Opportunity Analysis is a practical, data-driven tool designed to reveal the reality in our processes and quantify the impact of that reality so that we can design a path forward to reshape the process to a more desirable state. It is a proactive tool that allows senior leaders, physicians, managers, and staff members to uncover improvement opportunities in a very systematic and comprehensive manner.

An OA can be applied both reactively and proactively. For example, in reaction to a sentinel event involving a medication error, the medication administration system can be analyzed using the OA tool to identify and quantify gaps in performance. The most beneficial use of OA is when it is used proactively to improve system safety and efficiency to avoid adverse events. For instance, to build the business case for patient safety improvement and focus improvement efforts, quality department staff can use OA to calculate the total annual loss attributed to near-miss events. Department managers can use OA to evaluate systems that are causing budgetary cost overruns. OA can be used in improvement projects to root out and quantify waste. The underlying principle of OA is to define, for a given system, where we would like to be versus where we are at right now. Then, that gap is broken down into events that are preventing us from reaching our goals.

However, use of OA in health care organizations has its challenges. The data needed to complete an OA is not always easily obtained and this may be viewed as a barrier. Although the absence of such data should make us question and dig deeper—Why don't we have the data? If we did have it, what would it tell us?—the OA is looking at events that are occurring right now. These undesirable outcomes are harming patients, causing undue risk and resulting in excessive and unnecessary costs to the organization. The OA can have a dramatic impact on patient safety and the facility's financial bottom line and is supported by data to substantiate successes.

Discussion Questions

1. What are advantages and disadvantages of quantifying the cost of opportunities or failures in a health care organization?

2. How can OA be applied to patient safety improvement opportunities?

3. What are the risks of not recognizing the significant few events causing the greatest losses?

Key Terms

Opportunity analysis (OA)   Process flow diagram   Total annual loss

References

Latino, R. *Patient safety: The PROACT® root cause analysis approach.* Boca Raton, FL: CRC Press, 2009.

Leatherman, S., Berwick, D., IIes, D., Lewin, L. S., Davidoff, F., Nolan, T., & Bisognano, M. (2003). The business case for quality: Case studies and an analysis. *Health Affairs (Millwood), 22*(2), 17–30.

PART 3

REACTIVE AND PROACTIVE SAFETY INVESTIGATIONS

CHAPTER 7

ACCIDENT INVESTIGATION AND ANTICIPATORY FAILURE ANALYSIS

Sanford E. Feldman
Douglas W. Roblin

LEARNING OBJECTIVES

- Describe methods used in accident analyses to discover root causes and latent failures
- Identify techniques for evaluating how human errors contribute to accident evolution
- Understand how anticipatory failure analysis can be used to mitigate the risk of adverse patient events

Since the 1990s, health care organizations have been encouraged to use methods employed in private industry for investigating the cause of adverse events. These accident investigation methods, including **root cause analysis (RCA)**, can aid caregivers in identifying the underlying system faults that allow mistakes to occur in the first place. To solve a problem, one must first recognize and understand what is causing the problem. If the real cause of the problem is not identified, then corrective actions will merely address the symptoms and the problem will continue to exist. For this reason, identifying and eliminating **root causes** of adverse events is of utmost importance.

Root cause analysis is a structured approach for identifying and resolving problems. By isolating and correcting root causes, the risk of recurrence of similar patient injuries can be diminished. Traditional problem solving approaches in health care focused on the immediately obvious human error but rarely pursued investigation of the underlying causes. These causes include poorly designed or maintained medical equipment, deficiencies in information management, and inadequate work processes.

There are different root cause analysis methods, several of which are described in this book. Regardless of the terminology used to portray the process, all methods place emphasis on finding what needs to be changed in the system to effectively reduce the risk of adverse events. Discussion in this chapter is directed toward those individuals in a health care organization who are charged with reviewing adverse patient events. These people include physicians, quality and risk management staff, nurses, technicians, plant safety personnel, and others involved in the design, operation, and review of safe facility practices. This chapter provides an overview of accident analysis and implementation of sustained inquiry in support of ongoing patient safety advocacy.

The application of root cause analysis to the investigation of unintended patient injuries is discussed. Two examples of actual cases are described to illustrate how human errors, root causes and latent system failures can be isolated. Finally, methods for identifying and resolving problematic processes are discussed. Instead of waiting for accidents to happen, **anticipatory failure analysis** techniques can be used to make riskier patient care processes safer.

Accident Investigation

Industries such as petrochemical processing, nuclear power generation, and air transportation are complex socio-technical systems involving the coordination of many diverse human and mechanical elements. Many of these industries have established reputations for high reliability and have achieved outstanding records for safe operation (Rochlin, LaPorte, & Roberts, 1987; Weick, 1987; Roberts, 1993). Yet even in high-reliability enterprises, accidents inevitably occur.

Accidents are injury-causing events that occur unexpectedly and unintentionally (Reason, 1990). Investigation of accidents in manufacturing and transportation has led to the recognition that serious accidents cannot be explained simply as a consequence of operator or pilot error. Awareness of the contribution of latent failures in the industrial systems (equipment design or maintenance, organization and management of work processes, conflicting or ambiguous production goals) has grown with each succeeding study of a catastrophic accident.

An accident investigation is undertaken to isolate root causes that increased the risk that an accident would occur and to assess whether the organization might have had some control over the circumstances that led to the evolution of that accident. A framework for isolating root causes includes identification of the following:

- The sequence of events contributing to the accident

- Events within that sequence that represent active failures (errors)

- Points in the sequence that represent latent failures (root causes)

In Chapter Two of this book, Ternov provided a comprehensive discussion of the causes of human errors, how these active failures contribute to accidents, and why root causes and latent failures allowed the active failures to occur.

Root Cause Analysis

A root cause analysis begins with outlining the event sequence leading to the accident. Starting with the adverse event itself, the analyst works backward in time, finding and recording each pertinent event. In gathering this information it is important to avoid early judgment, blame, and attribution and to concentrate on the facts of the incident. As each of the actions leading to an event is clearly defined, the investigation team must ask "Why did it occur?" That analysis will contribute to a better understanding of the causal factors in the **error chain** (Bagian, Gosbee, Lee, Williams, McKnight, & Mannos, 2002). These factors are generally the active precipitating errors.

"How" questions bring the analyst to the root causes or system failures that allowed the active errors to lead to patient injury. During the identification of active errors and system failures, the investigation team may be prompted to search for additional information or to pursue the sequence of events even further back in time (Weingart, Wilson, Gibberd, & Harrison, 2000). Very often it is not enough to consider only those events that occurred immediately prior to the accident because there may be other causes, more remote in time or in the organization, which must be considered.

The root cause analysis concludes with recommendations for system improvements based on the findings of the investigation. Different methods of root cause analysis vary in emphasis on how the causal factors are unearthed and what changes in the system might be effective in reducing the risk of accidents.

Medical Accident Investigations

Just as nuclear power plants and airplanes are prone to accidents and disaster when infrastructure subsystems fail, so too are hospitals. Eagle, Davies, and Reason (1992) were among the first to apply the concepts of active errors and latent system failures in an analysis of a health care incident in which a patient died in an anesthesia mishap. Clinicians erred several times during administration of anesthesia to a 72-year-old man undergoing an elective cystoscopy. First, the initial surgeon determined that the procedure could be done under local anesthesia although the man had a history of confusion and agitation. The patient was switched to general anesthesia when another surgeon assumed care of the patient after admission. However, an adequate preoperative evaluation had not been completed and the anesthesiologist was unaware that the patient had vomited the evening prior to surgery. During the procedure, the patient vomited two liters of gastric contents and aspirated. He died of aspiration pneumonia in six days.

Latent system failures in the organization of patient care magnified the ultimate consequences of these human errors. First, double-booking of staff for surgery caused a last-minute change in the surgeon assigned to perform the cystoscopy. Second, the patient's history was maintained in two separate systems—the patient's incident of vomiting the previous night was recorded in a computerized system but not in the patient's paper medical record, which was the only source of information available to the surgical team (no computer terminals had been installed in the operating room).

Below are analyses of two intraoperative adverse events (Feldman & Roblin, 1997). A brief discussion of each case is followed by a listing of what the root cause analysis team identified as active failures and root causes.

CASE 1

A patient was scheduled for nonurgent surgical repair of an aortic aneurysm. During the early stage of the operation, the surgeon requested that a blood transfusion be started. This was not an urgent or emergent matter; the patient had not experienced significant blood loss. The circulating nurse went to a refrigerator in the operating room and removed a unit of blood from among several units stored there. She looked at the unit label, presumably noting the patient name, and then signed the attestation slip indicating that she recognized the unit as the one prepared for her patient. She handed the blood unit to the anesthesiologist, who immediately started the transfusion without signing the identity affirmation slip. A nurse from an adjoining operating room came to the same refrigerator seeking the blood unit prepared for her patient in the adjourning room who was undergoing a prostatectomy. She noted that the unit was not in the refrigerator and found that the unit she was seeking was, in fact, the one being infused into the patient undergoing the aortic aneurysm repair. The incorrect transfusion was discovered and stopped after only 40 to 50cc was infused. The patient who received the wrong unit of blood developed coagulopathy and intractable bleeding and later expired.

Active Failures

The death of this patient was precipitated by several active errors. The operating room nurse mistakenly identified the unit of blood selected from the operating room refrigerator as the unit intended for the patient undergoing repair of an aortic aneurysm. The anesthesiologist made a mistake in assuming that the correct unit of blood had been selected and violated safe practices by failing to sign an attestation regarding the accuracy of the blood selection.

Root Causes

The organizational policy that allowed storage of the blood for different patients in the same operating room refrigerator created the potential for a catastrophic event. This was a general design fault in the hospital's blood distribution system. This blood storage practice was previously considered safe because it was assumed that several independent persons checking the accuracy of blood selections as well as personally attesting to the accuracy would be an adequate defense against a transfusion administration error.

CASE 2

A patient was scheduled for elective surgery for arthroscopic repair of a torn meniscus of the right knee. The hospital leased a CO_2 gas insufflator for distention of the knee joint and an accompanying CO_2 laser beam instrument for use during the procedure. The leasing company provided a technician to assist in the operation of this equipment during surgery. The safety valve on the gas insufflator had been set to release at a low pressure of 2.2 psi. During the surgery there was some difficulty in obtaining adequate gas flow from the insufflator and the technician inadvertently occluded the pressure release valve. For some unknown reason, the company had recently redesigned the equipment and placed the pressure release valve in an easily accessible location. The full force of the insufflator, capable of inflating a heavy truck tire, caused CO_2 under pressure to massively dissect upward from the patient's knee joint, past the tourniquet, and through the peritoneal cavity and diaphragm to the chest. The patient's heart and lungs were compressed; cardiopulmonary failure ensued. After resuscitation and rapid thoracotomy, the patient survived but had severe permanent brain damage.

Active Failures

The injury to this patient was precipitated by several active errors in the operation of the gas insufflator. The most egregious error was the unsafe act of the technician when he occluded the insufflator's safety barrier (pressure release valve). It was also a mistake for the equipment company to have moved the pressure release valve to a location that made it more likely that tampering could occur.

Root Causes

Several latent failures made use of this insufflator an accident waiting to happen. First, the basic design of the insufflator was dubious because it was capable of delivering pressure far exceeding any requirement for its intended use in surgery. Second, the hospital had no procedure for reviewing the design or safe operation of leased equipment prior to its use. Third, training of the technician responsible for operating the insufflator was inadequate and resulted in the penultimate unsafe act.

Summaries of the root cause investigation findings from these two cases are illustrated in Figures 7.1 and 7.2.

The occurrence of a sentinel event—an accident considered to be particularly egregious in the intensity of its damage to a patient—is a signal that there may be a fault in the organizational policies and procedures that contribute to the event or a deficiency in protective safety procedures that might have prevented the event. The root cause(s) of these medical accidents can be isolated by the methods of analysis that are applied to investigation of accidents in other industries. Once the root causes and latent failures are identified, corrective action can be taken to reduce the likelihood of future adverse events.

Anticipatory Failure Analysis

Ideally, latent failures can be identified and corrected before a significant injurious patient incident occurs. Evaluating processes within the organization to identify where and how an accident might happen is a common activity within private industry. It is also important to conduct similar evaluations within a

FIGURE 7.1 Root Cause Analysis Results of the Death of Patient Following Blood Transfusion (Case #1)

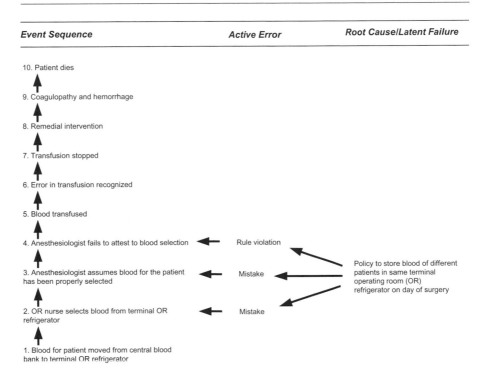

Event Sequence	Active Error	Root Cause/Latent Failure
10. Patient dies		
9. Coagulopathy and hemorrhage		
8. Remedial intervention		
7. Transfusion stopped		
6. Error in transfusion recognized		
5. Blood transfused		
4. Anesthesiologist fails to attest to blood selection	Rule violation	
3. Anesthesiologist assumes blood for the patient has been properly selected	Mistake	Policy to store blood of different patients in same terminal operating room (OR) refrigerator on day of surgery
2. OR nurse selects blood from terminal OR refrigerator	Mistake	
1. Blood for patient moved from central blood bank to terminal OR refrigerator		

hospital because of the comparable highly complex nature of patient care activities. As pointed out by Ternov in Chapter Two of this book, active errors are inevitable. Ongoing "what if" evaluation can improve recognition of potential accident trajectories.

A number of formal anticipatory failure analysis methods—sometimes called proactive risk assessments or hazard analyses—are already in use in private industry. There are over 100 anticipatory failure analysis methods in existence, but only a few are in general use and of those, fewer have been applied to health care settings (Lyons, Adams, Woloshynowych, & Vincent, 2004). In July 2001 The Joint Commission began to require accredited facilities conduct proactive risk assessments. The standard (LD.5.2.) required the following eight activities (Grissinger & Rich, 2002):

- Select at least one high-risk process.

- Identify steps where **failure modes** may occur.

FIGURE 7.2   Root Cause Analysis Results of Serious Disability
Following Elective Arthroscopic Knee Surgery (Case #2)

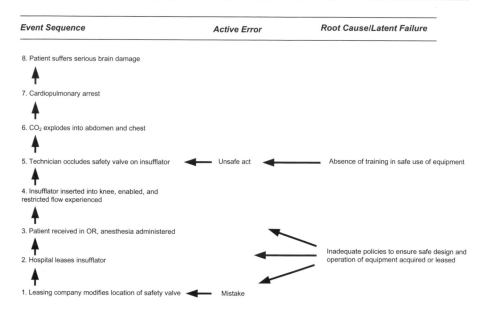

- Identify possible effects on patients.

- Conduct a root cause analysis to determine why failures may occur.

- Redesign the process to minimize the risk to patients.

- Test and implement the redesigned process.

- Monitor the effectiveness of the new process.

- Implement a strategy to maintain the process.

The Joint Commission did not mandate a particular proactive risk assessment model. Therefore health care organizations are using a variety of anticipatory failure analysis methods. Listed below are some of the more common methods that have been applied to health care processes:

- **FMEA (Failure Mode and Effect Analysis)** was developed by the U.S. military and it has been used in engineering, manufacturing, and by NASA. The FMEA identifies the following factors: How is care expected to be delivered? What could go wrong? Why would the failure happen? What are the consequences of the failure? (National Patient Safety Agency, 2006). This review starts with a diagram of the process and includes all components that could possibly fail and conceivably affect the safety of the process. FMEA is the most common model used by health care organizations to proactively improve the safety of a variety of high-risk processes. For instance, Burgmeier (2002) used FMEA to reduce risks and problems inherent in the blood transfusion process. Gowdy and Godfrey (2003) used FMEA to assess and prevent inpatient falls within a geriatric psychiatric unit. Ouellette-Piazzo, Asfaw, and Cowen (2007) used FMEA to prevent IV contrast misadministration in patients undergoing outpatient CT scans.

- **HACCP (Hazard Analysis and Critical Control Point)** is a systematic methodology evolved from team work by Pillsbury, NASA, Natick Laboratories of the United States Army, and the U.S. Air Force Space Laboratory Project Group. HACCP has since become the standard risk assessment approach within the food industry (Food and Drug Administration, 2009). The HACCP methodology involves defining a process through all stages and then considering every potential hazard (no matter how unlikely). Critical points in the process are identified and effective control-monitoring mechanisms established. HACCP has been used to review health care–associated infections (Richards, 2002) and to review the antenatal serum screening program for Down syndrome (Derrington, Draper, Hsu, & Kurinczuk, 2003a; Derrington, Draper, Hsu, & Kurinczuk, 2003b).

- **HFMEA®** (Healthcare Failure Mode and Effect Analysis) was developed in 2002, when the VA National Center for Patient Safety combined concepts, components and definitions from FMEA, HACCP, and root cause analysis into a single method. A HFMEA analysis consists of five consecutive steps: (1) define the topic; (2) assemble the multidisciplinary team; (3) graphically describe the process; (4) conduct a hazard analysis; and (5) describe actions and countermeasures (DeRosier and others, 2002). Since its introduction, HFMEA™ has been frequently applied in health care settings including projects involving drug administration and sterilization of surgical instruments (Esmail et al., 2005; Linkin et al., 2005).

- **FTA (Fault Tree Analysis)** is a failure analysis method suited to anticipatory study of potential hazards. When used in hazard recognition studies, FTA starts by hypothesizing a specific undesired event, which is graphically placed at the top of an inverted tree diagram. Branches containing potential precursors or causal events (that could lead to the top event) are drawn, extending downward from the top. Additional branching and sub-branching are continued down to several levels so as to reach basic causes or failures that need resolving. Marx and Slonim (2003) suggest that using FTA in probabilistic risk assessments is more robust than FMEA for modeling the complex interaction of multiple failures within a system.

- **HAZOP (Hazard and Operability Study)** is a hazard-seeking method popular in the chemical process industries (Goyal, 1993). HAZOP teams review the design and operation of processes and identify potential hazards or problems. Next, the consequences of the hazards or problems are evaluated by asking questions such as: Will someone be harmed? Who? In which way? How severely? Will the performance of the processes be reduced? In which way? How severely? What will the impact be? Will costs increase? If so, by how much? Will there be any cascading effects where this deviation leads to other deviations? If so, what are they? (McDonough, Solomon, & Petosa, 2004). When all hazards have been identified, the causes are sought and actions proposed to address each one.

In Chapter Eight of this book, Ternov briefly discusses Disturbance-Effect-Barrier analysis, an anticipatory failure analysis method that is used in some health care organizations in Sweden. Although all of these methods vary somewhat in scope and application, most anticipatory failure analysis activities share several common steps:

- Develop a model of the steps in the process that are potentially subject to failure.

- Ascertain what errors might occur at each step in the process. This requires "what if?" thinking or imaginative simulation of possible disasters.

- Evaluate the hazard potential of errors at each step.

- Isolate any latent system faults that might increase the hazard potential at each step.

- Decide what actions need to take place to lower the hazard potential at each step.

An excerpt from an FMEA on the process of ordering medications for hospitalized patients is illustrated in Figure 7.3. This example shows only one of the many process steps examined by the FMEA project team.

Just as airlines do not want to become famous for the highly efficient way in which they rescue the victims of their crashes, hospitals do not wish to be

FIGURE 7.3   One Process Step from FMEA on the Process of Ordering
Medication for a Hospitalized Patient

Process Step	Failure Mode (what could go wrong)	Potential Effects of Failure	Cause of Failure	Action Plans to Reduce/Prevent Failure	Expected Improvements
Physician orders medication for inpatient	Physician's written order is illegibly written	- Medication administration is delayed or omitted - Patient gets wrong medication or wrong dose of medication	Physician handwrites order	Short Term: - Reinforce RN behaviors through education and consistent discussion to question physicians if order is not clear. - Reinforce physician behaviors through education and consistent discussion to respect nurses who call for order clarification. - Regularly collect, aggregate, and present data to physicians on the number of times physician is called for order clarification due to illegible handwriting. Long Term: - Implement physician electronic order entry system. - Implement single sign-on software solution that makes system entry easy to encourage use by physicians.	- Reduction in medication order transcription errors. - Reduction in wrong medication/ wrong dose medication errors. - Decrease in the delay or omission of patient medication administration.

known for how well they respond to medical accidents (Wagenaar, 1996). Health
care organizations cannot afford the loss of reputation or the costs of litigation
that arise from adverse event injury to patients. Proactive error reduction efforts
are important. Accident prevention, not recovery from accident, is the hallmark
of a well-run industry. Every organization's patient safety improvement initiative
should include anticipatory failure analysis activities.

Conclusion

Hospital caregivers will make errors in the course of patient care delivery. These
slips, mistakes, and unsafe practices are not intended to cause injury and
are often responses to the immediate circumstances involving patient care.
Traditional quality improvement methods have in the past focused on human
error as a principal causal factor contributing to patient injury. Patient injuries
not attributed to human error were often dismissed as random, seldom occurring
situations.

Health care organizations are now turning to the accident investigation
methods and proactive risk assessment techniques that have been used by private
industry for years. By using root cause analysis techniques, clinicians are learning
that error-induced patient injuries often evolve from underlying hospital system
faults. By isolating these root causes and correcting them, the risk of future

incidents may be diminished. Anticipatory failure analysis methods provide caregivers with information that can be used to make processes more reliable and safe for future patients.

Retrospective root cause analysis and anticipatory failure analysis require a supportive culture within the organization. The commitment of senior management and a willingness to pledge resources are essential. Both management and staff should be familiar with general industry experience that identification and correction of hazards will prevent accidents, minimize injuries, and avert costs attendant to accidents and injuries. Health care organizations must adopt a culture of safety and reliability that places value on procedures, policies, and reward systems that promote error intolerance.

Discussion Questions

1. Describe the difference between root cause analysis and anticipatory failure analysis.

2. Search the literature related to root cause analysis and anticipatory failure analysis activities in health care organizations to identify how project teams are commonly formed and what departments are represented on the team.

3. What organizational strategies might be used to create and sustain attitudes and behaviors that support root cause analysis and anticipatory failure analysis activities in a health care setting?

Key Terms

Anticipatory failure analysis

Error chain

Failure mode

Failure Mode and Effect Analysis (FMEA)

Fault Tree Analysis (FTA)

Hazard Analysis and Critical Control Point (HACCP)

Hazard and Operability Study (HAZOP)

Healthcare Failure Mode and Effect Analysis (HFMEA)

Root cause

Root cause analysis (RCA)

References

Bagian, J., Gosbee, J., Lee, C., Williams, L., McKnight, S., & Mannos, D. (2002). The Veterans Affairs root cause analysis system in action. *Joint Commission Journal on Quality Improvement*, *28*(10), 531–545.

Burgmeier, J. (2002). Failure mode and effect analysis: An application in reducing risk in blood transfusion. *Joint Commission Journal on Quality Improvement, 28*(6), 331–339.

Derrington, M., Draper, E., Hsu, R., & Kurinczuk, J. (2003a). Can safety assurance procedures in the food industry be used to evaluate a medical screening programme? The application of the Hazard Analysis and Critical Control Point system to an antenatal serum screening programme for Down's syndrome. Stage 1: Identifying significant hazards. *Journal of Evaluation in Clinical Practice, 9*(1), 39–47.

Derrington, M., Draper, E., Hsu, R., & Kurinczuk, J. (2003b). Can safety assurance procedures in the food industry be used to evaluate a medical screening programme? The application of the Hazard Analysis and Critical Control Point system to an antenatal serum screening programme for Down's syndrome. Stage 2: Overcoming the hazards in program delivery. *Journal of Evaluation in Clinical Practice, 9*(1), 49–57.

DeRosier, J., Stalhandske, E., Bagian, J., & Nudell, T. (2002). Using health care failure mode and effect analysis: The VA National Center for Patient's Safety prospective risk analysis system. *Joint Commission Journal on Quality Improvement, 28*(5): 248–267.

Eagle, C., Davies, J., & Reason, J. (1992). Accident analysis of large-scale technological disasters applied to an anesthetic complication. *Canadian Journal of Anesthesia, 39*(2), 118–122.

Esmail, R., Cummings, C., Dersch, D., Duchscherer, G., Glowa, J., Liggett, G., & Hulme, T. (2005). Using healthcare failure mode and effect analysis tool to review the process of ordering and administrating potassium chloride and potassium phosphate. *Healthcare Quarterly, 8*(Spring), 73–80.

Feldman, S. E., & Roblin, D. W. (1997). Medical accidents in hospital care: Applications of failure analysis to hospital quality appraisal. *Joint Commission Journal on Quality Improvement, 23*(11), 567–580.

Food and Drug Administration. (2009, July 20). Hazard analysis & critical control points (HACCP). Retrieved from http://www.fda.gov/food/foodsafety/hazardanalysis criticalcontrolpointshaccp/default.htm.

Gowdy, M., & Godfrey, S. (2003). Using tools to assess and prevent inpatient falls. *Joint Commission Journal on Quality & Safety, 29*(7), 363–368.

Goyal, R. K. (1993). HAZOPs in industry. *Professional Safety, 38*(8), 34–37.

Grissinger, M., & Rich, D. (2002). JCAHO: meeting the standards for patient safety. *Journal of the American Pharmaceutical Association, 42*(5 Suppl), S54–5.

Linkin, D., Sausman, C., Santos, L., Lyons, C., Fox, C., Aumiller, L., … Lautenbach, E. (2005). Applicability of healthcare failure mode and effects analysis to healthcare epidemiology: Evaluation of the sterilization and use of surgical instruments. *Clinical Infectious Diseases, 41*(7), 1014–1019.

Lyons, M., Adams, S., Woloshynowych, M., & Vincent, C. (2004). Human reliability analysis in healthcare: A review of techniques. *International Journal of Risk and Safety in Medicine, 16*(4), 223–237.

Marx, D., & Slonim, A. (2003). Assessing patient safety risk before the injury occurs: An introduction to sociotechnical probabilistic risk modeling in health care. *Quality and Safety in Health Care, 12*(Suppl II), ii33–ii38.

McDonough, J., Solomon, R., & Petosa, L. (2004). Quality improvement and proactive hazard analysis models: Deciphering a new Tower of Babel. In P. Aspden, J. Corrigan, J. Wolcott, & S. Erickson (Eds.), *Patient safety: Achieving a new standard for care* (pp. 471–508). Washington, DC: National Academy Press.

National Patient Safety Agency. (2006). *Risk assessment programme overview*. Retrieved from http://www.nrls.npsa.nhs.uk/resources/?EntryId45=59813.

Ouellette-Piazzo, K., Asfaw, M. & Cowen, J. (2007). CT Healthcare Failure Mode Effect Analysis (HFMEA®): The misadministration of IV contrast in outpatients. *Radiology Management, 29*(1), 36–44.

Reason, J. T. (1990). *Human error: Causes and consequences*. New York: Cambridge University Press.

Richards, J. (2002). Risk management in infection control—HACCP, a useful tool? *Clinical Professional Development Infection, 3*(2), 59–62.

Roberts, K. H. (Ed.). (1993). *New challenges to understanding organizations*. New York: Macmillan.

Rochlin, G. I., LaPorte, T. R., & Roberts, K. H. (1987). The self-designing high-reliability organization: Aircraft carrier flight operations at sea. *Naval War College Review, 40*(4), 76–90.

Wagenaar, W. A. (1996). Profiling crisis management. *Journal of Contingencies and Crisis Management, 4*(3), 169–174.

Weick, K. E. (1987). Organizational culture as a source of high reliability. *California Management Review, 29*(2), 112–127.

Weingart, S., Wilson, R., Gibberd, R., & Harrison, B. (2000). Epidemiology of medical error. *British Medical Journal, 320*(7237), 774–777.

CHAPTER 8

MTO AND DEB ANALYSIS CAN FIND SYSTEM BREAKDOWNS

Sven Ternov

LEARNING OBJECTIVES

- Apply a systems theory model to improve learning from accidents
- Describe a method for retrospective incident analysis
- Describe a method for prospective patient safety improvement

Complex production systems, such as those used in health care, occasionally suffer from severe system breakdowns. These breakdowns can result in human injury or loss of life. By thoroughly examining such events, the hazards in the system can be identified and eliminated. The sad thing is that sometimes people have to die before the necessity for these changes are recognized. A better approach would be to identify and resolve system weaknesses before a breakdown occurs. In Chapter Seven Feldman and Roblin urge health care organizations to engage in both retrospective (root cause analysis) and prospective (anticipatory failure analysis) investigations. This principle is reinforced and expanded in this chapter. Two systematic techniques for conducting retrospective and prospective safety analyses are described: **MTO analysis** and **DEB analysis**.

MTO analysis (the abbreviation stands for Man-Technique-Organization) is a technique for identifying the underlying causes of accidents, derived from systems theory. MTO analysis is used for examining an incident which *has* occurred. It has been used by the Swedish National Board of Health and Welfare to examine medical mistakes. DEB analysis (the abbreviation stands for Deviation-Effect-Barrier) is designed specifically for use in complex socio-technical systems, as health care. The DEB analysis is used for examining a health care system for design flaws, *before* an incident happens.

Framework for Investigating Medical Accidents

The aim of investigating a medical accident is for the purpose of learning how to prevent similar and other accidents. The focus should be on *understanding* what caused the operator to make an active failure. To understand what made the operator perform in an unsafe way it is crucial to understand the *context* in which the mistake occurred. Which latent failures contributed to the error? Why did safety barriers not prevent the accident? To understand the context, a careful mapping of the accident must be done and it is important that this mapping shows the proper time sequence of events. Thus, analysis of a medical accident starts with gathering available data. The next step is to identify additional information that is needed to understand what went wrong. It is helpful to have a framework for structuring and analyzing this information is helpful.

Several accident investigation methods are described in the literature (Bagian, Gosbee, Lee, Williams, McKnight, & Mannos, 2002; Andersen & Fagerhaug, 2006; Aren et al., 2006). In this section, readers are introduced to just one—the MTO analysis method. As mentioned early in the chapter, the acronym MTO stands for Man-Technique-Organization. It exists under different names such as HPES (Human Performance Enhancement System) and ASSET (IAEA, 1990). It was adopted by the Swedish nuclear power industry and we have now adapted and applied it to health care accidents (Ternov & Akselsson, 2005). The steps of an MTO analysis are shown in the following list and described in subsequent sections.

1. Develop a preliminary map of the event
2. Conduct a preliminary cause analysis
3. Conduct on-site investigation and interviews
4. Review event mapping
5. Review cause analysis
6. Conduct barrier analysis
7. Identify situational factors

8. Identify latent failures

9. Identify absent or insufficient safety barriers

10. Develop an agenda for preventive actions

Form a Team

The MTO analysis is ideally conducted by a team of people from the health care organization where the accident occurred. The team should be organizationally aligned under administration, perhaps in the quality or risk management department. Because of the personal involvement of team members, investigation findings are more likely to result in organizational changes, contrary to what happens if an external expert supplies all the answers. The MTO analysis team should receive an introduction to the investigation method and, throughout the process, ongoing support from management and a facilitator.

Team members should be medical professionals (physicians, nurses, and technicians) and have certain personal qualifications. They should have high personal integrity and a genuine interest in error management. They should be able to think in terms of process and system and be analytical. They must be empathic, good listeners, and conduct themselves with dignity and respect for both the complexity of their task and the poor operators involved in the accident. They must be flexible and able to adapt easily to new information (not getting stuck in their own prejudices).

Establishing an MTO team takes quite some effort in both member selection and training. In Denmark we have trained all staff assigned to patient safety activities for all hospitals in a health care region (around 400 people). It was a one-day course with a half-day theoretical introduction and the rest of the time hands-on investigation training using real cases provided by the students.

Map the Event

The MTO analysis team begins the investigation process by reviewing written reports of the accident that were completed by involved staff as soon as possible after the occurrence. "Involved staff" are defined as those who committed an active failure and those otherwise involved in the actual situation of care, that is, the involved team. In addition, closest superiors to involved staff and heads of relevant departments (for example, chief of surgery, nursing director, and so on) should share their perspective.

An important part of information gathering is interviews conducted with relevant people in the organization. Interviews are often necessary for understanding the context in which the active failure took place. These interviews also provide a golden opportunity for the MTO analysis team to discuss patient safety risks with operators and management. The following should be considered when interviewing:

- Be well prepared.

- Always make an appointment.

- Never go behind the back of department management.

- Be very clear and specific as to the aim of the investigation.

- Do not schedule interviews too tightly (one hour per interview is a good guideline).

- Create a relaxed atmosphere; begin with small talk.

- Start the interview with an open mind.

- Skip the tape recorder; make notes instead.

- Interview as a rule only one person at a time, but allow a colleague to be present if the person being interviewed so desires.

Information gathered about the event allows the MTO analysis team to create a precise map of events leading up to the accident. The chronology of events is important. Therefore the team needs to know the dates and, if possible, the hour and minute of the event (hour and minute are not necessary if the event extends over several days). The event map is the first step in constructing an MTO analysis diagram. An example of an MTO analysis diagram that has yet to be filled in with accident investigation data is shown in Table 8.1. This diagram can be hand drawn or computer generated using spreadsheet software. In the cells across the top of the diagram, the chain of events that took place during the accident are detailed, one cell per event. Shown in Table 8.1 is a four-column diagram. A completed diagram has as many columns as needed to describe each event in the event chain.

Event mapping requires some experience. The most common error is to include too many actions in each cell. Only one step in the sequence of events should be stated per cell or the MTO analysis team will have difficulties during the analysis phase. If three distinctly separate actions are combined into one cell in the event map, the team could end up identifying three different causes for these actions. The rule during cause analysis, which occurs after event mapping, is "one cell—one cause."

Table 8.1   Example of a Blank MTO Diagram

Date/time
Event
Questions/ contributing causes
Situational factors
Safety barriers
Latent failures

Note: The diagram headings can be designed to the taste and need of the analyst.

Another common fault in creating an event map is to start the analysis too late in the sequence. For example, although the accident may have taken place in the emergency department, the MTO analysis should not be confined to this unit. Maybe the investigation should start a couple of days earlier when the patient first began to experience symptoms or at the time when the patient called an ambulance. The end point for the investigation is easier to define than the start point. If the accident causes a patient death, this is the end point. If not, corrective actions taken after the accident should be included in the analysis.

The row of "contributing causes" in the MTO analysis diagram in Table 8.1 serves a double function as denoted by the label "questions/contributing causes." During the investigation a lot of questions come to the minds of the team members; for example, "How could this happen?" or "Why did she do it like this?" These questions are noted in this row and then, when they are resolved during the personal interviews, the answers turn into direct causes.

Complete the MTO Analysis

A contributing cause represents the most immediate or obvious reason for the active failure. More than one contributing cause may be present for each active failure. To aid the team in identifying contributing causes, a taxonomy covering the major causes of medical mistakes has been developed. The taxonomy, shown in Table 8.2, is a simplified version of the HPES (nuclear power model MTO analysis).

Situational factors are defined as unforeseen, "unlucky" circumstances that play a major part in the evolution of the accident. It is often these unlucky circumstances that can explain why the process went wrong this one time even though the process was carried through in the usual way. Another way of putting it is that situational factors releases the risk represented by the latent failures.

The contributing cause(s) and situational factor(s) are noted on the diagram (Table 8.1) in the cells below the relevant active failure. The team may be tempted to stop the investigation at this stage and proceed to action. However,

Table 8.2   Taxonomy of Contributing Causes

Cause Categories	Examples of Problems in this Category
Oral communication	Oral communication from the sender is imprecise. Receiver does not acknowledge the message. Standardized vocabulary is not used. Unnecessary talk is not avoided. The sender and receiver did not "tune in" to each other (this takes a longer time if they are not already acquainted with one another).
Written procedures	The information in the procedure is given in the wrong sequence, or a sequence has been omitted. The text is difficult to understand, ambiguous, or too elaborate. The readability is poor (sentences too long, poor layout). The procedure mixes target groups. The procedure is written for both experienced and inexperienced users. Too many people are instructed to do the same thing and therefore nobody does it. The available instruction is outdated or otherwise invalid. It is not clear for which situation the procedure should be used. It is not clear who should use the procedure.
Workplace design/ physical environment	Maneuver gear or display is badly designed, hard to reach, or hard to read. Readability for important information is bad. Acoustical signals are inappropriately designed. Workplace design is inappropriate. Equipment is badly situated. There are too many people. Lighting is insufficient. Distracting noise is present.
Working environment	There is insufficient time for staff to prepare for work assignments. Not enough staff are allocated to work tasks or they are insufficiently trained for tasks. Planning of activities is not coordinated between departments. Staff members are easily distracted when performing simultaneous tasks.
Task supervision	Tasks are not properly defined for the operator. There is insufficient follow-up from the supervisor (for example, staff do not report when they are in trouble or when task is done). The level of training necessary to perform the task is not defined. Staff performance assessments are not done.
Training	Training of operator is insufficient. There is insufficient repetition of training. Educational goals are missing or goals are not related to the task. No follow-up assessment of educational effect is done.

it is important to complete the MTO analysis model; otherwise the latent failures will be missed. As we have seen, a medical accident is caused by a unique combination and interaction of latent failures and totally unforeseen situational factors, and these will probably not combine in the same way for many years to come. If latent failures are not identified and eliminated, actions will only safeguard against a similar accident but not cure the system. The cure is to eliminate latent failures. Safety barriers and latent failures are entered into the appropriate cells on the MTO diagram.

An illustration of a simple MTO analysis for an incident involving delayed diagnosis of appendicitis is shown in Table 8.3. Along the top row are the actions or events that took place in chronological order. In this example, action D ("misdiagnosis") was an active failure. One contributing cause was identified ("inexperienced physician"). One situational factor ("patient appeared to improve") was found and a safety barrier ("senior surgeon was supposed to examine patient") was identified that might either have prevented the erroneous action or the harmful influence on the system caused by the erroneous action. The contributing cause was eventually traced to a latent failure in the training system ("no mechanism in place to communicate 'standard operating procedures' to resident physicians"). An actual MTO analysis diagram can be five to ten pages in length.

Act on MTO Analysis Results

The learning from the MTO analysis must be put to use in order to improve safety; otherwise the exercise is a waste of time and money. The improvement **action plan** should be developed after internal discussions with the "**process owners**" in the facility. Often the number of identified latent failures and absent or insufficient safety barriers are greater than can be remedied at once. It may be necessary to prioritize where improvements will be made. The criteria to be considered when setting priorities include the frequency of safety occurrences caused by the latent failure and the severity of the occurrence. It should be borne in mind that latent failures can interact in nasty ways so that a number of seemingly "minor" latent failures may someday combine and cause an accident.

A latent failure that presents a great risk can sometimes be very expensive or difficult to remedy. An alternative is to circumvent the latent failure by designing a strong safety barrier.

A word of caution: A superficial analysis may give a counterproductive result. More procedures might be written, more operators might be instructed to comply with double checks, vigorous ad hoc training programs might be undertaken, and the administrative control concerning adherence to instructions

Table 8.3   Example of a Schematic Diagram from an MTO Analysis

A		B	C	D	E	F
1	Date/Time	May 5; 18:00	May 5; 19:00	May 5; 20:00	May 5; 22:00	May 6; 15:00
2	Event	Patient has had stomach pain for two days, temp of 38° C., nausea.	Patient calls ED and is told to come in for an examination.	Patient examined by physician, who diagnoses gastritis.	Patient sent home with instructions to return if condition gets worse.	Patient returns in ambulance in preshock due to peritonitis from ruptured appendix.
3	Contributing causes			Resident physician inexperienced.		
4	Situational factors			Slight improvement of patient during stay in ED.		
5	Safety barriers			The standard operating procedure is for the resident physician to call senior surgeon to examine patients with abdominal pain before patient leaves hospital.		
6	Latent failures			Proper training for resident physicians' work tasks not defined.		

might be tightened up (Rasmussen, 1980). The overall effect of this superficial analysis might be that instead of getting a safer system, one gets a fuzzier and more awkward system that is less reliable than the old one. This can be avoided by doing a proper MTO analysis. The cause-effect chain should be traced sufficiently backward to identify deficiencies in the quality system. Improvements in the quality system, as a result of an MTO analysis, will have an overall beneficial effect on system reliability instead of only preventing an accident that will likely (almost) never happen again.

Framework for Proactive Safety Improvements

Several **prospective risk assessment** methods intended to prevent accidents have been created. These methods include hazard and operability (HAZOP) studies, failure mode and effect analysis (FMEA), and tripod delta. These methods were developed and validated for use in technical complex systems. A few have been tried in health care, for instance failure mode and effect analysis (Spath, 2003; Abujudeh & Kaewlai, 2009) and probabilistic risk assessment (Marx & Slonim, 2003).

At the faculty of engineering, Lund University, we have developed and applied a method possibly better suited for complex socio-technical systems, the DEB analysis (Deviation-Effect-Barrier). It has been applied in health care and in air traffic control (Ternov & Akselsson, 2004). The principle is much the same as MTO analysis, but reverse. The DEB analysis can be summarized like this:

1. Choose a process to study.

2. Form an analysis team.

3. Map the process carefully.

4. Hypothesize deviations.

5. Validate hypotheses by observation, interview, or incident reports (if available).

6. Evaluate system effect of validated deviations.

7. Look for latent failures and safety barriers that need to be developed or redesigned.

8. Identify and implement error containment action plans.

The possible system effect of the disturbance is evaluated, latent failures that make the error possible are identified, and possible safety barriers that might be able to prevent harmful system effect of the error are looked for. The next section briefly describes the application of the DEB analysis method in a department of oncology at a university hospital.

DEB Analysis Case Study

To conduct this DEB analysis, two support analysts spent approximately five working days each in gathering the necessary data. This included process mapping and validation of hypotheses on process disturbances. Another two days were spent on report preparation on completion of the project.

Choose a Process to Study

The chosen process was the treatment of a patient with cytotoxic agents within one unit.

Form an Analysis Team

A group from the ward unit was established, consisting of two nurses (one of these was the head nurse for the unit) and a physician (oncologist) who had shown interest in the project. The group also included a pharmacist, who was supervisor for the cytotoxic agent preparation unit at the hospital pharmacy.

Map the Process Carefully

Because the chosen process was far more complicated than anticipated, the steps divided into the following subprocesses:

- Decision on treating a patient with cytotoxic agents

- Planning for treatment (when the patient arrives on the unit)

- Prescription (preparing the cytotoxic agent treatment chart [CAC])

- Preparation (at the pharmacy)

- Administering drugs to the patient

- Follow-up of ongoing treatment

- Planning for next treatment cycle

The whole process, including all the components in the subprocesses, were mapped in a diagram resembling the MTO diagram.

Hypothesize Disturbances

A number of hypotheses concerning possible disturbances in the process were generated. To perform this step, the team asked the following questions about each step in the process: What happens if we influence the process at this step too much? too little? wrongly? not at all?

Validate Disturbances

The hypothetical answers to the questions in the preceding step were validated by interviewing the process owners to determine if these disturbances could actually happen or have happened.

Evaluate System Effect of Validated Disturbances

In this step, possible consequences for negative impact on system stability were assessed; that is, what was the probability that a certain disturbance could create a system failure (serious accident) or only a minor process aberration? This step is closely integrated with the next step. The probability for a certain disturbance to cause system failure is of course much higher if no efficient safety barriers exist to counteract the harmful system influence of a disturbance.

Look for Latent Failures and Safety Barriers That Need to Be Developed or Redesigned

At this stage in the DEB analysis we are able to identify some major dangers in the system. One danger was that the most frequent, and the most serious, disturbances took place during the doctor's prescription on the CAC. For the most part, other types of prescription errors were regularly caught and remedied by the pharmacy preparation unit; however, CAC prescription errors tended to be missed. If the physician mixes up regimes and chooses the wrong one or misunderstands the dosage guidelines, this error (illustrated as a disturbance arrow on the diagram) had a high probability of shooting through the whole system without getting caught before it hit the patient.

The oncology nurse served as a safety barrier for CAC prescription-writing errors (the last possible one before the error hit the patient); however, this barrier appeared to have flaws. The CAC was often very poorly written, making it difficult for the nurse to act as a safety barrier. Further, the CAC layout was inappropriate, making it difficult for the nurse to get an overview of the day's medications. The nurse-safety barrier might work with experienced nurses but would be weakened with inexperienced nurses who may be unwilling to question a physician's prescription.

The group was also not happy to find that the nurse-safety barrier was an informal one (checking the correctness of the CAC was not a defined responsibility of the nurse). The nurses took on a responsibility that they had not been formally delegated to perform. This lack of formalization was a problem, too, concerning the interaction between the pharmacy chemotherapy preparation staff and the unit. The pharmacy staff did a lot of quality control of CAC content. Such checking was not a task formally delegated to the pharmacy unit, although it had been going on for quite some time. This might lead to a dangerous situation in which the physicians begin to rely on pharmacy double checks only to find that they are not taking place.

All in all, the DEB analysis disclosed 12 latent system failures and 6 flawed safety barriers, all with the potential of killing or seriously harming the patient on that day in the future when bad luck occurs.

Identify and Implement Error Containment Action Plans

The final DEB analysis report recommended several actions plans, including the following:

- Introduction of computer-aided prescriptions for the CAC

- Recommendations that responsibilities be clarified between the different actors in the system

- Implementation of double checks on important decisions

- Standardization of equipment (infusion pumps) in cooperating ward units

- Introduction of proper feedback loops concerning handling of blood tests

Because an incident-reporting system was not in place in this unit prior to the DEB analysis, it was very difficult for the group to quantify the study findings. Recommendations were made to put such a reporting system in place.

Conclusion

Latent failures and flawed safety barriers must be actively investigated after an accident; otherwise they are easily missed. The MTO analysis framework for accident analysis of medical accidents was presented. In the MTO analysis the chain of events leading to an accident is carefully mapped. Contributing causes, situational factors, latent failures, and deficient safety barriers are looked for in a systematic way.

A safe and reliable system for tomorrow cannot be based solely on analyses of yesterday's mistakes. Therefore, a proactive method for reliability analyses of processes in health care was presented (DEB analysis) together with a case study of its application. By studying the negative effects that human operators may exert on the system and the system's ability to absorb these negative effects, a "forgiving system" can be designed. Such a system will maintain its stability better than a nonforgiving system. It is imperative that health care systems be designed in a forgiving way to minimize the risk of medical mistakes and patient injury.

Discussion Questions

1. What are the similarities and differences between the MTO analysis and the root cause analysis process described in Chapter Seven?

2. What are the similarities and differences between the DEB analysis and the anticipatory failure analysis described in Chapter Seven?

3. Describe the advantages and disadvantages of MTO and DEB analysis as compared to the accident investigation techniques described in Chapter Seven.

Key Terms

Action plan

DEB analysis

MTO analysis

Process owner

Prospective risk assessment

References

Abujudeh, H., & Kaewlai, R. (2009). Radiology failure mode and effect analysis: What is it? *Radiology, 252*(2), 544–550.

Andersen, B., & Fagerhaug, T. *Root cause analysis: Simplified tools and techniques* (2nd ed.). Milwaukee, WI: ASQ Quality Press, 2006.

Aren, R., Iedema, M., Jorm, C., Braithwaite, J., Travaglia, J., & Lum, M. (2006). A root cause analysis of clinical error: Confronting the disjunction between formal rules and situated clinical activity. *Science & Medicine, 63*(5), 1201–1212.

Bagian, J., Gosbee, J., Lee, C., Williams, L., McKnight, S., & Mannos, D. M. (2002). The veterans affairs root cause analysis system in action. *Joint Commission Journal on Quality Improvement, 28*(10), 531–545.

International Atomic Energy Agency. *ASSET guidelines.* IAEA-tecdoc-573, IAEA, Vienna, Austria, 1990.

Marx, D. A., & Slonim, A. D. (2003). Assessing patient safety risk before the injury occurs: An introduction to sociotechnical probabilistic risk modeling in health care. *Quality and Safety in Health Care, 2*(Suppl II), ii33–ii37.

Rasmussen, J. (1980). What can be learned from human error reports? In K. Duncan, M. Gruneberg, & D. Wallis (Eds.). *Changes in working life.* London: Ashgate.

Spath, P. L. (2003). Using failure mode and effects analysis to improve patient safety. *AORN Journal, 78*(1), 16–37.

Ternov, S., & Akselsson, R. (2004). A method, DEB analysis, for proactive risk analysis applied to air traffic control. *Safety Science, 42*(7), 657–673.

Ternov, S., & Akselsson, R. (2005). System weaknesses as contributing causes for accidents in health care. *International Journal for Quality in Health Care, 17*(1), 1–9.

CHAPTER 9

USING DEDUCTIVE ANALYSIS TO EXAMINE ADVERSE EVENTS

Robert Latino

LEARNING OBJECTIVES

- Describe commonly used root cause analysis techniques
- Identify the difference between categorical and deductive investigation approaches
- Explain how a deductive analysis tool is used to identify root causes and appropriate corrective actions
- Describe how collection and analysis of data results in a more effective root cause analysis

Root cause analysis (RCA) is a systematic investigation technique that uses information gathered during an intense assessment of an accident to determine the underlying reasons for the deficiencies or failures that caused the accident. In 1996, The Joint Commission (TJC) began requiring hospitals use root cause analysis techniques to investigate sentinel events as a condition of maintaining accreditation (Anonymous, 1996). Although RCA techniques have been used in health care organizations for several years, there is still considerable variation in how the investigation process is conducted (Wu, Lipshutz, & Pronovost, 2008). Variation exists because there is no universally accepted method for conducting an RCA. This lack of uniformity has resulted in many different tools being used for adverse event investigations: 5 Whys, Ishikawa diagrams, prompt lists, and deductive analytic techniques. These tools are often viewed as equivalent accident investigation methods with equally comparable results and this is simply not true. Some tools improve the quality of investigation by broadening the scope and depth of inquiry.

In an industry where human error can mean the difference between life and death, it is essential that health care professionals use comprehensive investigation techniques to uncover and correct the fundamental causes of adverse events. Ineffective RCAs do not contribute to patient safety improvements. Are worthwhile event investigation techniques being used in your organization? If you agree with one or more of the statements below, it is time to consider a more comprehensive RCA approach.

- We lack quantifiable proof that RCAs have directly contributed to improved patient safety in our organization.

- Even after we have done an RCA, a repeat adverse event involving the same process is likely to occur.

- Though RCA increases patient safety awareness among the people involved in the event, there is little evidence that the knowledge gained during the RCA is spread throughout our organization.

- Since we have been doing RCAs, our rate of adverse patient incidents has not decreased significantly.

The technical differences of various accident investigation tools are explored in this chapter. The intent is to educate readers to the advantages and drawbacks of various RCA tools to enable facilitators of adverse event investigations to select the most effective analytic approach.

Adverse Event Investigation Techniques

Before describing RCA investigation techniques, terminology needs to be clarified. Much has been written about RCA methods and there are sometimes conflicting definitions. Take, for instance, the phrase *root cause analysis*. If you were to do an Internet search for the definition of this phrase, you would likely find hundreds of slightly different interpretations. At Wikipedia, a popular Internet site for seeking word definitions, root cause analysis is defined as "a class of problem solving methods aimed at identifying the root causes of problems or events" (2009). This broad and ambiguous description of RCA exists because no universally accepted definition exists. It is easy to understand why so many individuals and groups use RCA to describe their problem-solving approach.

For purposes of this chapter, key terms are defined. These definitions help readers understand the differences between various investigation methodologies and the impact that these differences have on the effectiveness of the RCA.

Dissecting the Terminology

To more precisely define RCA, the steps in the process must be dissected and clarified. The first step is to understand what happened. This step involves investigation, which in an RCA entails collection of data. Investigation is not the same as analysis. That comes later. Investigation deals with systematically observing and studying facts associated with the adverse event.

Analysis is the taking of collected data and reviewing it for a deeper understanding of the cause-and-effect relationships that lead to the adverse outcome. In RCA, analysis involves explaining the facts by breaking down the adverse event into its component parts and understanding the failure within the context of the overall system. To use the criminologist analogy, when forensic teams go to the crime scene they are charged with gathering evidence in an appropriate manner for the investigators and prosecutors to analyze. The forensic team deals with collecting the facts and the investigators then try to make sense of how the facts came to be. The collected facts lead to hypotheses about how they came to be, and then tests are conducted to validate or refute the hypotheses.

To piece together the facts in an RCA, a graphical depiction of the event is constructed. This visual display of the facts helps standardize the analysis and aids in communicating the final RCA results to others. In summary, the investigative phase of an RCA involves collecting data about what happened. This data is the "evidence" used to form opinions or hypotheses about how the adverse outcome came to be. Hypotheses that prove to be true are analyzed further for contributing factors, and unproven hypotheses are discarded.

Common RCA Tools

A tool is an instrument which conveys some advantage to its user in the execution of a task. Just as a carpenter would use a particular tool for a construction task, accident investigators use particular tools during an RCA. Health care organizations use different analytical tools to uncover the root cause of an adverse event. Tools for RCA vary from one another in how they organize the investigative reasoning process.

In this section, we describe the more popular tools as well as their benefits and drawbacks. Readers are encouraged to select the tools most likely to produce an effective RCA—one that results in proven and sustainable patient safety gains. The right tool applied in the right situation can make a significant contribution to the efficiency and effectiveness of an investigation.

The 5 Whys

Although there are varying forms of this simplistic tool, the most common form involves the analyst asking the question *why* five times to uncover the root cause. A visual representation of this analytic tool is found in Figure 9.1.

There is a reason the **5 Whys** approach is not encouraged by professional investigative agencies such as the National Transportation Safety Board. "Why" questions can be very limiting. When someone is asked *why* something happened, most often the response is a single answer. Contrast this with answers to the question, *how could* something happen? The response is more comprehensive. This difference is not merely a point of semantics. Phrasing of questions affects the analysis outcome. The appropriate use of questioning is discussed in later sections on deductive analysis tools.

A primary flaw with using the 5 Whys technique in an RCA is that failures rarely follow a linear pattern. The majority of situations involving an adverse patient outcome result from multiple factors that combine laterally (at the same time). Also, the 5 Whys technique misleads the analyst into thinking an adverse event results from only one root cause, when that is almost never true. The word "cause" is a misnomer because it is often used in a singular manner. For instance, television reporters at an accident scene often pronounce that investigators have yet to find the root cause—as if there were only one.

The 5 Whys approach is a path of least resistance but unfortunately this path leads to ineffective RCAs. It may be a useful troubleshooting tool for prob-

FIGURE 9.1   The 5-Whys Analytical Tool

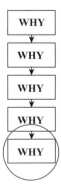

lems that require quick solutions, but it does not promote a comprehensive analysis of why a problem actually occurred. If an adverse outcome is attributed to a single cause and several causes in fact existed, the risk of a recurrent event is high.

The obvious advantages of the 5 Whys approach are that it is quick, inexpensive, and does not require extensive resources. Organizations must weigh these advantages against the risks associated with being wrong or not sufficiently comprehensive.

Ishikawa Diagram

The **Ishikawa diagram**, often called a fishbone or cause-and-effect diagram, is another popular analytical tool (Ishikawa, 1982). This general problem-solving tool gets its name from its founder and form (see Figure 9.2). The spine of the fish typically represents the sequence of events leading to the adverse outcome. The fish bones themselves represent major problem categories that may have contributed to the event.

The problem categories in an Ishikawa diagram change from user to user and event to event. Here are some of the more popular categories:

- The 4 Ms: Methods, Machines, Materials, Manpower

- The 6 Ms: Machine, Method, Materials, Maintenance, Man, Mother Nature (Environment)

- The 4 Ps: Place, Procedure, People, Policies

- The 4 Ss: Surroundings, Suppliers, Systems, Skills

FIGURE 9.2   Ishikawa Diagram

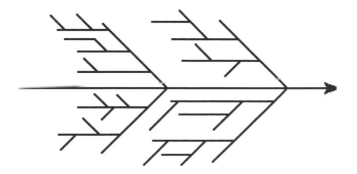

An Ishikawa diagram is often used to brainstorm all possible causes of an adverse outcome. RCA team members decide on the problem categories to be used and then theorize what factors within those categories may have caused the event. Once these factors are identified then the members ask *why* the factors occurred—similar to a 5 Whys analysis.

The visualization aspects of the Ishikawa diagram make it an appealing brainstorming technique, yet there are some drawbacks. There may be little effort to gather data to support or refute the cause hypotheses. Root causes may originate more from hearsay than actual facts. In addition, the process of identifying causes is categorical rather than a true cause-and-effect relationship. The RCA team must pick the problem categories to use for grouping ideas. If an important problem category is not included on the diagram, key causes of the event can be overlooked.

Prompt List

Problem categories on an Ishikawa diagram influence the scope of an adverse event investigation. Prompt lists serve a similar purpose. A prompt list is a series of questions grouped into themes drawn from risk management theory. The questions provide investigators with a process to help bring problems into focus and analyze them in an orderly way. An example is the tool developed by the Centers for Disease Control to use in performing an RCA of a sharps injury or near-miss event (2008). The tool prompts analysts to consider factors in 10 different categories that may have contributed to the event:

- Issues related to patient assessment

- Issues related to staff training or staff competency

- Equipment or device issue

- Work environment issues

- Lack of or misinterpretation of information

- Communication issues

- Appropriate rules, policies, or procedures, or lack thereof

- Failure of a protective barrier

- Personnel or personal issues

- Supervisor issues

RCA prompt lists often originate from regulatory groups. The lists contain details of what regulators are looking for and help ensure RCA teams comply with the expected scope and depth of inquiry. A prompt list commonly used by RCA teams in health care organizations is one developed by The Joint Commission. Accredited organizations are required to conduct an RCA following a sentinel event and the analysis must meet the minimum scope of investigation required for the particular type of event (Croteau, 2010). All factors listed on the TJC RCA framework are to be addressed (The Joint Commission, n.d.).

Like an Ishikawa diagram, prompt lists are a categorical RCA approach. In other words, the potential cause categories are predefined and it is up to evaluators to determine if any subsystems of these categories contributed to the adverse outcome. Though this may be an efficient RCA methodology, there are some important drawbacks. First of all, key contributing factors could be missed if the prompt list omits an important cause category.

In addition, the investigator must be well-versed in every factor encompassed by a cause category. For instance, the TJC RCA framework contains the category, human factors. There is an entire field of study around human factors engineering and causes of human errors which is only briefly summarized in Chapter Two. How many evaluators understand the difference between rule-based, skill-based, and knowledge-based errors and contributing factors? More than likely, analysis of human factors will cover only the questions posed by the prompt list and accompanying TJC instructional manuals.

RCA prompt lists created by regulatory or accreditation groups make it easier for health care organizations to document compliance with external requirements; however, this categorical approach is coming under increased scrutiny (Wu, Lipshutz, & Pronovost, 2008). There is scant evidence that patient care has gotten any safer even though health care organizations have been using the TJC RCA framework, or something similar, for over a decade (DeRosier, Taylor, Turner, & Bagian, 2007). A correctly completed RCA form may be helpful for complying with government regulations or accreditation standards, but analysts should not rely solely on the framework to guide the investigation. Prompt lists of causal factors and root causes can channel the analyst's thinking down certain paths.

Deductive Analysis Tools

These analytic tools provide a means for clarifying what actually happened without the limitations of a categorical approach. Fault trees are an example of a deductive tool that can be used to determine how the system failed (Office of

Nuclear Regulatory Research, 1981). Fault trees were initially developed as risk management tools to help identify and mitigate or eliminate the risk of failure in the new design of aircraft. Similar types of analytic tools include event trees, causal trees, and cause maps (Vincent, 2006).

Deductive analysis should be familiar to most health care professionals as this analytic approach is often used in research studies. Caregivers also use deductive analysis—a key element in critical thinking—to make patient management decisions. These same critical thinking skills should be used during investigations of adverse patient events.

In general, deductive analysis RCA tools follow a similar pattern. The RCA starts with identification of the adverse event to be investigated. The RCA team then identifies the immediate and proximal causes of the event. In the causal tree example in Figure 9.3 there are two immediate causes, but there could be many more. Both of these immediate causes were necessary to produce the adverse event. Each cause is analyzed until all root causes are identified. Deductive analysis constitutes reasoning from the general to the specific without the tunneling affect of categorical analysis tools.

A lack of logical thinking about cause-and-effect relationships is one of the barriers to an effective RCA (Okes, 2009). To overcome this problem, several industries are required by regulation to use deductive analysis tools when analyzing the cause of accidents. Many companies, including some health care organizations, are using software-based rather than paper-based tools. This helps to ensure consistent application of the RCA process for all accident investigations. Some of the commonly used software-based tools are proprietary and the deductive models used by these applications have unique brand names. In Table 9.1

FIGURE 9.3   Causal Tree

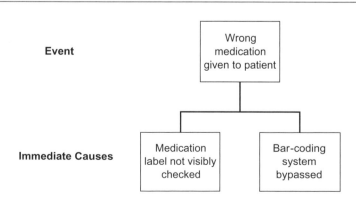

Table 9.1 Proprietary RCA Deductive Analysis Software Products

Name of Product	Company	Description of Approach
PROACT®	Reliability Center, Inc. http://www.reliability.com	This tool uses a logic tree to graphically depict potential hypotheses and subsequent validated causal paths to identify physical, human, and latent or systemic root causes.
RealityCharting®	Apollo Associated Services http://www.apollorca.com	This tool offers guidance and structure for RCAs and provides a graphic representation of interrelated causes and causal paths.
REASONS®	Decision Systems, Inc. http:// www.rootcause.com	This tool comprises elements of several RCA techniques—human factors analysis, barrier analysis, change analysis, Ishikawa diagrams, and fault trees.
TapRooT®	System Improvements, Inc. http://www.taproot.com	This tool uses what is described as a Root Cause Tree® to help investigators perform a systematic analysis of an incident to identify causal factors and root causes.

is a description of the mainstream RCA software products that reportedly employ a deductive analysis approach.

Although it is possible to use a paper-based process, there are several benefits to automation:

- Improved data organization

- Reduced analysis time

- Improved rigor

- Enhanced reporting capabilities

- Ability to clearly visualize cause-and-effect relationships

When evaluating whether to use the various investigation tools, analysts may find that the level of breadth and depth gained by deductive analysis is not required for all events.

Application of Deductive Analysis

Several software-based deductive analysis products are available. They are distinguished by differences in their embedded rules. As I am most familiar with the PROACT® product, it is used in this section to illustrate how deductive analysis thinking is applied during the RCA of an adverse patient event. My using PROACT as the model for discussion does not signify that other products (see Table 9.1) are any less effective. It is my hope that readers will explore all software applications to learn more about each product.

Overview of the Analysis Process

When an adverse outcome occurs it is important to gather information about the event. Going back to the detective analogy, it is hard to imagine that a detective or forensic team would not be dispatched to a crime scene to collect evidence. The perpetrator of the crime could not be brought to justice on the basis of hearsay evidence alone. Assumptions and unfounded information are also unreliable sources for conducting a root cause analysis. A concerted effort must be made to collect factual data.

The RCA team should meet and discuss what data needs to be collected to ensure a comprehensive analysis of the event. The 5 Ps of data collection, shown in Table 9.2, can help guide the team in selecting information necessary for analysis. Notice some data may be applicable to more than one category. For instance, monitoring strips might be considered a *Tangible*, but some people would put it in the *Paper* category. What is most important is to gather the data, not quarrel over categorizations.

Collection of data to validate RCA conclusions is a key difference between conducting an effective investigation versus one that merely seeks to comply with regulatory requirements. Time pressures and the natural human propensity to take the path of least resistance can cause an RCA team to overlook the data collection step. The organization's approach to RCA should *require* data collection be done to validate investigation conclusions. Data are vital in investigation and analysis. Hearsay and assumptions may be quicker ways of validating the RCA team's hypotheses, but these methods are likely to yield unsatisfactory

Table 9.2   The 5 Ps of Data Collection

PARTS	Anything tangible. Some examples: ● Equipment (new and failed) ● Tissue samples ● IV solutions ● X-rays ● Monitoring strips ● Medications ● Syringes ● Surgical devices ● Ambient air samples (testing for contamination of air) ● Fluid samples
POSITION	Positions in time and space. Some examples: ● Location of event in facility (for example, fall in bathroom near toilet on 1E, Room 104B) ● Location of event in relation to where other similar equipment was located (i.e., dialysis machines at different locations in same systems) ● Control panel readings (for example, position of dials on IV pump) ● Date and time of event and same for similar events to look for correlations regarding work shift or day of the week ● Environmental conditions (such as humidity, lighting, type of floor surface, temperature, noise level, and so on) ● Location of personnel at time of event and where they were supposed to be at time of event
PEOPLE	Potential people to interview. Some examples: ● Anyone involved in processes or the event ● Anyone who observed the event ● Individual(s) who discovered the event ● Individual(s) from departments involved in providing support for the processes (such as biomedical services, information management, procurement or materials management, transport services, and so on)
PARADIGMS	Personal belief systems. These are convictions that people believe and hold true about the event, despite facts that may be contrary. Paradigms are often extracted from interviews. Some examples of paradigm statements: ● We were understaffed. ● The staff member was inexperienced. ● It is the equipment manufacturer's fault. ● The patient was very frail. ● That is the way we always do it. ● I did not have time to follow the proper procedure. ● The doctor told me to do it that way. ● I was distracted.

(continued)

Table 9.2 *Continued*

PAPER	Anything on paper (written or electronic). Here are some examples: • Literature references • Applicable procedures, guidelines, protocols, and so forth • Maintenance histories • Shift assignment logs • Monitoring strips • X-rays • Design specifications and modifications • Training records • Operating room schedule • Purchasing records

FIGURE 9.4   PROACT Logic Tree

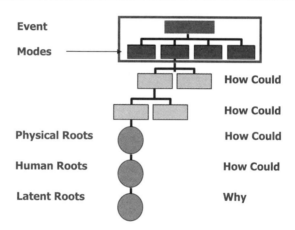

results. Health care professionals would never think of treating a patient without first knowing the facts about the patient's condition. The same rigor should be applied to the treatment of system problems causing adverse events.

Once data are gathered, the RCA team is ready to use deductive thinking which is facilitated by the PROACT software. The PROACT logic tree (shown in Figure 9.4) is an expression of cause-and-effect relationships that queued up in a particular sequence to cause an adverse outcome to occur. These cause-and-effect relationships are validated with hard evidence—data gathered during the investigation. Data drives the team's analysis of the event, not the loudest subject matter expert in the room.

The logic tree starts off with a description of the facts associated with an event. These facts comprise what is called the Top Box (the Event and the Modes). **Modes** are the manifestations of the failure and the Event is the final consequence that triggered the need for an RCA. Once the Top Box is constructed, the team proceeds with the questioning of *how could* the Modes have occurred? People may have been conditioned to ask the question *why* during such analyses, however the logic tree tool starts off with the question *how could*. The goal is to identify all the possibilities (not just the most likely) and then use evidence to back up what did and did not occur. Often what is found to have *not* happened is equally as important as what *did* happen.

This questioning process is reiterative as the team follows the cause-and-effect chain backwards. Questions are asked and answered with hypotheses and evidence used to validate the results. This continues until the team uncovers the human roots—points where a human made a decision error. Human roots represent errors of omission or commission by an individual. Either the person did something that should not have been done or did not do something that should have been done. At this point the RCA team explores the question of *why* someone made the decision that was made.

This is an important spot in the analysis because the team is seeking to understand why someone thought the decision made at the time was correct. In this part of the analysis, the questioning switches to *why* to better explore a set of answers particular to an individual or group. The answers from this questioning result in identification of latent root causes—the organizational systems that allow people to make the best decisions. The latent roots represent the rationale for the decision that triggered the consequences to occur at the time of the decision. These conditions are called latent because they are always there in the organization, lying dormant until triggering some human action that results in sequences of physical root causes to occur. If unbroken this error chain continues to the point it produces an adverse outcome requiring an immediate response.

The PROACT logic tree approach clearly links cause and effect, requires evidence to back up what people say, and encourages understanding and recognition of the system flaws that contribute to poor decisions on the front lines.

Deconstruction of the Logic Tree

The above overview of the PROACT logic tree is deceptively simple, whereas in reality there are many rule sets built into the decision process supported by the software application. Just as many of the clinical decision support tools used by health care professionals require software support, so do complex RCA deductive analysis tools. In the following section, rule sets found in the PROACT logic tree are further explained. Keep in mind that other software-based RCA deductive analysis products contain similar, but slightly different rule sets.

A surgical fire is used to illustrate application of the PROACT logic tree. This case involves a 65-year-old man with advanced adenocarcinoma of lung. He underwent laser bronchoscopy to stop the bleeding from a tumor obstructing his right main stem bronchus. During the procedure, an endotracheal fire occurred. The bronchoscope and endotracheal tube were swiftly removed. The patient was then reintubated and irrigated with normal saline. The patient survived this event and later died from his cancer. Surgical fires are considered sentinel events by The Joint Commission and an RCA must be done (Croteau, 2010).

Define the Problem

The problem statement is found in the Top Box, which is comprised of the Event plus the Modes. The RCA team must accept that anything in the Top Box is a fact; otherwise the foundation of the analysis will be rocky. This is where data comes into play. The team should have data to support the facts put in the Top Box.

The Event statement is the last effect in the cause-and-effect chain. The Event is the reason an in-depth RCA is being done. The Mode(s) are the immediate causes of the Event. The Top Box for this event is illustrated in Figure 9.5.

FIGURE 9.5   Surgical Fire Incident Top Box

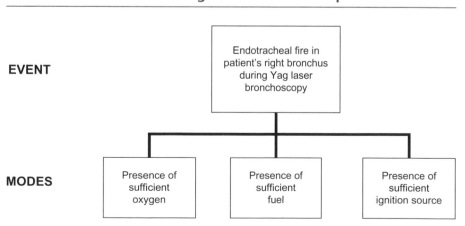

Three Modes of the Event are represented in the example. The Modes are identified by effectively asking, how did the patient experience a fire in the right bronchus while undergoing laser bronchoscopy (the Event)? The answers are very broad at the top of the logic tree, with the Modes representing all possibilities in the fewest number of boxes. In this example, the team concluded that only three responses were possible: presence of sufficient oxygen, presence of sufficient fuel, and presence of a sufficient ignition source.

Drill Down

Once the Top Box is completed to the satisfaction of the RCA team, the facts are explored and hypotheses regarding how the event happened are formulated. A hypothesis is an educated guess based on the known facts at the time. To ensure that the RCA results in worthwhile improvement recommendations, it is important that decisions made in the investigation and analysis phase are based on facts not hearsay or assumptions. The PROACT logic tree supports the development of fact-based conclusions.

Collected data are used to document and validate hypotheses in the logic tree. Each hypothesis entered into the PROACT logic tree has a corresponding spreadsheet-style verification log that identifies the hypothesis, the data collection or verification method used, the data results or outcome, the person responsible for gathering the verification data, the start and completion dates for data collection. This verification log provides important backup to the logic tree created by the investigation team. When reporting the RCA results, the log provides evidence that the root cause conclusions are based on data, not assumptions.

The investigation proceeds down the logic tree, moving from the general to the specific. "How could this happen" questioning generates more hypotheses to explore. If a hypothesis is proven incorrect based on the outcome of verification, the logic tree path stops at this point and is noted as "not true" with an "X" on the hypothesis. However, a leg of a logic tree may also end because the condition noted was known and acceptable for the circumstances. For instance, in our example, oxygen and ignition sources were found to be present because obviously there was oxygen in the atmosphere and also a laser used for the procedure. There would be no value in pursuing these two conditions deeper as they were expected so they are left on the logic tree as true but the leg ends at that point. In the surgical fire example, the investigation continued down the path of "presence of sufficient fuel" because it was unknown as to what the fuel source could have been. The questioning at this point continues with, how could sufficient fuel have been present? The logic tree branch represented in Figure 9.6 illustrates the three answers to this question.

FIGURE 9.6　Drill Down of Modes in Surgical Fire Incident

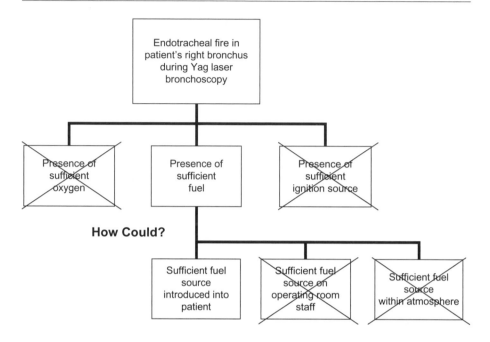

In the ideal world, there would always be facts—hard evidence—to validate every decision made by the RCA team. Yet, facts are sometimes hard to come by. To overcome this problem, the PROACT logic tree uses a weighting scale to measure the investigators' confidence in the verification techniques and outcomes. A **confidence factor** is assigned to the evidence, using a scale of 0 to 5. The highest rating, 5, indicates the team is absolutely certain the evidence confirms the hypothesis is true. The lowest rating, 0, indicates the team is absolutely certain the evidence confirms the hypothesis is not true. The other numbers represent shades of uncertainty where there is no conclusive evidence and the team must subjectively apply a weight to express a confidence factor. Typically, the team continues to explore a hypothesis with a confidence factor of 3 or higher. A hypothesis with a lower confidence number is considered to be a low probability and is not explored any further. The numeric confidence factor rating of each hypothesis is noted on the logic tree and also in the verification log.

The questioning process continues with all hypotheses that have proven to be true (or designated as a high probability based on evidence collected). Using the surgical fire example, presume the RCA team concludes that the broncho-

FIGURE 9.7   Body of the Logic Tree for Surgical Fire Incident

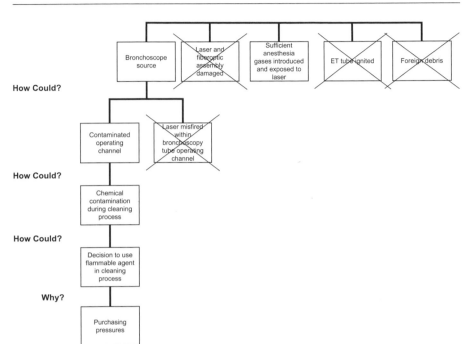

scope itself and the anesthesia gas were the sources of fuel for the fire. The body of the continued logic tree is found in Figure 9.7. All hypotheses with an "X" were proven to be not true (confidence factor of zero) based on evidence collected. In the boxes shown beneath one of the verified hypotheses—bronchoscope source—are answers to *how could this happen* questioning.

Notice that the RCA team switched to *why* questions to examine the decision error. Asking *how could* someone have made a decision could produce thousands of possibilities and waste a great deal of analytical time. It is better to ask a person *why* he felt his decision was appropriate at the time he made it.

In this case scenario, the RCA team found that management decisions were influenced by purchasing pressures. To hasten drying after sterilization in the Steris machines, bronchoscopes were being flushed with alcohol. There were an insufficient number of Steris machines to meet demand and no back-up autoclavable scopes were available. The need to control equipment and inventory costs had influenced purchasing decisions that eventually led to physical causes, which produced an undesirable effect.

Remember, the logic tree is merely a graphic representation of the investigative and deductive analysis thought process of the RCA team. The software provides documentation of the team's conclusions.

The PROACT methodology rule set differentiates between physical root causes, **human root causes**, and **latent** or systematic root causes. **Physical root causes** are the observable consequences of decision errors. When someone makes a poor decision it results in something physical or observable. For instance, in the surgical fire example, the central sterile manager allowed a flammable agent to be used in the cleaning of bronchoscopes. This decision caused a fuel source to be introduced which led to a fire. Human root causes are decision errors. They are errors of omission or commission by a human. In this scenario the manager's decision would be a human root cause (see Figure 9.8).

Latent root causes are the reasons why people believed they were making the appropriate decision at the time the decision was made. Latent root causes are synonymous with organizational and systemic root causes. Decisions are usually made with good intent and an expectation of a good outcome. However, the information considered when making a decision can be flawed. It may be inaccurate, untimely, or inadequate. The flawed information systems that contribute to poor decisions need to be identified and corrected.

Once the root causes are identified, the RCA team can look back at the entire logic tree and see the direct correlation from the systems (latent roots) which influenced the decisions (human roots) which triggered a series of consequences (physical roots) until a patient experienced harm. The completed logic tree in Figure 9.9 illustrates the investigative and deductive analysis thought process of the RCA team. It is presented for illustration purposes only and does not include all findings (see Figure 9.9).

An often debated question is how deep should the RCA team drill down? There are no universally accepted standards. The bigger concern is stopping the investigation too soon, not being too thorough. Only the RCA team can decide where to stop the investigation; ideally at the deepest, significant underlying causes where the most value will be gained from improvement actions.

The PROACT logic tree should not be confused with predetermined decision or causal factor trees that provide a series of pick list options for analysts to choose from. These one-size-fits-all models pose the same analytic questions for every incident and convey a false impression that the correct answer must be contained in the pick list. The drawbacks of an automated categorical approach are the same as paper-based prompt lists. To paraphrase Eliyahu Goldratt, author of *The Goal*, an RCA expert is not someone that gives you the answers to your problems, but rather someone that asks you the right questions and forces you to realize that you know the answers yourself.

FIGURE 9.8   Physical, Human, and Latent Root Causes

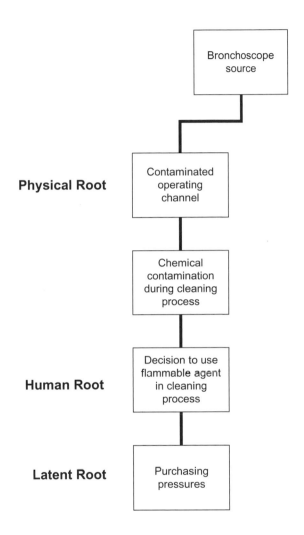

Why Use Deductive Analysis?

Adding deductive analysis to the RCA process expands the breadth and depth of the investigation. When this occurs, the underlying system problems are more likely to be identified so that appropriate corrective action can be taken. If the RCA team investigating the surgical fire had only used the 5 Whys analysis

FIGURE 9.9   Completed Logic Tree for Surgical Fire Event

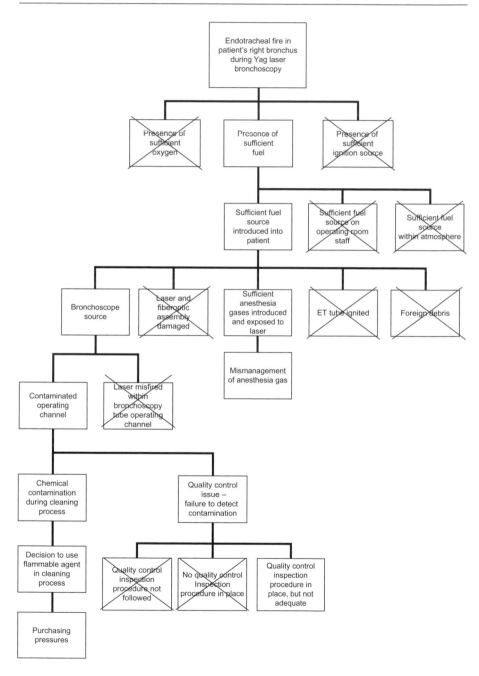

FIGURE 9.10   Surgical Fire Analysis Results Using the 5-Whys Method

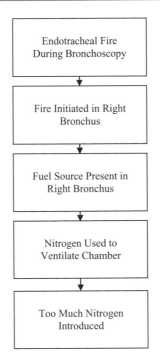

approach the scope of the evaluation would have been narrow. The diagram in Figure 9.10 illustrates the linear and limited thinking of why-why questioning. The root causes of the surgical fire event would not have been identified by using the 5 Whys method.

Ishikawa (1982) advocated the cause-and-effect diagram as a tool for breaking down potential causes into more detailed categories so they can be organized and related into factors that help identify the root cause. However, cause-and-effect diagrams were not purposely designed for use in accident investigations. In a study comparing Ishikawa diagrams and current reality trees, a deductive analysis tool, groups using cause-and-effect diagrams were less likely to identify a specific and reasonable root cause. Groups using the deductive analysis tool were more successful at identifying root causes and systemic problems (Doggett, 2005).

Prompt lists of questions sorted into broad categories, such as The Joint Commission RCA model, can be equally limiting. Identification of causal factors and root causes of an event should be unbiased and dictated by the cause-and-effect chains of what actually happened. By using a deductive analysis approach the facts of the case guide the team's decisions, not predefined cause categories and questions.

Conclusion

The health care workforce wants good patient outcomes. When things do not go as planned, the causes must be uncovered and eliminated. To achieve this goal, investigation and analysis of adverse events must be thorough. Significant events almost never result from one single cause. Most adverse events involve multiple, interrelated frontline factors as well as system issues. The analysis methods used in an RCA should encourage an unbiased and in-depth evaluation of this complexity.

A commonly used RCA analysis tool, 5 Whys, leads investigators to conclude that only one root cause exists. And because hard evidence is not normally required to validate this string of logic, that one cause could likely be wrong. Even if the one root cause is correct, almost certainly the RCA team will have missed many other contributing factors.

The Ishikawa diagram, though more exploratory than the 5 Whys technique, is a brainstorming tool that relies primarily on the team's intuition rather than hard evidence to support the facts. Because the Ishikawa diagram is categorical, it is not strictly based on cause and effect. If a relevant category is not included on the diagram, the RCA team may overlook some physical, human or latent root causes.

Prompt lists are often used to guide questioning when regulators expect accident investigators to ask certain questions. Such lists, whether embedded in a paper-based RCA framework or in deductive analysis software, can cause RCA teams to look in a particular direction instead of following the facts wherever they may lead (as in true cause-and-effect thinking). Categorical tools such as prompt lists can sometimes cut inquiries short—people keep investigating until a familiar cause is found to which the cure is known (Rasmussen, 2003).

Deductive analysis is an RCA technique that investigates from the general to the specific to determine *how* a system failed and *why* wrong decisions were made. The analysis essentially "rewinds the video" of what happened, starting with the event and reeling backwards from that point on (just like a detective's investigation). When RCA team members reason about cause and effect in an effective manner, significant benefits can be realized.

Sequencing methods, like the PROACT logic tree and other deductive analysis software, are very helpful for investigating adverse health care events.

Tools to support hypothesis formation are of particular help with investigations that are complex in their detail. Such methods also support the tasks of reviewing and managing complex investigations by providing a measure of transparency. Not only can the whole analysis be seen at a glance, the RCA team can quickly and easily add, amend and rearrange data. Paper-based deductive analysis tools are less accessible, making it more difficult to share the knowledge gained from the RCA.

Understandably, health care organizations must weigh various factors when selecting RCA investigation methodologies. However, the most important consideration should be patient safety. For several years health care organizations have primarily used simple 5 Whys thinking and categorical investigation approaches, yet patients are still experiencing adverse outcomes. It is time for greater use of deductive analysis techniques to uncover and fix latent root causes. By correcting system issues that result in undesirable decisions and behaviors health care organizations will better protect patients from unintended harm.

Discussion Questions

1. Explain the difference between an investigation and an analysis.

2. Describe the advantages and drawbacks of categorical and deductive analysis RCA approaches.

3. Discuss the benefits of collecting evidence and data during an RCA.

Key Terms

5 Whys

Confidence factor

Human root cause

Ishikawa diagram

Latent root cause

Mode

Physical root cause

References

Anonymous. (1996). Policy for evaluating occurrence of "sentinel events" established. *Joint Commission Perspectives, 16*(1), 6.

Centers for Disease Control. (2008). *Workbook for designing, implementing and evaluating a sharps injury prevention program.* Retrieved from http://www.cdc.gov/sharpssafety.

Croteau, R. J. (Ed.). (2010). *Root cause analysis in health care: Tools and techniques* (4th ed.). Oakbrook Terrace, IL: Joint Commission Resources.

DeRosier, J. M., Taylor, L., Turner, L., & Bagian, J. P. (2007). Root cause analysis of wandering adverse events in the Veterans Health Administration. In A. Nelson & D. L. Algase (Eds.), *Evidence-based protocols for managing wandering behaviors* (pp. 161–180). New York: Springer.

Doggett, A. M. (2005). Root cause analysis: A framework for tool selection. *Quality Management Journal, 12*(4), 34–45.

Ishikawa, K. (1982). *Guide to quality control* (2nd rev. ed.). Tokyo: Asian Productivity Organization.

Office of Nuclear Regulatory Research. (1981). *Fault tree handbook.* Washington, DC: U.S. Nuclear Regulatory Commission.

Okes, D. (2009). *Root cause analysis: The core of problem solving and corrective action.* Milwaukee, WI: ASQ Quality Press.

Rasmussen, J. (2003). The role of error in organizing behaviour. *Quality and Safety in Health Care, 12*(5), 377–383.

The Joint Commission. (n.d.). Framework for conducting a root cause analysis and action plan. Retrieved January 10, 2010 from http://www.jointcommission.org/NR/rdonlyres/C8CE68F6–85D7–4EA4-B3E0–895FC1075EE6/0/rcawordframework.doc.

Vincent, C. (2006). *Patient safety.* New York: Churchill Livingstone.

Wikipedia. (2009, December 17). Root cause analysis. Retrieved January 9, 2010 from http://en.wikipedia.org/wiki/Root_cause_analysis.

Wu, A. W., Lipshutz, A. K. M., & Pronovost, P. J. (2008). Effectiveness and efficiency of root cause analysis in medicine. *Journal of the American Medical Association, 299*(6), 685–687.

PART 4

HOW TO MAKE
HEALTH CARE
PROCESSES SAFER

CHAPTER 10

PROACTIVELY ERROR-PROOFING HEALTH CARE PROCESSES

Richard J. Croteau
Paul M. Schyve

LEARNING OBJECTIVES

- Understand how and why processes fail
- Describe characteristics of high-risk processes that increase the risk of failure
- Identify common prospective analysis methods to evaluate process risks
- Describe actions to reduce errors and mitigate the effects

In health care, the occurrence of a sentinel event is compelling. A response is demanded, driven in some cases by guilt, shame, or fear of retribution; in other instances by a need to understand and correct the problem. That response can be limited to placement of blame and removal of the offending party. Or through the process of a root cause analysis, people can achieve an understanding of the factors that enabled the event to occur. Such an analysis may lead to process redesign to reduce the risk of that type of event in the future. However, even a root cause analysis, with all its potential for reducing risk, can itself be limited by the "blinder" effect of the specific event. The best root cause analyses look not only at the factors surrounding the specific event, but also at the entire process that was involved and its support systems. The goal of a good root cause analysis should be to minimize overall risk associated with that process, not just recurrence of the event that prompted the investigation. The event itself serves only as a flag: "Risky process here!" It signals an opportunity to reduce overall risk and provides the motivation to do so. Having served that purpose, the event, although potentially useful as a reference point, is no longer necessary to the analysis and redesign of the overall process.

So why wait for a sentinel event before improving processes? Surely we can identify processes that are high risk through our own and others' experience. The purpose of this chapter is to explore the possibilities for proactively assessing and minimizing risk. These activities are perhaps less compelling than responding to an actual event unless one sees this activity in the context not of a single event, but of the overall, unacceptably high frequency of sentinel events in all of health care. Add to that the far higher frequency of less serious adverse events and of "near misses" and "close calls" that cause patient discomfort and emotional distress and introduce inefficiency and added cost to the health care delivery system.

Anatomy and Physiology of a Process

Aspiring clinicians are taught extensively about the human body: what can go wrong with it and what can be done to protect it. They learn these lessons in order to prevent things from going wrong and to treat the body when things do go wrong. But these curricula have included little or nothing about what can go wrong with the process of providing that care. Clinicians study the recipients of health care but not the anatomy, normal physiology, pathology, prevention, and treatment of what they personally do as health care professionals.

Let's try to understand what health care professionals do by using a model that clinicians are already familiar with: structure (anatomy), function (physiology), dysfunction (pathology), treatment (health promotion, disease prevention, active treatment, palliation, and rehabilitation), and maintenance (follow-up care) as these concepts apply to health care processes. The analogy may suffer somewhat because of the way we relate to the participants. In studying disease, the immediate participant is the patient. And we have, for the most part, tended not to blame the patient for his or her disease. Health care processes, on the other hand, involve a number of participants whom we still have a tendency to blame when the process breaks down. Perhaps it would be instructive for the moment to suspend the concept of blame in our thoughts about the function or dysfunction of health care processes.

The dictionary definition of a process, "a systematic series of actions directed to some end" (Random House, 1993), provides some insight into the structure, function, and potential risk points of a process that can be useful in formulating an approach to **proactive risk reduction**. *Systematic* implies regularity or consistency; *series* tells us that there is some order, that the parts are related in some way. *Actions* are things to be done, forcing the question, By whom or what? (This is where we sometimes wander down the path to blame and retribution.) *Directed* suggests intent, design, or plan to achieve some end (the desired outcome). The anatomy then is the totality of the parts of the process—the actions or steps—their sequence and connections. As with the human body or a machine, a part can fail (a bone can break, a tire can blow out) but the effect of the failure is most often determined by how the parts interact, how the function of the process (or body, or machine) is affected. The physiology of a process is how it functions; how the parts work together to produce the desired effect. Each step in the process requires an input—delivered on time, complete, and in usable form—and yields an output—a product of that step in the process. This output is often the input for another step in the process.

How Processes Fail

Given the structure and function of a process, what kind of pathology might we expect to see? Consider a relay race with four runners, each making one lap around the track, each in top physical condition, each a well-trained, experienced runner. What can go wrong? A trip. A cramp. Did I mention the baton? Oh yes, in a relay race, continuity is important. The baton represents the deliverable to be handed off from one runner to the other. The winning team is not necessarily the one with the fastest individual times; it is often the one with the most efficient and reliable **hand-offs**. It is the interaction between the racers that most often determines the outcome. And an error in transferring the baton is much more likely than a runner tripping or getting a leg cramp!

So what does this mean for our process? Certainly the anatomy can be flawed; that is, a step in the process is poorly designed. If the process is designed from the outset to do something different from the desired result (that is, a primary design flaw that could be considered a congenital defect in the process), the results will be more or less consistently undesirable. But far more often, the failure of a process to achieve its designed objective has to do with the design of the linkages between steps in the process: how the steps relate to one another—the hand-offs. It is the interrelationships that are themselves prone to failure and that propagate the effects of a failure to other parts of the process, often in ways that are unexpected (side effects) or not immediately evident (long-term effects).

There are, of course, factors outside the process itself that can influence the outcome. And though these may not be subject to our direct control, they can nonetheless be identified and their influences on our process understood and protected against. Such an external factor may be a special cause of variation in the process under review and therefore generally cannot be controlled through redesign of the process itself (Gitlow, Gitlow, Oppenheim, & Oppenheim, 1989). However, such a special cause may, and often should, lead us to assess and redesign factors external to the process that are under our control or to redesign our process to protect it against those factors that are not under our control.

Whether any cause is common or special depends on the frame of reference. That is, the concepts of "common" and "special" are not attributes of a cause but rather express the relationship of a specific cause to a specific process. For example, a patient's death may result from the loss of electrical power during a surgical procedure. Although this undesirable variation in outcome is the result of a special cause in the operating room, the special cause is, in turn, the result of a common cause in the organization's system for preparing for a utility failure. In fact, often a special cause of variation in one process will be found to be the result of a common cause of variation in the larger system (that is, larger set of processes) of which the immediate process is a part.

This analysis leads to the conclusion that the identification of a special cause for a sentinel event is only the first step in a full evaluation of the event. The second step is to identify the larger system whose common cause variation is the source of the special cause. This larger system then becomes the focus for improvement, because only it can be redesigned to eliminate the common cause of the adverse event. The component process cannot correct a special cause in itself.

Continuation of this analytical process, as depicted in Figure 10.1, will eventually lead to factors that are outside the control of the organization itself. The external environmental factors—whether physical, social, economic, political, or other—may correctly be identified as the ultimate root causes. However, these factors are largely beyond the control of the individual organization. The organization's corrective actions should focus on its own internal systems because only they can be redesigned to reduce risk; in this case by acknowledging the realities of uncontrollable external environmental factors, anticipating their impact on the organization, and redesigning to protect against the effects of those external factors.

What does this mean for health care organizations? All clinical processes in the organization are part of larger systems in the organization. Thus, special cause sentinel events that occur in the care of patients are frequently the result of common causes in organizational systems. For example, when individual physicians are admonished to avoid prescribing medications that lead to adverse drug-drug interactions, they may try very hard to do so. But the large number

FIGURE 10.1   Levels of Analysis

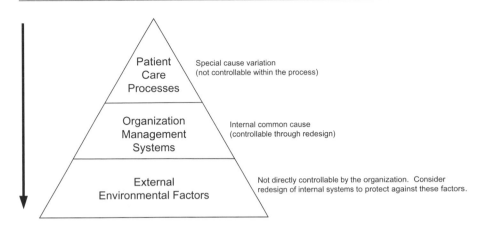

of possible drug-drug interactions and the constantly growing knowledge base in this area make it impossible for physicians to remember all of the possible interactions. Errors in memory will occur.

The individual physician prescribing process is likely to be improved only when it is seen as part of the larger medication use system that involves the pharmacy, nursing, and information management. One solution some organizations are using is a computer-based order entry system linked to a real-time expert system that provides feedback to the physician about potential adverse drug-drug interactions, enabling better-informed clinical judgment (Bates et al., 1998). The solution to the problem has been found by addressing the common cause in the design of an organization's information management system, not by focusing on the special cause of error in the clinical process; that is, the physician's faulty (human) memory.

For the health care organization, identification of a special cause for a clinical sentinel event should automatically lead to a search for the common cause(s) in the system(s) of which the process is a part. It is the larger system, not the process, that must be redesigned to reduce the likelihood of future sentinel events. Errors by individual physicians, nurses, and pharmacists should generate evaluations of the organizational systems in which they work and which support their work. These systems include the following:

- The credentialing and privileging processes for physicians and other licensed independent practitioners and the hiring and competency review processes for others

- The continuing education of staff

- The management of information, including facilitation of communication, accessibility of knowledge-based information, and linkage of information sources

- The design and maintenance of the environment in which clinical activities occur

- The measurement of system performance with respect to both processes and outcomes

It is the responsibility of the organization's management and clinical leaders to focus attention on systems that can be redesigned for improvement, rather than on processes and people who cannot control causes outside of themselves.

Why Processes Fail

The characteristics of a high-risk process that tend to increase the risk of a process failure include the following:

- Variable input

- Complexity

- Inconsistency

- Tight coupling

- Human intervention

- Tight time constraints

- Hierarchical culture

Variable Input

The nature of the input to the process can greatly influence the reliability of the process, ultimately affecting the output (results) of that process. Specifically, a process that receives a variable input is more prone to dysfunction because the process itself must be modified to accommodate the input variation. In health care processes, the patient—who is the principal input—is highly variable.

Table 10.1 Probability of Success in a Process

Number of Steps	Probability of Success of Each Step			
	0.95	0.99	0.999	0.9999
1	0.95	0.99	0.999	0.9999
25	0.28	0.78	0.98	0.998
50	0.06	0.61	0.95	0.995
100	0.006	0.37	0.9	0.99

Complexity

Complex processes are more prone to failure than simple ones. This seems obvious, yet we in health care have tended to design very complex processes, often of necessity given the nature of the work, but sometimes, it would seem, deriving satisfaction from the complexity itself and comforted by the assumption that nothing will go wrong. The more steps in a process and the greater their interdependence, the greater the complexity of the process. The more complex the process, the greater the chance of unanticipated and undesirable side effects and unrecognized long-term effects. Table 10.1 illustrates the problem (Berwick, 1998). For example, if the rate of error in each step is 1% (the "0.99" column in the table), then if there is only one step in the process, the likelihood of an error occurring in the process is 1%; if there are 25 steps, the likelihood of an error in the process is 22%; for 50 steps the likelihood of an error is 39%; and for 100 steps it is 63%! And now, consider that the risk of unintended consequences is increased not only by complexity of the process itself but also by complexity of the context—the related processes and supporting systems—in which it operates. How resilient is the process to variation in its inputs or to changing needs for the outputs of the process or to modification of organizational support systems? Will these contextual changes even be identified before a failure occurs? These failure modes involving context can be just as significant and are just as worthy of proactive assessment as internal process failures.

Inconsistency

The tendency for a process to fail is also diminished in relation to the consistency with which it is carried out; that is, the degree to which it is standardized. Efforts in recent years to standardize health care processes through the introduction of practice parameters, protocols, **clinical pathways**, and so forth have been met with limited enthusiasm among practitioners and are only slowly affecting the actual delivery of care. Achieving process consistency while retaining the ability to recognize and accommodate variation in the input (for example, the patient's severity of illness, comorbidities, other treatments, and preferences) is one of the major challenges to standardization in health care. Process variation to meet individual patient needs and preferences is an essential principle of modern medicine; variation to meet individual practitioner preferences need not be. When individuals perform in isolation, standardization of process is the usual and natural consequence of the human tendency to routine—we are, indeed, creatures of habit. But most health care is not provided by one individual in isolation. Rather, it is provided by a treatment team. When a team is involved—with the necessary transitions in care and coordination—standardization will be advantageous because it will achieve better overall results more safely. Assuming each is a *good* practice, it doesn't matter which of multiple processes is selected as the basis for standardization; it is the standardization that can enable greater safety in team functioning.

Tight Coupling

Given that a process is a series of actions, and recognizing that process failure very often occurs at the interface between the steps (actions) in a process, the characteristics of the relationships between actions become important. The relationship between the steps in a process is called coupling and is commonly described in terms of the tightness or looseness of the coupling (Perrow, 1984). A **tightly coupled process** is one in which the steps follow one another so closely that a variation in the output of one step cannot be recognized and responded to before the next step is under way. Thus the next step is dealing with an input (the output of the preceding, closely coupled step) that it may not have been designed to handle, and therefore may itself fail. This helps to explain the phenomenon of "cascade of failure" that often amazes the casual observer following a sentinel event. How could so many things have gone wrong at once? The answer, of course, is that the process was not designed to stop the chain of events once the initial failure occurred.

Human Intervention

Any process that depends heavily on the intellectual and physical intervention of humans will be more prone to failure than a process that does not have such dependency, such as automated activities. This is the case as long as things are going smoothly. Automated processes function better than human processes in a routine mode but often don't do as well when things start to go wrong (Reason,

1997). Human judgment is still superior to a machine in dealing with an unanticipated contingency and adjusting the process to avoid harm. This distinction becomes important in defining the ideal roles of humans and technology, respectively, in complex processes. The strengths and weaknesses of each are, happily, complementary. The heavy dependence on human intervention in health care processes has recently led to reconsideration of the meaning of "reliability" in this context. The traditional definition of reliability is no variation. Weick and Sutcliffe point out that a more practical definition for health care, as well as other high-risk activities that are heavily dependent on human intervention, would be the ability to handle unforeseen situations in ways that forestall unintended consequences (Weick & Sutcliffe, 2007). This requires a level of cognition and adaptation for which humans (so far) are superior to machines. It is often the person who "creates" safety for the individual patient in the health care process (Cook, 1998).

Tight Time Constraints

Time truly is of the essence in so much of what we do, and especially so when dealing with acute illness or injury. Tightening the time constraints for human participation in a process tightens the coupling between steps, thus allowing less opportunity to identify, analyze, and respond appropriately (safely) to variation and thereby increasing the likelihood of failure. Health care processes often seem to have a certain inertia. Once in motion, they tend to keep moving, adding to the time pressure, further limiting opportunity to analyze a variation and plan an ideal response. Very loose time constraints can also increase the likelihood of failure, probably because of the human propensity for boredom or distraction.

Hierarchical Culture

The airline industry's **crew resource management** studies demonstrated clearly that the relationships among participants in a complex process, specifically the manner and degree to which they communicate with one another, can affect the overall reliability of the process (Helmreich, Wilhelm, Gregorich, & Chidester, 1990). Generally, a group of individuals interacting as a team, without constraints on communication based on rank or role, will function more reliably, both in stable and unstable situations, than a group that is constrained by hierarchical conventions such as, "The captain is always right; don't question the captain." The MedTeams project described in Chapter Fourteen of this book illustrates how the lessons learned in the airline industry are now being applied to health care teams.

Medical Management of the Health Care Process

If the analogy used above is valid, then the approach to "healthier" (that is, safer) health care processes should follow the model for medical management: diagnosis, treatment, and follow-up (essentially the measure-assess-improve cycle). Proactive medical management of health care processes, as for health promotion and disease prevention, holds the promise of greater benefit for the resources consumed compared with simply reacting when something bad happens.

Diagnosis

A proactive approach to reducing risk means starting with a prospective risk assessment or diagnostic evaluation. Prospective risk assessment recognizes that things can and do go wrong and looks for those possibilities before they manifest themselves. What are the processes that pose the greatest risk to patients? How do those processes fail? What is it that most often goes wrong? Why? What other things might go wrong in the process? What are the **failure effects**? And, ultimately, how could the patient be affected? These are the types of questions that are asked in Failure Mode and Effect Analysis (FMEA), an analytical method used for decades in engineering to identify and reduce hazards (Juran & Godfrey, 1999). This technique examines a system's individual components and their interrelationships to determine the variety of ways each component and linkage between components could fail and the effect of a particular failure on the stability of the entire system.

An important aspect of this prospective analysis is the determination of why certain failures might occur; that is, identifying the root causes of potential failure modes. The failure modes are not viewed as causes in themselves but as symptoms. In the case of an actual sentinel event, one of these failure modes might be the proximate or immediate cause identified at the start of the root cause analysis, perhaps a human error or equipment failure. Later in the analysis, we identify the underlying systemic factor(s) that enabled the proximate cause to occur. Using FMEA, people can identify weaknesses in a system design and predict what might happen as a result of those weaknesses. FMEA is especially useful in analyzing a new design or redesign, such as that which might be proposed following root cause analysis of a sentinel event. Another important application of this powerful analytical tool is in judging the effect of an uncontrollable external failure. For example, what would be the impact on the organization's internal systems and, ultimately, its health care processes and outcomes if a natural disaster—a tornado or earthquake, say—knocked out power and contaminated the water supply while flooding the emergency department with injured victims?

Realistically, FMEA cannot identify all possible failure modes or all of the effects of a failure (direct, indirect, or long-term), and it has limited efficacy in dealing with multiple-failure modes. In complex systems such as are prevalent in health care, nothing can be truly error-proof. There will always be unexpected, unintended consequences that will not be linear (for example, small changes at one point in the system can result in big changes elsewhere in the system). No prospective risk assessment method, including FMEA, can guarantee uniformly good outcomes, but they can help to reduce the risk of bad outcomes when systematically applied.

Another related prospective analytical approach is called Fault Tree Analysis (FTA) (Juran, 1999). Whereas FMEA starts with the identification of possible failures in the steps of a process or in the interactions between steps and then looks downstream for the effects and upstream for the causes, FTA starts with the identification of a potential effect—a hypothetical sentinel event, if you will— and works backward. A root cause analysis approach is used to pick the most likely process failures that could produce that effect. The analyst then works further back to identify the underlying systemic factors that could be modified to reduce the likelihood of that outcome.

A useful technique for testing a new process design is "worst-case" analysis. This involves a trial of the new process (on paper or using computer simulation) assuming the maximum likely variation in those factors that are generally uncontrollable, such as the input to the process and the external environment in which the organization functions. For example, a hospital is designing a new emergency angiography unit. The facility, staffing, and procedural specifications are established. Then the worst-case scenario is hypothesized: What would happen if a 400-pound patient with active tuberculosis presented with a cold leg at 2 AM on a Sunday morning? Clearly an unlikely scenario, but such a hypothetical "stress testing" of the new process can unmask weaknesses that might otherwise go unnoticed until an equally unlikely situation actually occurred.

Determining the Treatment

When designing systems, engineers start with the premise that anything can go wrong, and they write volumes on analysis and prevention of potential failures. Health care professionals, on the other hand, tend to work from the premise that if they are competent and committed in doing their jobs, nothing will go wrong (and if something does go wrong, it probably could not have been prevented). Given this attitude, health care professionals tend to write about failure only in retrospect. We do root cause analyses of what went wrong rather than prospective analysis of what might go wrong. Most of the psychological barriers to effective risk reduction disappear when the analysis anticipates rather than follows the failure. Although the movement toward root cause analysis in response to sentinel events is necessary and will result in significant contributions to our understanding of medical errors, even greater advances will result from a cultural reorientation that acknowledges fallibility of systems, processes, and people. By encouraging prospective analysis of potential failures and supporting system redesign to minimize adverse outcomes, significant patient safety improvements can be realized.

An error—a failure in one or more steps of a process or in the transitions between steps—can lead to an undesirable outcome. Therefore, actions to reduce the likelihood of errors should be pursued whenever possible. The problem, of course, is that despite our best efforts, things will still go wrong. The next challenge, then, is to further design our processes to accommodate this reality by building in safeguards to protect against a bad outcome even if an error occurs. Such treatment or protective design takes two forms: (1) preventing the error from reaching the patient, and (2) mitigating the effects of an error that reaches the patient.

Preventing the Error from Reaching the Patient

If an error occurs in step 3 of a five-step process, and in step 4 someone recognizes the resulting variation in its expected input and (a) sounds an alarm and (b) interrupts the process, the error can then be corrected without an adverse result for the process as a whole (other than, perhaps, a minor delay while the error is being corrected). For example, a computerized medication order entry system may identify an unusual dose (perhaps the result of a misplaced decimal point), provide immediate online feedback to the ordering practitioner, and accept a corrected order, all before the patient receives the first dose. This represents a design that includes a means for recognizing an antecedent error, communicating the fact of the error, and modifying (temporarily halting) the process to deal with the error while protecting against an adverse outcome.

It is usually safer not to act (at least for a while) than to act incorrectly. Therefore, a process that is designed to detect failure and to interrupt the process flow is preferable to a process that continues on in spite of the failure. In a more general sense, we should favor a process that can, by design, respond automatically to a failure by reverting to a predetermined (usually safe) default mode. Very often it is simply enough to "pause" the process to allow for human intervention to assess and deal with the contingency. Modern software design with its warnings and required confirmations for high-risk actions such as "Delete all files? Y/N" is an example of a process interruption intended to minimize hasty actions that we may later regret. Likewise, a "time-out" in the operating room before initiating surgery to confirm the patient's identity, the type of procedure to be performed, and the site of the procedure can interrupt the process before a wrong-patient, wrong-procedure, or wrong-site surgery occurs.

In systems design, the term **redundancy** refers to a backup mode or a secondary means of accomplishing what the primary system was supposed to do. Requiring two nurses to independently check the label on a unit of blood against the patient's identification band is a type of system redundancy. To be maximally effective, the redundant systems should be independent of one another and not subject to the same external influences. If the systems are not independent of each other, the backup may be disabled by the failure of the primary system. If the primary and secondary systems are subject to the same external influences, the cause of a primary system failure would in all likelihood cause the backup (redundant) system to fail also. In this transfusion example, if both nurses check the blood container label against the same source document identifying the patient's blood type, and that document is in error, then both nurses will make the same mistake (for the same reason). To make matters worse, human redundancy, as in the transfusion example, is further complicated by the all too common assumption that the other person won't make a mistake (that is, the "nothing will go wrong" presumption) that results in a cursory and potentially inaccurate redundant check.

Even when systems are well designed, redundancy will always increase the complexity and, therefore, will itself add to the risk of a failure. The failure of a redundant system will usually not be evident until the backup process is needed. Thus, redundant systems should be subjected to regular testing and maintenance. An obvious example is the necessary periodic testing of the emergency power supply for a hospital, a redundant system that one hopes will not fail when it is needed.

Mitigating the Effects of an Error
The second form of protective design involves mitigating the effects of an error on the patient. For example, if a medication error has not been identified before the patient receives an incorrect dose, a well-designed system would ensure that the patient was monitored closely for the effects of the medication, any adverse effects would be quickly identified, and antidotes and other supportive medications and equipment would be readily available to mitigate the effects of the error.

Simplification

We have often been admonished to K.I.S.S.—keep it simple, stupid. A simple process is one that fully addresses the need without any extraneous parts or motion. But we must be careful not to confuse simplification with taking shortcuts. When people take shortcuts, even breaking safety rules at times, there are often no immediate consequences. Without consequences the perpetrators are relieved of the burden imposed by the rules and their behavior is thereby reinforced. This kind of process simplification is obviously undesirable but may not be evident until revealed by a sentinel event unless the organization conducts some type of prospective risk assessment. A recent study of shortcuts in the use of bar-coded medication administration systems offers a good example of the frequency, causes—especially, faulty integration into workflow processes—and risks of shortcuts (Koppel, Wetterneck, Telles, & Karsh, 2008).

Technology

Finally, in selecting a treatment for a process found to be at risk of a failure, the role of technology must be carefully considered. Technology is a tool—actually an extensive, very powerful set of tools, but tools nonetheless. These tools should be seen as complementary to human intervention, not competitive. Computers and other technology lack the ability to make allowances for incomplete or incorrect information, an important requirement for dealing with complex situations (Reason, 1997). Human judgment is still superior to a machine when dealing with an unanticipated contingency and adjusting the process to avoid harm. Technology is more effective than humans in enhancing process consistency and in receiving, storing, and processing information. Technology does not take shortcuts. It is not influenced by emotion. And it has the advantage of being a long-term improvement, in contrast to **risk-reduction strategies** that, say, focus on staff retraining. More information on the topic of technology and patient safety is found in Chapter Thirteen.

Implementing the Treatment

Once you've chosen the system redesign that is intended to reduce the chances that an error will occur or reach the patient if it does occur, or mitigate the effect of an error if it does reach the patient, then it is time to consider how to best implement the change. In doing so, it is important to understand that the effect of a well-thought-out risk-reduction strategy may not always be what was intended. A "paper" analysis of the new design may be instructive and a lot less expensive than a premature implementation of a well-intended but faulty design. An example of a perfectly good "bad" idea was revealed during the planning for the Apollo moon landing. In an early model of the lunar module, the design team recommended an innovative approach to vehicle stability on an unpredictably uneven landing surface. Risk assessment had identified the possibility of failure of one of the four landing legs to fully extend prior to the controlled descent to the lunar surface. That was the failure mode. The effects analysis confirmed that such a (single-leg) failure would result in a "neutral stability" situation if the landing occurred on a perfectly smooth horizontal surface. "Neutral stability" means that although the vehicle might land in an upright position, even a slight irregularity of the surface, minor shift of weight distribution within the vehicle, or any number of other variables could cause the vehicle to fall over. This would be a mission-critical failure: there would be no way to launch the ascent stage of the vehicle back into lunar orbit if this presumed failure actually happened.

The solution: a fifth leg. With five legs evenly positioned around the periphery of the descent stage, a single-leg failure would result in a stable situation—the center of gravity would remain within the outline of the remaining four legs. Ingenious. But wait. More legs means more legs could fail. What if two legs failed? As long as they were not adjacent to one another, the vehicle would still be in a stable situation, and the odds of two adjacent legs failing was felt to be vanishingly small. What a great idea!

But now let's look at the implications of this redesign. A fifth leg is quite problematic for engineers trying to design a vehicle whose propulsion systems require a high degree of symmetry in the payload they are moving. This is clearly a more complex design and therefore more prone to failure. It has other implications of great importance to a space vehicle. Legs are heavy. A 20% increase in the weight of the landing gear will require additional thrust capability from the descent stage engine. This means the engine may have to be heavier, and the liquid propellant supply will certainly have to be increased. This increased payload for the lunar module would add 10 times that weight to the Saturn launch vehicle in additional propellant requirements.

The lesson: things aren't always as good as they seem. It is particularly difficult to reject a clever solution to a vexing problem, especially when it is your own idea. But history is cluttered with good ideas gone bad. Thorough analysis and testing of any new or redesigned process or system will enhance its risk-reduction potential and decrease the likelihood of unintended consequences. The recommended approach is to first assess the potential effectiveness of a risk-reduction strategy on paper through application of failure mode and effects analysis, fault tree analysis, and other analytical techniques, with particular attention to potential side effects and long-term effects of the proposed process changes. Whenever possible, simulation testing should be considered. Simulation allows us to experience the implications of a redesign, albeit in a less complex environment without real risk to patients. It can reveal potential unanticipated side effects of variation in the process and, in the case of computer simulation, has the further advantage of allowing things to play out in compressed time to reveal long-term effects.

At some point the new or redesigned process will be implemented. Consider pilot testing as a prudent alternative to full-scale implementation. It can reveal much about the real-life effectiveness of the new process.

Follow-Up

Be sure to guard against the assumption that the absence of immediately obvious negative side effects means that the correct measures have been taken. Remember, the reason for making changes in the first place was to reduce the likelihood of an infrequent adverse outcome. To objectively conclude that the redesign is effective requires more than simply observing the absence of sentinel events. For this reason, the measures of effectiveness should focus more on process than on outcomes. Objective measurement of the consistency, completeness, timeliness, and intermediate outputs of selected steps in the new process will provide greater assurances about the effectiveness of the changes and the suitability for full-scale implementation.

Finally, once the new or redesigned process is fully implemented, attention must be paid to maintaining the process and protecting it against the ravages of time and the inevitable changes in the community of processes and supporting systems of which it is a part. This will require documenting the new process, training staff in the new process and its redesigned system support, providing ongoing (preferably online) access to information about these new processes and systems, and continued monitoring of the new process. Examples of effectiveness measures for various processes are found in Chapter Four of this book.

Let us focus for a moment on documenting the new process. We all dislike documentation when there seems to be no immediate payback—documentation for documentation's sake. The risk is that failure to fully document a new or redesigned process can have its own unanticipated and unintended consequences. Remember the nightmare (and costs) of attempting to hunt down every Y2K bug in our older, undocumented software programs. Failure to have documented these programs 20 years previously could have resulted, at the very least, in a variety of inconveniences, perhaps much worse. Process documentation is itself a proactive risk-reduction strategy not only for the short term (for example, to educate staff in the new process) but also for the long term in order to enable future root cause analyses of potential or actual sentinel events.

Finally, where humans play a role in the process there will be a tendency to revert back to old ways. Appropriate technological support and, ideally, the involvement of leadership to induce a change in organization culture supportive of the new approach to safety will provide the greatest assurance of long-term success (Reason & Hobbs, 2003).

Exhibit 10.1 provides a checklist for organizing proactive risk-reduction activities. Recognizing that certain health care processes pose higher risks to patients than others, both in frequency and severity of adverse outcomes, it seems reasonable to focus these activities where the risks are greatest. Several suggestions for identifying such high-risk processes are offered in the figure, including a decision to implement a new service or modify an existing one. Integrating the risk-reduction activities described in this chapter into the design and redesign of health care processes will, over time, reduce the incidence of sentinel events in health care as it has in so many other fields. This checklist is provided as a tool to facilitate this integration.

EXHIBIT 10.1

CHECKLIST FOR PROACTIVE RISK-REDUCTION ACTIVITIES

❑ Identify a high-risk process.

  ❑ History of adverse outcomes

  ❑ Identified in the literature as high risk

  ❑ Has several characteristics of a high-risk process (see bulleted list under "Why Processes Fail" in this chapter)

  ❑ New process

  ❑ Proposed redesign (such as in response to a sentinel event)

❑ Create a flowchart of the process as designed.

❑ Assess the actual implementation of the process (different locations, shifts, and so on).

❑ Identify where there is, or may be, variation in the implementation of the process; that is, what are the failure modes?

❑ For each identified failure mode, what are the possible effects?

❑ Assess the seriousness (that is, the "criticality") of the possible effects (for example, delay in treatment, temporary loss of function, patient death).

❑ For the most critical effects, conduct a root cause analysis to determine why the variation (the failure mode) leading to that effect occurs.

❑ Redesign the process or underlying systems, or both, to minimize the risk of that failure mode or to protect the patient from the effects of that failure mode.

❑ Conduct a failure mode and effect analysis on the redesigned process with special attention on how the redesigned steps will affect other steps in the process and whether they will continue to do the beneficial things that the previous design could do.

❑ Consider simulation testing of the redesigned process.

❑ Consider a pilot test of the redesigned process.

❑ Identify and implement measures of the effectiveness of the redesigned process.

❑ Implement a strategy for maintaining the effectiveness of the redesigned process over time.

Conclusion

Risk-reduction strategies can be categorized and arranged according to the increasing likelihood of successful long-term effects, as follows:

1. Punitive actions directed at individuals

2. Counseling and retraining of individuals or groups

3. Process redesign

4. Technical system enhancement

5. Cultural change

Unfortunately, the ease with which these types of changes can be successfully implemented is in reverse order of their efficacy.

Risk-reduction strategies that include punitive actions directed at individuals and counseling and retraining of individuals or groups are the quickest to enact.

Unfortunately, these are the least effective in achieving long-lasting change. Process redesign and technical system enhancement are far more labor-intensive risk-reduction strategies, but the likelihood of sustainable improvements is far greater.

Health care organizations need not wait for sentinel events to occur in order to reduce process errors. We can start today. We know a great deal already about where the risks are in health care, and we are learning more every day. The tools are available for analyzing high-risk processes. The techniques for designing safe processes are also known, waiting only to be adapted to health care. It is time for a reality check. We are not perfect. We must design accordingly.

Discussion Questions

1. Select a health care process. What are the possible safety-related errors that could occur during this process.

2. For the safety-related errors identified in question 1, what process characteristics increase the risk of these errors?

3. For the health care process selected in question 1, what actions can be taken to minimize or prevent safety-related errors?

Key Terms

Clinical pathway	Hand-off	Risk-reduction strategy
Crew resource management	Proactive risk reduction	Tightly coupled process
Failure effect	Redundancy	

References

Bates, D., Leape, L., Cullen, D., Laird, N., Petersen, L., Teich, J., & Seger, D. (1998). Effect of computerized physician order entry and a team intervention on prevention of serious medication errors. *Journal of the American Medical Association, 280*(15), 1311–1316.

Berwick, D. M. (1998, November). *Taking action to improve safety: How to increase the odds of success.* Conference presentation, Enhancing Patient Safety and Reducing Errors in Health Care, Rancho Mirage, CA.

Cook, R. I. (1998, November). *Two years before the mast: Learning how to learn about patient safety*. Conference presentation, Enhancing Patient Safety and Reducing Errors in Health Care, Rancho Mirage, CA.

Gitlow, H., Gitlow, S., Oppenheim, A., & Oppenheim, R. (1989). *Tools and methods for the improvement of quality*. Homewood, IL: Richard D. Irwin.

Helmreich, R., Wilhelm, J., Gregorich, S., & Chidester, T. (1990). Preliminary results from the evaluation of crew resource management training: Performance ratings of flight crews. *Aviation, Space, and Environmental Medicine, 61*(6), 576–579.

Juran, J. M., & Godfrey, A. B. (1999). *Juran's quality handbook* (5th ed.). New York: McGraw-Hill.

Koppel, R., Wetterneck, T., Telles, J., & Karsh, B. (2008). Workarounds to barcode medication administration systems: Their occurrences, causes, and threats to patient safety. *Journal of the American Medical Informatics Association, 15*(4), 408–423.

Perrow, C. (1984). *Normal accidents: Living with high-risk technologies*. New York: Basic Books.

Random House. (1993). *Random House unabridged dictionary* (2nd ed.). New York: Random House.

Reason, J. (1997). *Managing the risks of organizational accidents*. Aldershot, UK: Ashgate.

Reason, J., & Hobbs, A. (2003). *Managing maintenance error: A practical guide*. Aldershot, UK: Ashgate.

Weick, K. E., & Sutcliffe, K. M. (2007). *Managing the unexpected: Resilient performance in an age of uncertainty* (2nd ed.). San Francisco: Jossey-Bass.

CHAPTER 11

REDUCING ERRORS THROUGH WORK SYSTEM IMPROVEMENTS

Patrice L. Spath

LEARNING OBJECTIVES

- Describe common work redesign strategies for managing the risk of errors
- Identify process improvements that prevent or mitigate the effects of errors
- Recognize the role of patients and family members in patient safety improvement

In the mid-twentieth century, with the discovery of sulfonamides, penicillin and other antibiotics, antitubercular drugs, and the polio vaccine, people began to think that medicine had the potential to successfully treat all disease. In the 1950s and 1960s an explosion of new medical technology further fueled society's optimism over conquering disease. In this climate the errorless imperative evolved in which both health professionals and society demanded that mistakes not be made (Fagerhaugh, Strauss, Suczek, & Wiener, 1987). Although the errorless imperative is a nice ideal, increases in medical technology have actually heightened the chance of error because health care practitioners must learn highly specialized skills. The decline in infectious diseases has been countered by an increase in such chronic conditions as heart disease, cancer, and respiratory disorders. These health problems tend to require more technology and complex medical interventions that, in turn, intensify the risk of error (Shepherd, 2004). The fact remains that health care practitioners are only human and not perfect, and there are no guarantees that mistakes won't be made and patients won't occasionally be injured.

Errors can occur in all aspects of health care services. During the diagnostic phase practitioners can fail to order indicated tests, misread lab results, or fail to act on the results of diagnostic findings. During the treatment phase a technical error can occur in preparation or performance (for example, miscalculation of dose, delivery of treatment to the wrong patient, or mishap during surgical procedure). Treatment can be mistakenly delayed, or inappropriate care can be provided. During the preventive phase of health care, practitioners can inadequately monitor patients during prophylactic treatments or provide insufficient follow-up. Communication errors and equipment failures can occur at any time.

Over the past fifty years, behavioral scientists have studied the nature, varieties, and causes of human error in hopes of discovering what can be done to reduce errors or mitigate their effects. In Chapter Two, Ternov described why people err on occasion, emphasizing that although a human is usually involved when accidents occur in a professional setting such as health care, the causes of the error are likely to be out of the individual's control. Thus, the personal approach to error management—individual training and punishment—has not proven to be a long-lasting patient safety improvement strategy. The balance of scientific opinion clearly favors finding and eliminating the error-producing factors in tasks, the workplace, and the organization (Dekker, 2006). Accident prevention requires an understanding of what is happening and why it is happening. Armed with this situational understanding, practitioners can then formulate appropriate task, workplace, and organizational improvements.

Anesthesiology has already begun to apply this situational approach to error management, with resulting improvements in ergonomics, operating room layout, monitoring interfaces, and other systemwide refinements (Cooper & Gaba, 2002). An increasing number of proactive efforts are also under way to find and correct error-producing factors before an anesthesia-related accident occurs. Thanks to new anesthesia techniques, drugs, and enhanced training, anesthesia mortality risk has declined from approximately 1 death in 1,000 anesthesia procedures in the 1940s to 1 in 10,000 in the 1970s and to 1 in 100,000 in the 1990s and early 2000s (Li, Warner, Lang, Huang, & Sun, 2009).

Although accident investigation techniques have been used for many years in private industry, there is scant information on developing accident prevention recommendations. For example, the 1,992-page *Management Oversight and Risk Tree (MORT) Accident/Incident Investigation Manual* only contains two paragraphs about making recommendations for improving safety in energy facilities (Johnson, 1985). Only one of the eight chapters in *Root Cause Analysis in Health Care: Tools and Techniques* (Croteau, 2010) describes how to develop solutions. Ludwig Benner Jr., a longtime industrial safety consultant, has observed that about 90% of the person-hours in an accident investigation are typically devoted to determining what happened and preparing a report of those findings versus about 10% in recommendation development. He suggests this ratio should be more in the range of a 50-50 to 60-40 split (Hendrick & Benner, 1987).

Conventional wisdom suggests that a well-done root cause analysis will result in the development of worthwhile improvement recommendations. However, this does not always occur (Wu, Lipshutz, & Pronovost, 2008). The purpose of this chapter is to familiarize health care practitioners with general error-reduction strategies and many specific process changes that have proven to be successful in both industrial and health care settings. Several general work system improvements designed to reduce or mitigate the effects of human error are contained in the first section of this chapter.

One of the more popular error-reduction strategies is automation. Though automating tasks can potentially diminish common slips or mistakes, automation itself introduces a different class of hazards into the health care workplace. How automation can improve patient safety and how to overcome common implementation challenges are covered in Chapter Thirteen. Because the processes involved in medication administration are very risk prone, an entire chapter has been devoted to the subject of medication safety improvement (Chapter Fifteen). Several additional examples of medication process improvement techniques can be found in Chapter Fifteen.

The recommendations included in this chapter are not intended to represent the entire universe of improvement choices. In fact, almost monthly there is another published research report describing what works and what doesn't work to improve patient safety. The suggestions in this chapter can serve as an effective starting point when developing redesign recommendations during an accident investigation or for proactive error reduction purposes. Readers are cautioned against indiscriminate adoption of any process change. The unique circumstances of each organization must be taken into consideration, as well as the impact on collateral processes (Brach, Lenfestey, Roussel, Amoozegar, & Sorensen, 2008). Haphazard process improvement is tantamount to tampering, and tampering can lead to chaos with an eventual increase in errors (Deming, 1982). Experience in the nuclear power industry has shown that some preventive "fixes" actually played a major role in causing subsequent accidents (Reason, 1997).

Error Management Strategies

High-reliability industries, such as aviation, air traffic control, and nuclear power, learned long ago the fallacy of relying on human perfection to prevent accidents. Like health care, these industries believe in training, rules, and high standards, but they don't rely on them to prevent accidents. They look to their systems (Van Cott, 1994).

If the health care industry is to improve patient safety, systems and processes must be designed to be more resistant to error occurrence and more accommodating of error consequence. To achieve this goal, we must first understand the error environment and where errors are most likely to occur. Information for this evaluation can be based primarily on observation (by walk-throughs or talk-throughs) or experience (examination of past incidents and errors). Once the error environment is understood, organizations can better match expected error-causing situations with appropriate redesign solutions. It is impossible to eliminate all error risk; however, process improvements that preferentially deal with error occurrence first and error consequences second are recommended.

Two types of process redesign can affect error occurrence. The first is known as **error elimination**, in which the process is changed so that an error is impossible to make. An example is the anesthesia machine that was redesigned so that the connector for the oxygen tank could not fit into the nitrous gas tank, thus making it impossible for the anesthesiologist to make a connection error. At times, deleting the error-prevalent task from the process can subsequently eliminate mistakes. For example, in 1996 it was discovered that hospital nurses were making significant errors in the administration of concentrated potassium chloride solutions (United States Pharmacopoeia, 1996). Many hospitals subsequently removed this medication from the floor stocks as suggested by the U.S. Pharmacopeia and the Joint Commission, thereby taking the nurse out of the process entirely (The Joint Commission, 1998).

If error elimination is not possible or feasible, then the next best choice is to reduce error occurrence through process redesign. For example, with just a simple change in the notification process for positive fecal occult blood tests, the internal medicine practice at the University of Virginia Health Systems, Charlottesville, Virginia, was able to improve follow-up from 77% in the one-year pre-intervention period to 100% in the year after the intervention was implemented fully (Plews-Ogan et al., 2004).

The third approach to process redesign is to eliminate the consequences of errors. Given that mistakes will occasionally happen, the process can be designed to catch errors before eventual patient harm occurs. An example of a process redesign intended to catch errors is the use of radio frequency identification technology (RFID) to detect retained objects inadvertently left in a patient's surgical wound. An RFID reader is used in conjunction with RFID beacons sewn into surgical sponges, laps, and towels. A wand scanning device is waved over the patient before the surgical wound is closed to enable detection of retained objects that may have been missed by manual count methods (Marcario, Morris, & Morris, 2006).

If errors and consequences cannot be completely eliminated, consider process improvements intended to reduce the effect of errors. This may be achieved through application of process design features that prompt actions to mitigate the consequences of an error. For example, laboratory technicians have been trained to immediately flush their eyes with water if they've been splashed with a toxic substance. Unfortunately, few patient care processes have similar automatic interventions designed to mitigate the consequence of errors. Perhaps, as suggested by Lori B. Andrews, lead researcher in a recent study of medical adverse events, "We've misled ourselves into thinking that errors are infrequent, so we don't incorporate the potential for error as part of the ongoing process" (Blecher, 1997).

Several general work system improvement principles have come out of human factors studies. These principles suggest how the working conditions of health care professionals can be changed to eliminate or reduce error occurrence (Karsh, Holden, Alper, & Or, 2006; AORN Foundation, 2007; Grout, 2007). These changes can also be useful in eliminating the consequence of errors and mitigating the effects of an error. Not surprisingly, these principles are similar to the process reliability improvement tactics described in Chapter Three. The work system improvement principles are:

- Simplify the process; reduce hand-offs
- Standardize
- Reduce reliance on memory
- Improve information access
- Use constraints and forcing functions
- Design for errors
- Adjust work schedules
- Adjust the environment
- Improve communication
- Decrease reliance on vigilance
- Provide adequate safety training

- Choose the right staff for the job

- Engage patients and family members

Simplify the Process

Simple processes are easier for people to understand and errors are easier to recognize and correct before an accident occurs. Many errors come from slips in transfers of materials, information, people, instructions, or supplies. Processes with fewer hand-offs are at less risk for mistakes. For example, Children's Hospital and Regional Medical Center, Seattle, Washington, reduced the risk of errors in administration of total parenteral nutrition (TPN) by reducing the process steps from 70 to 46 steps and improving communication among the care team (Anonymous, 2006). The original process for ordering TPN required coordination between a pharmacist, a dietician, and a physician and it took a long time and many phone calls to agree on the order. Decisions depended on lab results which were often not available when the different care providers saw the patient. The overall process was slow and error prone. The process redesign not only reduced the total process time from 12 hours down to 7 hours, but it also resulted in few mistakes.

Process simplification is a lean technique that improves efficiency as well as reducing the chance for errors. More examples of how processes can be simplified to improve patient safety are covered in Chapter Twelve.

Standardize

If a task is done the same way every time—by everyone—there is less chance for error. Areas in which unnecessary variation may be found include drugs, equipment, supplies, work processes, and the location of equipment and supplies. Lack of standardized practices contributed to the following event (Meisel, 2005):

> An ambulance was dispatched to help an elderly woman whose heart was beating irregularly. Although the patient was awake and her blood pressure was normal, the paramedics on the scene detected a worrisome cardiac rhythm on their monitor: The heart was beating too fast, and each beat appeared widened on the screen. The patient's condition was consistent with a serious and sometimes fatal heart rhythm called ventricular tachycardia. One of the paramedics called a local hospital, and a doctor there told him to administer intravenously 100

milligrams of a potent anti-arrhythmic drug, intravenous lidocaine hydrochloride. In the cramped ambulance, the medic grabbed a 2-gram syringe of lidocaine in concentrated form, which must be diluted in a bag of saline and dripped into the vein slowly. Thinking he had a different vial, the paramedic quickly injected the entire syringe into the patient. The woman went into cardiac arrest and died.

Ambulances would be safer for patients if they were all organized in the same way, with cardiac meds on the left and respiratory meds on the right. Syringes could all be prefilled and even color-coded with standard adult and pediatric dosages.

The Hospital Corporation of America (HCA) used standardization techniques to improve patient care and coordination among physicians, nurses, technicians, and others involved in delivering babies. Highly specific, checklist-driven protocols and procedure documentation templates were created for use by caregivers. By standardizing the care provided to obstetric patients, HCA improved perinatal outcomes, reduced the primary cesarean delivery rate, and lowered the incidence of maternal and fetal injuries (Clark, Belfort, Byrum, Meyers, Perlin, 2008).

Like simplification, process standardization is also a lean technique. More examples of error reduction through the use of process standardization are covered in Chapter Twelve.

Reduce Reliance on Memory

With the seemingly unlimited information needed to perform a particular job, people's memory limits can easily be exceeded. Easy-to-use information retrieval systems can help to reduce errors caused by memory overload. Checklists, protocols, clinical pathways, preprinted physician orders, and computerized decision aids are common examples of point-of-care reminders that can reduce people's reliance on memory.

To standardize the treatment of patients at risk of venous thromboembolism (VTE), practitioners at Nebraska Methodist Hospital in Omaha created an assessment tool for surgical and medical patients (Figure 11.1). The assessment results help clinicians manage patients appropriately with both pharmacologic and nonpharmacologic therapies.

Accompanying the assessment tool is a preprinted order form that reminds physicians of appropriate treatments based on the patient's VTE risk score. The paper-based physician order sheet (Figure 11.2) also includes contraindications

FIGURE 11.1 Thrombosis Risk Assessment for Surgical and Medical Patients

NMH Thrombosis Risk Assessment for Surgical & Medical Patients			

Score 1	Score 2	Score 3	Score 5
❑ Minor Surgery ❑ Age 41–60 ❑ History of prior major surgery (<1 month) ❑ Obesity (BMI > 30) ❑ Pregnant, or postpartum < 1 month ❑ Oral contraceptive or hormone replacement therapy ❑ Inflammatory bowel disease ❑ Leg swelling, ulcers, stasis, varicose veins ❑ COPD ❑ Pneumonia/respiratory failure ❑ History of MI, CHF Class I,II ❑ Rheumatoid or other Inflammatory arthritis	❑ Minor Surgery (>45min) ❑ Laparoscopic surgery (>45min) ❑ Age > 60 ❑ Malignancy ❑ Patients who are immobile or anticipated to be immobile > 72hr* ❑ Lower limb immobilization (cast, etc) ❑ Central venous access *Immobility defined as lack of patient ambulation of at least 100 ft a minimum of 3 times daily	❑ Severe infection or sepsis ❑ History of DVT/PE ❑ Inherited or acquired hypercoagulable states** ❑ Active cardiac dysfunciton (CHF class III,IV; MI within 1 month, cardiomyopathy) ❑ Nephrotic syndrome (≠ renal failure) ❑ Systemic lupus or similar autoimmune disease (ie collagen vascular disease) Signature: _____ Date: ___	❑ Elective major lower extremity arthroplasty ❑ Hip, pelvis, or leg fracture ❑ Multiple trauma ❑ Acute spinal cord injury (paralysis) ❑ Stroke with paralysis ❑ Use of paralytics or continuous sedation

** includes: activated protein C resistance; factor V Leiden, prothrombin variant 20210A, antiphospholipid antibodies (lupus anticoagulant and anticardiolipin antibody); deficiency or dysfunction of antithrombin, protein C, protein S, or heparin cofactor II; dysfibrinogenemia; decreased levels of plasminogen and plasminogen activators; HIT, hyperhomocystinemia; myeloproliferative disorders such as polycythemia vera and primary thrombocytosis

(Check each box above that applies and add score for total) **Total Risk Score:** _____

Potential exclusions for use of pharmacologic prophylaxis		
❑ Active bleeding ❑ Coagulopathy ❑ Active GI ulcer ❑ Patients with high bleeding risk	❑ Recent history of cerebral, GI, GU hemorrhage ❑ History of hemorrhagic stroke within 6 months ❑ Recent intracranial/intraocular surgery ❑ **Spinal tap/epidural anesthesia within 24 hrs** ❑ **Indwelling epidural catheter**	❑ Uncontrolled hypertension ❑ Aspirin, NSAID, or platelet inhibitor use ❑ Thrombocytopenia (including HIT) ❑ Allergy to heparin, enoxaparin/LMWH, or pork products

Source: Nebraska Methodist Hospital, 2010. Used with permission.

to the use of TED stockings or sequential compression devices. After implementing the assessment tool and preprinted order form, Nebraska Medical Center reported a decrease in the incidence of deep vein thrombosis in surgical and medical patients and fewer pulmonary emboli in surgical patients (Nygaard et al., 2009). Studies have shown that making physicians aware of the appropriate treatment, using point-of-care reminders, improves adherence to accepted practices (Pathman, Konard, Freed, Freeman, & Koch, 1996).

OSF St. Francis Medical Center in Peoria, Illinois, reduced the incidence of pressure ulcers from 9.4% in 2001 to 0.6% as of September 2008 (American Hospital Association, 2009). To achieve this success, they implemented a policy of turning patients every 2 hours, required documentation of patient turning and conducted regular chart audits with each unit's results regularly published. Pressure-redistributing mattresses were purchased for use with high-risk patients. In addition, several decision aids and reminders were built into the system, including:

- Play part of the "Roll Over Beethoven" over the hospital speaker system every two hours during the day and evening as a reminder to nurses to reposition their patients

FIGURE 11.2 Physician Orders for VTE Prophylaxis

Physician Orders (Check specific order and sign below)

Risk Score	Incidence of DVT	Recommended Prophylaxis Regimen for Each Risk Group **Order one of the following**
Low Risk (Score = 0–1)	2%	Aggressive mobilization. ☐ Ambulate _____
Moderate Risk (Score = 2)	10–20%	☐ Heparin 5000 units SC q12h ------OR--------- ☐ Enoxaparin 40mg SC daily ------OR--------- ☐ Intermittent pneumatic compression device
High Risk (Score = 3–4)	20–40%	☐ Heparin 5000 units SC q8hr ------OR--------- ☐ Enoxaparin 40mg SC daily ------OR--------- ☐ Intermittent pneumatic compression device + elastic stockings
Highest Risk (Score ≥ 5)	40–80%	☐ Heparin 5000 units SC q8hr + intermittent pneumatic compression device + elastic stockings ------OR--------- ☐ Enoxaparin 40mg SC daily + intermittent pneumatic compression device + elastic stockings ------OR--------- ☐ Enoxaparin 30mg SC BID + intermittent pneumatic compression device + elastic stockings ------OR-------- *(Enoxaparin dose suggested for orthopedic, major trauma, acute spinal cord injury)* ☐ Warfarin _____ mg _____ (Goal INR 2–3) ------OR--------- ☐ Enoxaparin 40mg SC daily *(Medical, non-critical care patients only)* ☐ Intermittent pneumatic compression device + elastic stockings *(If anticoagulation contraindicated)*
Prophylaxis Exceptions		☐ Pharmacologic contraindication ☐ Compression device/elastic stocking contraindication ☐ Currently receiving therapeutic anti-coagulation (warfarin, heparin, enoxaparin, direct thrombin inhibitor) ☐ No treatment at this time due to _____
		☐ No change in previously ordered prophylaxis is necessary

Reference: Seventh ACCP Conference on Antithrombotic Therapy. Chest 2004
This is meant to be a treatment guideline, however, treatment for each patient needs to be individualized.
Contact pharmacy for enoxaparin dosing in patients with renal impairment or extreme high/low body wight

Patient Label

_____ **MD Signature**

_____ **Date**

File in Medical Record   Form 180–558
      (Approved 5/03/05, Revised 5/2006)

Contraindications to TED or Sequential Compression Device (SCD)
If any of the following are present, contact physician for further instructions

Local Leg Conditions (device may cause discomfort, impair healing, or increase risk of other complications)
Dermatitis
Recent vein ligation
Gangrene
History of skin grafts
Severe artherosclerosis or other ischemic vascular diseases
Massive edema of legs or pulmonary edema from congestive heart failure
Extreme deformity of legs
Suspected or pre-existing deep vein thrombosis or pulmonary embolism *(applies to SCD only)*

Reference: Product labeling of SCDs and TEDs by Kendall

Source: Nebraska Methodist Hospital, 2010. Used with permission.

- Send nurses a page message every two hours to prompt them to reposition their patients
- Place "Save Our Skin" signage on at-risk patient doors

Improve Information Access

Good decisions require good information. People must have ready access to relevant and complete information or faulty decisions can occur. Grimshaw and

Russell (1993) found that the guideline implementation strategies most likely to be effective were those that delivered patient-specific advice at the time and place of a consultation.

Better communication of information among caregivers is the goal of the recommendations of the American Academy of Orthopaedic Surgeons (AAOS) for eliminating wrong-site surgery (2010). According to its advisory statement, a surgeon should place his or her initials on the operative site in a way that cannot be overlooked and in a manner that will be clearly incorrect if transferred onto another body area prior to surgery. Once the patient has been moved into the operating room, the surgical team should pause to take a "**time-out**" to communicate about the specific patient and procedure.

Not only must information be accessible, it must also be up to date. The importance of having up-to-date information during patient hand-off communications is emphasized by the Joint Commission's National Patient Safety Goals. Accredited organizations are to ensure the process for transitioning patient care from one caregiver to the next includes up-to-date information regarding the patient's care, treatment and services, condition and any recent or anticipated changes. To accomplish this, organizations often develop a standardized approach to hand-off communication to ensure consistency. The standardized approach would include a description of the following elements (Joint Commission Resources, 2008):

- The situations in which the standardized hand-off applies (for example, physician-to-nurse, nurse-to-nurse, physician-to-physician)

- People who are expected to be involved in the communication

- Information to be communicated (for example, patient's diagnoses and current condition, recent and anticipated changes in condition or treatment, situations to watch for)

- Mechanism for caregivers to ask and respond to questions

- Process for documenting hand-off communications

Use Constraints and Forcing Functions

Constraining functions, such as the "Are you sure?" **prompt** that follows hitting the delete key in a computer program, make it more difficult to commit errors. Forcing functions, such as being unable to start your car when in reverse gear, are an effective method for error-proofing processes. An example of a constraining function that was shown to reduce medication errors in a residential care is described by Chappell, Dickey, & DeLetter (1997). Researchers found that caregivers who used prefilled seven-day medication dispensers to administer residents' medications had fewer omission errors than those who used the traditional prescription bottle method of dispensing. Caregivers using prescription bottles committed 113 omission errors during the three-week study period, compared with only 21 omission errors by the group using dispensers. Researchers also observed that the medication dispensers prompted caregivers to order prescription refills in a timelier manner than caregivers using the traditional bottle method. The medication dispenser acted as a constraint that reduced errors.

Forcing functions, as defined by Norman, "are a form of physical constraint: situations in which the actions are constrained so that failure at one stage prevents the next step from happening" (Norman, 1988, p. 131). Bar-coded patient identification and disposable blood bag combination locks are two forcing functions being used in blood transfusion services to eliminate transfusion errors caused by failure to comply with traditional unit-recipient identification protocols (Wenz, Mercuriali, & AuBuchon, 1997).

Forcing functions are often integrated into the computer-user interface. For example, at some facilities clinical staff is unable to schedule an MRI procedure without first confirming the patient has no contraindications such as a metallic implant. This technique creates a "time out" to reduce the risk that a patient will be harmed inadvertently as a result of his or her care. To make sure patients on opiate medications also receive stool softeners or laxatives, one hospital added a forcing function to the computerized order entry system. When the physician orders an opiate, the system automatically defaults to a stool softener ordering screen. At this point the physician can opt out; however they must document their reason for doing so (Luria, Muething, Schoettker, & Kotagal, 2006).

Design for Errors

Design systems that encourage error detection and correction before an accident occurs. At Fairview Health Services in Minneapolis, pharmacists are empowered by the medical staff to modify ordered doses of certain drugs based on patient status. After instituting this process change, the appropriateness of benzodiazepine dosing for patients over the age of 65 went from 25 to 100% in a two-week time period. Similar medication dosing improvements have occurred in other drug classes (Meisel, 1998). Pharmacists are provided with medical staff–approved protocols and are allowed to automatically intervene when a physician orders an inappropriate medication dose.

Studies of problem detection in aviation and nuclear power both found that misassessments of the situation at hand were only corrected when fresh perspectives entered the situation (Patterson, Woods, Cook, Render, 2007). **Independent double checks** are a way to add a fresh perspective by having one practitioner cross-check the work of another. Research has shown that people find approximately 95% of mistakes when checking the work of others (Campbell & Facchinetti, 1998). Adding independent double checks to high-risk processes greatly reduces the chance of an error reaching the patient.

However, not all double checks are equally effective in preventing errors. For example, an error in calculating the dose of a medication is more likely to be detected if the second person performs all calculations independently, without having seen the prior calculations (Institute for Safe Medication Practices, 2003). Thus, the double checks must be carefully designed to maximize the visibility of errors. In addition, health care organizations must be careful about overreliance on double-checking to prevent mistakes. If a facility is not selective in its double-checking requirements caregivers may consider the pervasive requirement to be a superficial routine task and not check independently.

Another potential process design problem is related to the equipment used by caregivers. Equipment can contribute to adverse events by either directly causing the accident or contributing to human errors that cause accidents. Even if equipment malfunction is the direct cause of the accident, malfunctions can often be traced back to human error (poor training or maintenance). The equipment-related event described below illustrates the human component of equipment failures (Prielipp, Lewis, & Morell, 1998):

A 40-year-old man underwent uneventful aortic valve replacement surgery and was transported to the intensive care unit (ICU) and placed on a Bourns Bear 2® ventilator. Within 40 seconds of initiation of mechanical ventilation, the patient became hypotensive (BP = 60/40 mmHg). Initial urgent evaluation focused on a presumed bleeding source or possible cardiac or aortic valve complication. Fortunately, following arrival and evaluation by an experienced respiratory therapist and attending intensivist, it was noted that the ventilator was malfunctioning. The patient was immediately removed from the ventilator and hand ventilated with 100% FiO_2 until he could be placed on another ventilator.

Analysis of the incident revealed that the ICU personnel routinely worked with only two models of ventilators and were very comfortable with troubleshooting problems rapidly in those devices. The Bear 2 ventilator was a backup and only used in situations of intense ICU activity and maximal patient census. Few of the ICU staff had experience using this equipment. Thus, the contributing factor in this equipment failure was staff lack of training and education necessary for maintaining expertise and proficiency in a rarely used piece of equipment. The exhalation value malfunction that occurred in the Bear 2 ventilator is a known problem, but only to those familiar with the equipment. The latent failure in this event was the organization's decision to use old equipment for backup purposes without ensuring that staff proficiency was maintained for these rarely used devices.

In evaluating the circumstances surrounding accidents or near misses involving equipment, investigators have identified common hazardous situations or problems that existed prior to the incident (Sawyer, 1996):

- Staff training has been slow and arduous.

- Only a few staff members seem to be using the device.

- Staff tends to modify the equipment and takes shortcuts.

- Staff refuses to use the device.

- Staff finds installation of accessories difficult, confusing, or overly time-consuming.

- Alarms and batteries often fail.

- Incorrect accessories sometimes are installed.

- Parts often become detached.

- Equipment displays are difficult to read or understand.

- Equipment controls are poorly located or labeled.

- Alarms are difficult to hear or distinguish.

- Alarms are very annoying.

- Equipment operation is illogical and confusing.

If one or more of these device-related situations is known to exist in your organization, it should be viewed as a warning signal. Be sure to investigate and correct the problem before an untoward incident occurs. In the Bear 2 ventilator equipment malfunction, only a few personnel knew how to use the device. Fortunately, those people were available and acted quickly. However, the situation could have been avoided altogether if the early warning signs had prompted further investigation and action.

Adjust Work Schedules

Practices such as failing to provide a sufficient number of staff members for the job (increasing workload) and frequently altering work shifts of employees (increasing fatigue) may ultimately lead to errors in human performance. Rogers, Hwang, Scott, Aiken, & Dinges (2004) found that nurses who work overtime were three times as likely to make an error if they worked shifts lasting 12.5 hours or more. Similar findings have been reported by Scott, Rogers, Hwang, & Zhang (2006) in a study of the work patterns of critical care nurses to determine if an association exists between the occurrence of errors and the hours worked by nurses. They found that longer work duration increased the risk of errors and near errors and decreased nurses' vigilance.

The relationship between errors and short staffing or long work hours has not always been substantiated by researchers. For instance, in a study of process errors by pharmacists in retail pharmacies, more errors were found to be made when pharmacists are less busy (40–105 scripts per shift) as compared to shifts in which pharmacists are busier (106+ scripts per shift) (Grasha & Schelle, 2001). The Texas Board of Nursing Examiners reviewed the number of working hours and fatigue experienced by nurses under investigation for nursing practice errors. The overwhelming majority of the nurses reported working for only one employer and working 40 hours a week or less at the time of the practice incident (Thomas, 2005).

The Institute of Medicine (IOM) report, *Keeping Patients Safe: Transforming the Work Environment of Nurses* (IOM, 2004), provides a review of research literature on this topic. Based on this review, experts recommend that to reduce error-producing fatigue, nursing staff members should not provide direct patient care more than 12 hours in any given 24-hour period or in excess of 60 hours in any seven-day period.

Whether work schedules can be adjusted or not, there are several steps that health care organizations can take to reduce cognitive overload on people—thus reducing their risk of making a mistake. People must be physically and psychologically fit to complete their job tasks, otherwise mistakes can occur. Individuals who are physically ill or under psychological duress should work limited hours or be discouraged from working until they are able to safely complete their work duties.

Be sure staff members periodically take a break from work and audit the quality of the breaks. The absolute number of breaks or the amount of time on any one break is not the major issue; it is the ability of individuals to have a quiet time away from the hustle of the workplace. People make fewer mistakes and are better able to identify and correct errors when they have an opportunity to periodically "recharge."

Fatigue due to overwork and a lack of rest reduces productivity and efficiency and is a contributor to error. Some experts suggest that chronic fatigue has a detrimental effect on performance equivalent to a blood alcohol level of .10. Fatigue must be taken seriously. Fatigued health care workers are a hazard. Monitoring of personnel for excessive fatigue is a good idea. An increase in the incidence of process errors (mistakes made and corrected) is one of the signs of worker fatigue and a general lack of rest. Excessive overtime is a known precursor to human error. It is a source of overload on people in the workplace. Consider placing limitations on overtime or spacing the intervals between overtime shifts to help reduce negative effects.

The Joint Commission considered including **fatigue management** requirements in their 2007 and 2008 National Patient Safety Goals. Other safety improvement issues were prioritized as more important and the proposed fatigue management requirements did make it to the final list of safety goals. Although health care organizations are not required at the present time to formally address issues of worker fatigue, it is recommended that senior management commit to developing an organizational culture that addresses the importance of fatigue and engages everyone in the organization in developing strategies to cope with it. This engagement should include (Spath, 2006):

- Involvement of employees in developing shift schedules, since they best understand the rhythm of the work and how it affects them

- Hosting of mandatory education programs for managers and employees on how to manage fatigue and to promote individual coping strategies such as improving diet, exercise, sleep habits, and relaxation to mitigate fatigue

- Collection and evaluation of data on the safety effects of any changes to shift schedules or workplace organization that might contribute to cognitive overload for employees

Adjust the Environment

Human factors engineers have long recognized the error-producing factors in work environments; for example, noise, poor lighting, glare-producing surfaces, heat, clutter, electrical interference, humidity, and moisture. Staff members working in less-than-ideal situations are more likely to make errors. Use the checklist in Exhibit 11.1 for conducting observational audits to identify human performance problems related to workstation design, workspace layout, equipment, supplies, and procedures.

EXHIBIT 11.1

CHECKLIST FOR AUDITING THE SAFETY OF THE PHYSICAL ENVIRONMENT

Look for:

❏ Sensory components of the environment that make it more difficult for people to conduct work (they should be able to see, hear, touch and feel what they need to do their jobs)

❏ Light, noise, environmental distractions, crowding, temperature, humidity, and other features of the physical workspace that contribute to unsafe working conditions

❏ Components of the physical environment that make equipment and technology difficult to use (for example, heat, humidity, poor lighting, power surges, dust, noise, and distracting sounds)

❏ Department or unit physical layouts that increase distractions and interruptions for people doing final checks of their work

❏ Workspaces that are not clean, orderly, and free of clutter

❏ Sources of distractions and noise that affect the concentration and attention of people

---

The environment also creates hazardous situations for patients. For instance, Simpson, Lamb, Roberts, Gardner, & Grimley-Evans (2004) reported that wooden carpeted floors were associated with the lowest number of fractures per 100 patient falls in nursing homes. Other environmental hazards that contribute to patient falls include: bed rails, footwear, lighting, lack of walking aids such as hand rails, and lack of assistive devices (Hignett & Masud, 2006).

Improve Communication

To reduce mistakes, avoid indirect communication among the work team and cut down on the number of communications per task. Often, determining the most appropriate patient care action requires effective sharing of information among the health care team and collective decision making. Patient hand-offs among caregivers are a particularly critical time for effective communication.

According to The Joint Commission, 70% of sentinel events in 2005 were caused by poor communication, with approximately one-half of those events occurring during patient hand-offs (The Joint Commission, 2006).

One type of risky hand-off involves transporting hospitalized patients from the nursing unit to other areas of the hospital for tests or treatments. Some hospitals have adopted a "ticket to ride" process to ensure vital information about the patient is clearly communicated to transporters and the receiving providers (Pesanka et al., 2009; Ray, 2009; West, 2009). The process varies somewhat among hospitals; however it commonly involves the use of a one- or two-page form for recording the patient's allergies, fall risk, and any special needs such as impaired senses, positioning requirements, or oxygenation needs. This document is completed by the nurse and accompanies the patient off-unit so that critical patient safety information is readily available should problems arise or the patient is away from the unit longer than expected.

In Chapter Fourteen of this book, Risser and others describe techniques for improving how health care team members establish and maintain a common understanding of patient and operational issues through communication improvements.

Decrease Reliance on Vigilance

Errors are commonplace events however very few errors actually progress to complete a chain of events leading to a patient injury. Why? Because people catch and fix most mistakes before a patient is harmed. In a study of nursing activities at five California hospitals, researchers found that nurses identified and corrected an average of one process failure every 1.23 hours (Tucker & Edmondson, 2003). The failures ranged from missing items (such as supplies, information, or medications) to computer data entry errors.

Unfortunately, health care organizations have in the past relied heavily on people finding and fixing mistakes and not enough on designing safer systems. Yet, relying on caregiver vigilance as the primary strategy for preventing mishaps is problematic. James Reason's research in the cause of accidents has led him to conclude that people's ability to find and correct errors can be worn down through attrition by coping with minor events (Reason, 2008). When people are expected to devote too much of their attention to a problem or situation, they are apt to become forgetful or complacent in their vigilance.

At a minimum, work system redesigns should make errors more visible so they can be quickly corrected. An example is the use of colored indicators on identification bands of patients having surgery at Cincinnati Children's Hospital. The hospital recognized the need to ensure that all patients wear a proper indicator identifying whether they received a preoperative antibiotic. A patient wristband is placed over the patient identification band on the same wrist to remind the clinician to check whether the patient received preoperative antibiotics when he or she checks the patient identification wristband (Hines et al., 2008). In addition, other preoperative antibiotic reminders, such as stickers, all use the same color: orange.

Provide Adequate Safety Training

Make employees aware of the potential hazards relevant to their job and the given strategies for avoiding them. If faced with an unsafe situation, staff members must know what steps to take and they must be empowered to act. After a patient died of a massive fluid overload following hysteroscopy surgery to remove a uterine fibroid, practitioners at Beth Israel Hospital in New York found that the surgeon had failed to heed several warnings from the circulating nurse and scrub nurse about the patient's lack of fluid output (Patterson, 1998). One of the policy changes made subsequent to the incident is that the circulating nurse must notify the surgeon and the anesthesiologist when input of the distention medium exceeds output by 1,500 mL. The surgeon is expected to terminate the procedure as soon as hemostasis can be obtained. Failure by the surgeon to terminate the procedure is grounds for summary suspension. If this policy had been in place prior to the patient's surgery, the death may have been avoided.

All staff working at Virginia Mason Medical Center, Seattle, Washington are taught to "**stop the line**" (cease any activity that could cause further harm) and make an immediate report to a patient safety specialist when faced with a situation likely to cause patient harm (Furman & Caplan, 2007). Nurses in some intensive care units are empowered to abort the insertion of a central line if the operator fails to adhere to all elements of the insertion checklist (Pronovost et al., 2006).

Likewise, staff must be prepared to act in case of a life-threatening emergency. Thomsen and Bush (1998) studied management strategies for patients who experience an **adverse reaction** to radiographic contrast materials. Although the incidence of reactions is low (0.2 to 0.4% of patients receiving nonionic low-osmolar contrast media, 1 to 2% of patients receiving ionic high-osmolar contrast media), the authors suggest that radiologists and their staff remain sufficiently trained and prepared to take immediate action should a reaction occur. Periodic drills or rehearsals are especially important for those situations that rarely happen to ensure that practitioners maintain their skill proficiencies.

A number of health care organizations are using scenario-based **simulation training** to enhance the skills and safe practices of caregivers (Jha, Duncan, & Bates, 2001). This training involves more than just practicing resuscitation techniques on a computerized mannequin. For instance, simulation modalities are being used to teach and enhance interprofessional team training. One model that is commonly used is the AHRQ and the Department of Defense's **TeamSTEPPS® system**, which stands for Team Strategies and Tools to Enhance Performance and Patient Safety (AHRQ, n.d.).

Choose the Right Staff for the Job

For any job or task, it is important to identify people with the abilities necessary to perform the job safely. Staff members must also be adequately trained in the competencies necessary to perform the job and their readiness confirmed prior to work execution. Organizations should have written policies and procedures that include competency standards for each patient care area and a method for measuring individual performance against these competency standards. Facilities should have mechanisms for rapid deployment of competent personnel when any labor-intensive event occurs, for example, multiple admissions or discharges or an emergency health crisis for an individual patient.

Float staff should be assigned only to those areas for which they have received orientation. Likewise, the float staff must have demonstrated competency to care for patients in that area; otherwise they should not be given full responsibility for a patient assignment. For example, a nurse who has not been oriented to, and demonstrated the ability to manage, a ventilator should not be assigned responsibility for the care of a patient on a ventilator.

Engage Patients and Family Members

Training patients to be more assertive and involved in the medical encounter has been shown to be effective in increasing patient involvement in their own care and in producing better health outcomes (Kaplan, Greenfield, & Ware, 1989; Stewart et al., 2000). Involving patients and family members in safety improvement is a logical extension of this partnership (Spath, 2008).

In March 2002, the Centers for Medicare and Medicaid Services together with The Joint Commission launched a national campaign to urge patients to take a role in preventing health care errors by becoming active, involved, and informed participants on the health care team (The Joint Commission, 2010).

When a patient asks questions about their medications or a test that has been ordered, the patient is serving as a point-of-care reminder. Such questions remind caregivers to recheck or validate that the right thing is being done. Most errors that occur in health care are system-related and not attributable to individual negligence or misconduct. More effective safeguards (checks and balances) can prevent unintended mistakes. Patients can be one more safeguard against untoward events by paying attention to the care being provided to them. They can let practitioners know if a possible error is being made. Patients can also help by ensuring that all clinicians have pertinent health information to provide safe care. Unfortunately, information the patient shares with one provider is not always passed on to the next provider caring for the patient. Patients can help prevent mistakes by keeping practitioners informed of their needs and their specific health issues. They can help prevent medication errors from occurring or procedures or treatments being performed on the wrong person.

In addition, patients' perception of safety increases when more information is shared (Wolosin, Vercler, & Matthews, 2006). When nurses say, "I'm checking your ID band against the number assigned on the medication to ensure you are receiving the correct medication. We will need to do this quick check whenever you receive medication," it communicates to the patient that the process is a safety step. If the patient is engaged in even a brief interaction, such as asking the patient to say his or her name out loud while the nurse reads the name on the label, it can reaffirm the organization's commitment to patient safety.

The response of health care professionals to patients' questions, concerns, and feedback directly influences how comfortable patients are with speaking up. If a patient asks that the nurse confirm the accuracy of the medications being dispensed or that the surgeon recheck the operative site, the subtle inference is that patient is challenging our professionalism. Such challenges can be uncomfortable and thus we may be reluctant to encourage patients to speak up. Health care professionals must admit that human errors will occur despite everyone's best efforts. Overconfidence in the abilities of caregivers can actually cause harm. Securing the patient's participation as one of the safeguards in health care delivery helps to build a system that is more resistant to errors.

Involving patients and their family members in medical error reduction and safety improvement requires more than simple education. Recent data show that patients want to be more involved in their care and they worry about the chance of a medical error (Peters, Slovic, Hibbard, & Tusler, 2006). Health care professionals must create opportunities for involvement and show people how to take advantage of these opportunities (Storri & Hookway, 2005). Successful participation of the public in patient safety improvements will require changes in attitudes and behaviors on the part of patients and caregivers alike.

Multiple Improvements Are Needed

Human errors can occur for a number of reasons. Errors can be directly attributed to system and process design and environmental and personnel factors. To reduce or eliminate human error occurrence in a risk-prone process, more than one work system improvement is necessary. For instance, an improvement team at Exempla Lutheran Hospital, Denver, Colorado, implemented several work redesigns to reduce problems involving chemotherapy treatments for adult patients in the oncology unit (Hines et al., 2008, p. 53):

- Change the location of chemotherapy preparation to reduce staff interruptions during preparation

- Standardize chemotherapy orders and provide access to up-to-date references

- Create a standardized chemotherapy preparation checklist for pharmacists and nurses

- Create a chemotherapy medication administration record that is sequenced the same as actual administration

A variety of work system improvements must be enacted to minimize the occurrence and limit the consequences of human error. There is no quick one-time fix that is likely to be effective. In the more than 10 years since publication of the Institute of Medicine report *To Err Is Human* (1999), the research on patient safety has exploded and organizations now have access to many recommended safety improvement practices. Listed in Exhibit 11.2 are sources of work redesign and safety improvement ideas and materials to engage patients in safety improvement activities.

EXHIBIT 11.2

SOURCES OF WORK REDESIGN AND PATIENT SAFETY IMPROVEMENT IDEAS AND PATIENT ENGAGEMENT MATERIALS

- Advancing Excellence in America's Nursing Homes
  www.nhqualitycampaign.org

- AHRQ Health Care Innovations Exchange
  www.innovations.ahrq.gov

- AHRQ WebM&M
  http://webmm.ahrq.gov

- Australian Commission on Safety and Quality in Health Care
  www.safetyandquality.gov.au

- Consumers Advancing Patient Safety
  www.patientsafety.org

- Council on Surgical and Perioperative Safety
  www.cspsteam.org

- Institute for Healthcare Communication
  www.healthcarecomm.org

- Institute for Healthcare Improvement
  www.ihi.org

- Institute for Safe Medication Practices
  www.ismp.org

- Medicare Quality Improvement Community
  www.medqic.org

- Mistake-Proofing the Design of Health Care Processes
  www.ahrq.gov/qual/mistakeproof

- National Initiative for Children's Healthcare Quality
  www.nichq.org

- National Patient Safety Agency (UK)
  www.npsa.nhs.uk

- National Patient Safety Foundation
  www.npsf.org

- Pennsylvania Patient Safety Authority
  www.patientsafetyauthority.org

- Promising Practices sponsored by the Robert Wood Johnson Foundation
  www.rwjf.org/qualityequality/pp.jsp

- The Joint Commission
  www.jointcommission.org

- VA National Center for Patient Safety
  www.patientsafety.gov

- WHO Collaborating Centre for Patient Safety Solutions
  www.ccforpatientsafety.org/

Don't fall into the trap of "magic bullet thinking." Work system improvements by themselves do not automatically result in a safer environment for patients (Davidoff, 2010). Leadership is needed to create incentives for adopting new practices, open channels of communication among caregivers, and keep people focused on the goal (Bosk, Dixon-Woods, Goeschel, & Pronovost, 2009).

Conclusion

In a perfect world there would be no errors, and the operation of a health care facility would be under complete control at all times. There would be no unplanned, undesirable events and no accidents, incidents, or inefficiencies. Unfortunately, such perfect control does not exist in any organization that I know of. Every human action taken in the provision of health care services is an opportunity for error. An action may be a visible act, such as raising the patient's bedrails; an internal process, such as reading the patient's health record; or even a lack of activity, such as omitting the procedural step of checking the patient's allergy history.

The problem of errors in health care is recognized as a major health-quality issue. It will not disappear from public concern. In the 1990s a body of research on the prevalence and etiology of medical errors emerged, informed in part by the experience of the aviation and nuclear power industries and by students of human factors engineering. Today, a review of human error analysis in the health care literature reveals a growing number of studies that define types of human error, methods for analyzing errors, and strategies for reducing or mitigating the effects of human errors in medicine. Learning more about the error environment in your organization is far more important than determining who made the mistake. Focus improvements on the way things are done on the job, rather than the individuals doing the job. Corrective action should first be sought through modification of systems and processes, not through placing blame.

Discussion Questions

1. What are the common types of mistakes you encounter in your daily life? What error management strategies described in this chapter would work best to prevent these mistakes?

2. What are five safeguards that health care professionals rely on to prevent process errors or catch errors before patients are harmed?

3. In the *Sentinel Events Alerts* issued by The Joint Commission (www. jointcommission.org), what are common causes of adverse events and what strategies does it suggest for preventing these events?

Key Terms

Adverse reaction

Constraining function

Error elimination

Fatigue management

Independent double check

Prompt

Simulation training

Stop the line

TeamSTEPPS® system

Time-out

References

AHRQ. *(n.d.)* National implementation of TeamSTEPPS. *Retrieved from* http:// teamstepps.ahrq.gov/.

American Academy of Orthopaedic Surgeons. (2010). *Information statement: Wrong-site surgery*. Retrieved from http://www.aaos.org/about/papers/advistmt/1015.asp.

American Hospital Association. (2009, April). Save our skin: Preventing pressure ulcers. *Hospitals in Pursuit of Excellence*. Retrieved from http://www.ahaqualitycenter.org.

Anonymous. (2006). Getting lean not mean: Morale, leadership, and integration issues surrounding LEAN in the laboratory: An interview with Dr. Joe Rutledge and Joanne Simpson. *Laboratory Errors and Patient Safety*, *2*(5), 1–8.

AORN Foundation. (2007). *Human factors in health care tool kit: Team training using human factors to enhance patient safety*. Retrieved from http://www.aorn.org/PracticeResources/ToolKits/HumanFactorsInHealthCareToolKit/.

Blecher, M. (1997). Accident scenes. *Hospital & Health Networks 71*(10), 46–48.

Bosk, C., Dixon-Woods, M., Goeschel, C., & Pronovost, P. (2009). Reality check for checklists. *Lancet, 374*(9688), 444–445.

Brach, C., Lenfestey, N., Roussel, A., Amoozegar, J., & Sorensen, A. (2008). *Will it work here? A decisionmaker's guide to adopting innovations.* Prepared by RTI International under Contract No. 233–02–0090. Agency for Healthcare Research and Quality (AHRQ) Publication No. 08–0051. Rockville, MD: AHRQ.

Campbell, G., & Facchinetti, N. (1998). Using process control charts to monitor dispensing and checking errors. *American Journal of Health-System Pharmacists, 55*(9), 946–952.

Chappell, H. W., Dickey, C., & DeLetter, M. (1997). The use of medication dispensers in residential care homes. *Family and Community Health, 20*(10), 10.

Clark, S. L., Belfort, M. A., Byrum, S. L., Meyers, J. A., & Perlin, J. B. (2008). Improved outcomes, fewer cesarean deliveries, and reduced litigation: results of a new paradigm in patient safety. *American Journal of Obstetrics and Gynecology, 199*(2), 105.e1–105.e7.

Cooper, J., & Gaba, D. (2002). No myth: Anesthesia is a model for addressing patient safety (editorial). *Anesthesiology, 97*(6), 1335–1337.

Croteau, R. J. (Ed.). (2010). *Root cause analysis in health care: Tools and techniques* (4th ed.). Oakbrook Terrace, IL: Joint Commission Resources.

Davidoff, F. (2010). Checklists and guidelines: Imaging techniques for visualizing what to do. *Journal of the American Medical Association, 304*(2), 206–207.

Dekker, S. (2006). *The field guide to understanding human error.* Hants, UK: Ashgate.

Deming, W. E. (1982). *Out of the crisis.* Cambridge, MA: MIT Press.

Fagerhaugh, S., Strauss, A., Suczek, B., & Wiener, C. (1987). *Hazards in hospital care: Ensuring patient safety.* San Francisco: Jossey-Bass.

Furman, C., & Caplan, R. (2007). Applying the Toyota Production System: Using a patient safety alert system to reduce error. *Joint Commission Journal on Quality and Patient Safety, 33*(7), 376–386.

Grasha, A. F., & Schelle, K. (2001). Psychosocial factors, workload, and risk of human error in a simulated pharmacy dispensing task. *Perceptual and Motor Skills, 92*, 53–71. Retrieved from http://pharmsafety.org/extras/PsychWrkload.pdf.

Grimshaw, J. M., & Russell, I. T. (1993). Effect of clinical guidelines on medical practice: a systematic review of rigorous evaluations. *Lancet, 342*(8883), 317–322.

Grout, J. R. (2007). *Mistake-proofing the design of health care processes.* Washington, DC: Agency for Healthcare Research and Quality.

Hendrick, K. M., & Benner, L. (1987). *Investigating accidents with STEP.* New York: Marcel Dekker.

Hignett, S., & Masud, T. (2006). A review of environmental hazards associated with in-patient falls. *Ergonomics, 49*(5–6), 605–616.

Hines, S., Luna, K., Lofthus, J., et al. (2008, April). *Becoming a high reliability organization: Operational advice for hospital leaders.* (Prepared by the Lewin Group under Contract No. 290–04–0011.) AHRQ Publication No. 08–0022. Rockville, MD: Agency for Healthcare Research and Quality. April 2008. Retrieved from http://www.ahrq.gov/qual/hroadvice/hroadvice.pdf.

Institute for Safe Medication Practices. (2003). The virtues of independent double checks—they really are worth your time! *ISMP Safety Alert! 8*(5), 1.

Institute of Medicine. (1999). *To err is human: Building a safer health system.* Washington, DC: National Academy Press.

Institute of Medicine. (2004). *Keeping patients safe: Transforming the work environment of nurses.* Washington, DC: National Academy Press.

Jha, A. K., Duncan, B. W., & Bates, D. W. (2001). Simulator-based training and patient safety. In Making health care safer: A critical analysis of patient safety practices. Evidence Report/Technology Assessment, No. 43. AHRQ Publication No. 01-E058, July 2001. Agency for Healthcare Research and Quality, Rockville, MD. Retrieved from http://www.ahrq.gov/clinic/ptsafety/.

Johnson, W. G. (1985). *Accident/incident investigation manual* (2nd ed.), DOE/SSDC-45/27. Washington, DC: U.S. Department of Energy.

Joint Commission Resources. (2008). *Handoff communication: Toolkit for implementing the NPSG.* Oak Brook Terrace, IL: Joint Commission Resources.

Kaplan S., Greenfield S., & Ware, J. E. (1989). Assessing the effects of physician-patient interactions on the outcomes of chronic disease. *Medical Care, 27*(Suppl), S110–S127.

Karsh, B. T., Holden, R. J., Alper, S. J., & Or, C. K. L. (2006). A human factors engineering paradigm for patient safety: Designing to support the performance of the healthcare professional. *Quality and Safety in Health Care, 5*(Suppl I), 59–65.

Li, G., Warner, M., Lang, B., Huang, L., & Sun, L. (2009). Epidemiology of anesthesia-related mortality in the United States, 1999–2005. *Anesthesiology, 110*(4), 759–765.

Luria, J. W., Muething, S. E., Schoettker, P. J., & Kotagal, U. R. (2006). Reliability science and patient safety. *Pediatric Clinics of North America, 53*(6), 1121–1133.

Marcario, A., Morris, S., & Morris, D., (2006). Initial clinical evaluation of a handheld device for detecting retained surgical gauze sponges using radiofrequency identification technology. *Archives of Surgery, 141*(7), 659–662.

Meisel, S. (1998, December 9). *Reducing adverse drug events.* Conference presentation, National Forum on Quality Improvement in Health Care, Orlando, FL.

Meisel, Z. (2005, November 5). Re: Ding-a-ling-a-ling: Ambulances can be dangerous places [Online forum comment]. Retrieved from http://www.slate.com/id/2129684/.

Norman, D. A. (1988). *The design of everyday things.* London: MIT Press.

Nygaard, A., Nelson, A. S., Pick, A., Danekas, P., Massoomi, F., Thielsen, J., & Ryschon, K. (2009). Inter-rater reliability in the evaluation of a thrombosis risk assessment tool. *Hospital Pharmacy, 44*(12), 1089–1094.

Pathman, D. E., Konard, T. R., Freed, G. L., Freeman, V. A., & Koch, G. G. (1996). The awareness-to-adherence model of the steps to clinical guideline compliance. The case of pediatric vaccine recommendations. *Medical Care 34*(9), 873–889.

Patterson, P. (1998). Fine levied after hysterectomy death. *OR Manager 14*(12), 6.

Patterson, E., Woods, D., Cook, R., & Render, M. (2007). Collaborative cross-checking to enhance resilience. *Cognition, Technology and Work, 9*(3), 155–162.

Pesanka, D., Greenhouse, P., Rack, L., Delucia, G., Perret, R., Scholle, C., Johnson, M., & Janov, C. (2009). Ticket to ride: Reducing handoff risk during hospital patient transport. *Journal of Nursing Care Quality, 24*(2), 109–115.

Peters, E., Slovic, P., Hibbard, J. H., & Tusler, M. (2006). Why worry? Worry, risk perceptions, and willingness to act to reduce medical errors. *Journal of Health Psychology, 25*(2), 144–152.

Plews-Ogan, M., Nadkami, M., Forren, S., Leon, D., White, D., Marineau, D., Shorling, J., & Schectman, J. (2004). Patient safety in the ambulatory setting: A clinician-based approach. *Journal of General Internal Medicine, 19*(7), 719–725.

Prielipp, R. C., Lewis, K., & Morell, R. C. (1998). Ventilator failure in the ICU: Déjà vu all over again. *Anesthesia Patient Safety Foundation Newsletter, 13*(3). Retrieved from http://www.apsf.org/resource_center/newsletter/1998/fall/09vent.html.

Pronovost, P., Needham, D., Berenholtz, S., Sinopoli, D., Chu, H., Cosgrove, S., Sexton, B., & Goeschel, C. (2006). An intervention to decrease catheter-related bloodstream infections in the ICU. *New England Journal of Medicine, 355*(26), 2725–2732.

Ray, L. (2009). Patient safety: A "ticket to ride" protects patients off the unit. *Nursing 2009, 39*(5), 57–58.

Reason, J. T. (1997). *Managing the risks of organizational accidents.* Aldershot, UK: Ashgate.

Reason, J. T. (2008). *The human contribution: Unsafe acts, accidents and heroic recoveries.* Aldershot, UK: Ashgate.

Rogers, A. E., Hwang, W. T., Scott, L. D., Aiken, L. H., & Dinges, D. F. (2004). The working hours of hospital staff nurses and patient safety. *Health Affairs, 23*(4), 202–212.

Sawyer, D. (1996). *Do it by design: An introduction to human factors in medical devices.* Washington, DC: Center for Devices and Radiological Health, Food and Drug Administration.

Scott, L. D., Rogers, A. E., Hwang, W. T., & Zhang, Y. (2006). Effects of critical care nurses' work hours on vigilance and patients' safety. *American Journal of Critical Care, 15*(1), 30–37.

Shepherd, M. (2004). A systems approach to medical device safety. In J. Dyro (Ed.). *Handbook of Clinical Engineering* (pp. 246–249). The Netherlands: Elsevier.

Simpson, A., Lamb, S., Roberts, P., Gardner, T., & Grimley-Evans, J. (2004). Does the type of flooring affect the risk of hip fracture? *Age and Ageing, 33*(3), 242–246.

Spath, P. L. (2006). Running on empty. *For the Record, 18*(10), 30–32.

Spath, P. L. (2008). *Engaging patients as safety partners: A guide for reducing errors and improving satisfaction.* Chicago: AHA Health Forum.

Stewart, M., Brown, J. B., Donner, A., McWhinney, I. R., Oates, J., & Westin, W. W. W. (2000). The impact of patient-centered care on patient outcomes. *Journal of Family Practices, 49*(9), 796–804.

Storri, J., & Hookway, J. (2005). Preventing infection in hospital—should patient involvement be central to current hand hygiene strategies? *Clinical Governance Bulletin, 5*(5), 6–8.

The Joint Commission. (1998). Medication error prevention—potassium chloride. *Sentinel Event Alert,* Issue 1. Oakbrook Terrace, IL: The Joint Commission.

The Joint Commission. (2006). Improving handoff communications: Meeting National Patient Safety Goal 2E. *Joint Commission Perspectives, 6*(8), 9–15.

The Joint Commission. (2010, January 28). Facts about Speak Up™ initiatives. Retrieved from http://www.jointcommission.org/GeneralPublic/Speak+Up/about_speakup htm

Thomas, M. B. (2005). Study examines working hours and feelings of fatigue by reported nurses. *Texas Board of Nursing Bulletin, 36*(4), 2–3.

Thomsen, H. S., & Bush, W. H., Jr. (1998). Adverse effects of contrast media: Incidence, prevention, and treatment. *Drug Safety, 19*(10), 313–324.

Tucker, A. L., & Edmondson, A. C. (2003). Why hospitals don't learn from failures: Organizational and psychological dynamics that inhibit system change. *California Management Review, 45*(2), 55–72.

United States Pharmacopoeia. (1996). USP quality review: intravenous potassium predicament. Issue 56. Bethesda, MD: U.S. Pharmacopoeia Convention.

Van Cott, H. (1994). Human errors: Their causes and reduction. In Bogner, S. (Ed.) *Human error in medicine*. Mahwah, NJ: Erlbaum.

Wenz, B., Mercuriali, F., & AuBuchon, J. P. (1997). Practice methods to improve transfusion safety by using novel blood unit and patient identification systems. *American Journal of Clinical Pathology*, *107*(4; Suppl 1), S12–S16.

West, J. C. (2009). Ticket to ride: How useful is this new handoff tool? *Journal of Healthcare Risk Management*, *29*(1), 28–33.

Wolosin, R. J., Vercler, L., & Matthews, J. L. (2006). Am I safe here? Improving patients' perceptions of safety in hospitals. *Journal of Nursing Care Quality*, *21*(1), 30–38.

Wu, A. W., Lipshutz, A. K. M., & Pronovost, P. J. (2008). Effectiveness and efficiency of root cause analysis in medicine. *Journal of the American Medical Association*, *299*(6), 685–687.

CHAPTER 12

IMPROVE PATIENT SAFETY WITH LEAN TECHNIQUES

Danielle Lavallee

LEARNING OBJECTIVES

- Describe the lean philosophy and core concepts
- Apply lean improvement tools to create safer health care processes
- Identify common mistake-proofing techniques
- Recognize the role of senior leaders in supporting a lean organization

"No new idea springs full-blown from a void. Rather, new ideas emerge from a set of conditions in which old ideas no longer seem to work" (Womack, Jones, & Roos, 2007). This observation describes the evolution of the Toyota Production System in the Japanese automotive industry in the 1950s. The statement also captures the essence of challenges facing the U.S. health care system. We are finding that old ideas of health care delivery are no longer effective in meeting today's safety and quality expectations. Health care organizations must adopt new delivery principles and practices.

In mid-1980 a research team at the Massachusetts Institute of Technology, led by James Womack and Daniel Jones, explored manufacturing processes in the automotive industry. Toyota Motor Company stood apart from other automotive competitors. Not only did Toyota make automobiles with fewer defects than other manufacturers, their production process required less on-hand inventory, a smaller amount of capital investment, and fewer suppliers. In addition, the company was perfectly meeting customer demand. The researchers coined the phrase *lean manufacturing* to describe the unique attributes of the

Toyota Production System. Simply put, Toyota was able to provide a customer-focused product while using fewer resources (Womack et al., 2007).

Since introduction of lean manufacturing concepts, industries outside of automotive production—including health care organizations—have begun to implement lean philosophies and methodologies (Feinstein, Grunden, & Harrison, 2002; Sirio et al., 2003; Nelson-Peterson & Leppa, 2007). The influx of new process improvement methods comes at a critical time for the health care industry as quality and patient safety is being questioned (Institute of Medicine, 1999). Increasing complexity and disjointed health care systems are often cited as root causes for medical errors and poor quality (Savary & Crawford-Mason, 2006). Lean methods promote simple and standardized processes with less chance for mistakes. Organizations adopting lean philosophies create a culture for continual assessment and improvement of patient services. Becoming a lean organization is a long-term commitment to continual evaluation and improvement of processes within the health care system.

This chapter provides an overview of lean principles and describes methods for successfully incorporating these principles into the health care culture to enable reduction of errors. Examples of how lean methods have been used to reduce medical errors and create safer systems are described.

Going Lean

Although lean methods originated in manufacturing, application of these methods spans all industries. Lean philosophy promotes continual pursuit of process improvements to better meet customer needs. For health care, lean philosophy implies continuous pursuit of optimal patient care. Organizations adopting a lean approach strive to deliver the best possible patient-focused care. This is achieved by removing process steps that do not provide direct value to the patient or, in many cases, to the care provider. Lean implementation requires a systems perspective in which current processes and practices are evaluated from the patient viewpoint. The systems perspective helps to ensure continuous flow of information and patients throughout the entire continuum of care. The objective is to create health care delivery processes that:

- Are simple and direct
- Are user-friendly
- Make problems obvious
- Provide a rewarding working environment for staff

- Encourage immediate problem resolution

- Are waste free

- Exceed patient expectations

The initial step for improving a health care process is to understand what patients value most about the process. Processes are viewed from this customers' perspective when evaluating current practice. A lean organization is continuously striving to enhance patient value-added processes by eliminating wasteful steps—tasks that do not benefit patients. Categories of waste and examples from the hospital setting are listed in Table 12.1.

Consider the following process steps illustrating a typical patient visit to a diagnostic laboratory service for blood tests.

1. Patient presents to reception and signs in.

2. Patient takes a seat and waits to be called.

3. Receptionist calls patient to registration.

4. Patient registers for appointment, updates insurance and personal information as needed.

Table 12.1   Categories of Waste and Hospital Examples

Type of Waste	Examples in a Hospital Setting
Delays	Waiting for bed assignments, waiting for treatments, waiting for medications, waiting for orders, waiting for test results
Overprocessing	Excessive paperwork and documentation, requesting unnecessary lab tests, use of intravenous medications in place of oral medications
Inventory	Patient records waiting for physician signatures, excess medication in stock, storage of old or outdated equipment, surplus supplies kept "just in case"
Transportation	Excess movement of patients, transportation of labs, transportation of medications
Motion	Searching for patient records, looking for medications, providing care to patients not located in close proximity
Overproduction	Mixing intravenous medications in anticipation of need, completing paperwork in anticipation of admissions
Defects	Medication errors, lost specimens, preventable patient falls and infections, inaccurate labeling of test results, failure to recognize deterioration of patient's condition

5. Patient reseated and waits for laboratory technician.

6. Laboratory technician calls patient to specimen collection room.

7. Patient has blood drawn.

8. Patient leaves the laboratory.

In this example the patient is kept waiting at many of the process steps. Delays have become a normal and accepted part of health care delivery (why else would we have created waiting rooms?). Yet excessive waiting is the least valued aspect of health care from the patient perspective. In the laboratory testing example, several wasteful delays are apparent. The improvement team evaluating this process would identify the root cause of delays and make process changes intended to provide continuous flow of patients and information through the laboratory experience.

Process errors, or defects, are also considered waste. Errors that occur during health care delivery are not valued by patients. Although most mistakes are not life-threatening, many require tasks be redone to produce desired results. For instance, if the laboratory technician uses the wrong technique when drawing a patient's blood, the patient will experience the bother of a return trip to the laboratory. If the error is avoided, the patient is not inconvenienced and employees spend less of their time fixing mistakes. A lean health care process is a safer and more satisfying experience for everyone involved.

Building Lean Processes

Three core concepts are the basis of the lean philosophy: **standard work**, **user-friendliness**, and **unobstructed throughput**. By integrating these core concepts into health care delivery, organizations can provide patient care when it is needed and in the quantity needed. In addition, errors in the care delivery system become obvious so that they can be addressed and corrected in real time.

Standard Work

Standard work is a critical component of error-free patient care. Standard work is a process that has been broken down into a series of clearly defined tasks and is performed the same way every time by each individual involved in the process (Kenney, 2008). Standardization reduces the likelihood of errors by ensuring that specific steps are consistently followed in the delivery of care. When errors do occur, they become more obvious once the process is standardized. For instance, an example of standard work is the "Five Rights" of medication administration. In this process, prior to administering a medication the nurse confirms the patient's identification, the correctness of the medication to be given, the administration route and timing, and the medication dose. When this standard work is followed, errors that may have occurred upstream in the process can be immediately recognized and corrected to prevent patient harm.

In addition to making problems more obvious, standardization creates a foundation for future process improvements. Consistent performance of a process allows for more precise evaluation of practices and identification of improvement opportunities. It is impossible to accurately understand current practices and process risks when the people involved have their own unique way of doing the work. In addition, when a process is not standardized it is difficult to identify changes that will improve the efficiency or safety of the process. Furthermore, lack of standardization complicates staff training and everyone's perception of how work is to be done.

User-Friendliness

To maintain standard work, processes must be easy for people to carry out. User-friendly processes allow for patient care to be provided when it is needed in the quantity necessary every time. To achieve this, processes must be simple and direct and supplies for completing tasks must be readily available. When tasks are too complex or supplies unavailable, staff members may develop work-arounds to make the job more user-friendly. These work-arounds can lead to errors. Medication and supply "stashes" created by nurses to ensure that needed materials are close at hand are common work-arounds that cause unsafe patient care situations (Pape, 2006).

Unobstructed Throughput

The third core lean concept, unobstructed throughput, is a health care delivery process free of bottlenecks. This is achieved when each process step is balanced to create a continuous flow from one task to the next. When process constraints cause an imbalance, workflow can be affected such that people on one end of the process are operating above capacity, creating queues of patients, while the people on the other end of the process are operating below capacity. Consider, for example, an outpatient anticoagulation clinic that monitors patients on anti-coagulation therapy. The process steps must be balanced to ensure continuous flow of patients to avoid unnecessary waiting by patients and clinical staff. If the main steps to the process include (1) patient registration, (2) lab draws by a phlebotomist, (3) consultation with a clinician, and (4) checkout, it will be necessary to ensure that no constraints occur or are minimized. In many situations all services may be conducted within the same physical space. Imagine, however, if phlebotomy services were on a different floor in the building. Once registered, patients would be required to leave the clinic area and go to another location for blood tests and then return to the clinic area to see the clinician. This situation could easily cause a bottleneck of patients waiting for blood work and clinicians waiting for patients. In addition to being an inefficient process, this constraint could increase the risk of errors if the phlebotomist is rushing to get patients' lab work completed. Further, if the bottleneck in the laboratory causes patients to be late for their clinic appointment, their visit with the clinical team may be cut short.

Process constraints are identified by mapping out the entire process from a systems perspective. This process map, known as a value stream, highlights areas where breakdowns occur and problems exist. Constraints in the process are targeted for elimination or for improvement. In the preceding example, the constraint could be eliminated by adding a phlebotomist to the clinical team in the clinic or through adoption of point-of-care diagnostic blood testing devices. This would eliminate the process delay caused by patients traveling to a different area for laboratory services.

Though the lean philosophy is most often associated with efficiency improvements and reduction of production costs, application of the core concepts also has a significant impact on patient safety. By using lean process improvement tools, described in the next section, health care organizations can lessen the risk of patient care mistakes.

Lean Improvement Tools

Creating standardized work processes that are user-friendly and focused on patient value is a health care imperative. This section details specific tools used in lean organizations to continuously improve the quality and safety of patient care. Commonly used lean tools to be described include:

- 5S methodology
- Visual controls
- Kanbans
- Mistake-proofing

These tools are used to standardize work processes and create a user-friendly work environment that provides unobstructed process throughput.

5S Methodology

Clutter, lack of space, and inability to find needed supplies are just a few issues that plague the health care system. Though seemingly trivial, these concerns can be the root cause of process errors and defects. Implementation of **5S**, a systematic methodology for organizing standard work, provides a solid foundation for an error-free patient care environment. Listed in Table 12.2 are the Japanese words denoting the five implementation phases of this process improvement tool: *Seri* (Organize), *Seiton* (Orderliness), *Seiso* (Cleanliness), *Seiketsu* (Standardize), and *Shitsuki* (Discipline). 5S is a philosophy and a way of organizing and managing the workspace by eliminating waste (Hirano, 1995). To maintain the 5S acronym in the English translation, the five phases are often referred to as: Sort, Straighten, Scrub, Standardize, and Sustain (Zidel, 2006).

Execution of 5S (sometimes called a 5S event) begins with application of the first S, *seri* (sort). At this step people identify which items in the workplace are necessary. Unnecessary items are either disposed of or relocated. This step is in response to the common practice that when new supplies or technology are adopted, outdated or broken materials are stored nearby in case they are needed in the future. The results of this practice are evident—workplace closets and drawers filled with old computer equipment, overstocked blood pressure cuffs, obsolete labels, outdated patient education materials and forms, out-of-date reference manuals and the like. This practice leads to workplace crowding and makes it difficult for people to identify items currently in use. Such complexity perpetuates an environment prone to errors.

In applying *seri*, staff is involved in selecting items that may no longer need to be stored in or near the work area. These items are systematically tagged and placed in a holding zone for staff comment prior to the items being removed or discarded. Uniform tags are used in this sorting step to list pertinent item

Table 12.2 Five Phases of the 5S Lean Improvement Tool

Japanese	English	Translation
Seri	Sort	Get rid of what you don't need
Seiton	Straighten	Organize what is kept
Seiso	Scrub	Clean the area
Seiketsu	Standardize	Establish procedures
Shitsuki	Sustain	Maintain improvements

FIGURE 12.1   Equipment Red Tag for 5S Exercise

Department/Unit: **Sterile Processing**	Tag Number: **00001**

Category (Check One)	**X** Equipment ☐ Office Materials ☐ Medication ☐ Measuring Instrument ☐ Books ☐ Supplies ☐ Patient Items ☐ Furniture ☐ Other

Tag Date: **Dec. 1, 2008**   Tagged By: **D. Smith**

Classification (Check one)   ☐ Hazardous   **X** Non Hazardous

Item Name: **Supply Cart**
 Fixed Asset Code: Serial #

Quantity: Value: $

Reason Tagged (Check one)   ☐ Not Needed   ☐Beyond Expiration Date   ☐ Borrowed
 ☐Use unknown ☐ Not used in 6 mo   ☐Not used on unit **X** Defective Equipment

Disposition by: Authorized persons name: **M. Brown**   Dept: **Operative Services**

Disposition by: (Check one)   ☐ Discard   ☐ Move to storage   ☐ Return to Lender
 ☐ Use   **X** Repair   ☐Replace   ☐Move to Holding Area   ☐ Other.

Department: **Operative Services**   **Tag Locator**   Tag #: **00001**

information (for example, location found, frequency of use, manufacturer or item number and cost). In Figure 12.1 is an example of a tag that would be placed on an item during the sorting phase.

Once the sorting and tagging phase is complete, all employees using the workspace are given an opportunity to recommend the disposition for each item. Items used routinely should be kept accessible within the immediate work area. Items deemed necessary but used infrequently should be moved away from the primary workspace but in an accessible location. Items no longer needed should be removed from the work area. These items can either be discarded, relocated to another area that uses the item, or donated to another organization. After employees have provided input, items are catalogued and final disposition is approved by a manager with appropriate authority.

The second S, *seiton* (straighten), focuses on organizing those items judged to be retained in the workspace. Creating standard homes for all items ensures that staff members will be able to quickly find what they need. When supplies do not have a defined home people expend valuable time searching for needed patient care items (McLaughlin, 2003). This situation can be a safety concern if nurses and physicians cannot quickly find equipment and supplies to care for a patient experiencing a cardiac arrest. All routinely used items and those needed for emergency situations should have standard homes. Ideally, these standard homes can be made as consistent as possible from unit to unit. Variations in workspace layout and equipment storage in different patient care units create an unsafe condition for employees working in more than one unit. Visual controls and kanbans, discussed later in this section, can make it easier for people to see where items are stored in the various work areas.

When creating standard homes for items kept in the workspace, the rule of thumb is that a newcomer to the area should be able to, within 30 seconds, locate what they need to do a task. This goal can be achieved through the use of reference guides for supplies, appropriate labeling and signage. Straightening the workspace helps staff obtain the equipment and supplies required to efficiently complete a job.

Once only needed items are stored in the work area and these items have standard homes, the third S, *seiso* (scrub), is completed. This involves cleaning the workspace and performing other needed scrubbing such as painting and repairs. Health care delivery areas that are cluttered, dusty, or in disrepair are not valued by patients. Furthermore, these work environments negatively affect staff morale.

The fourth S, *seiketsu* (standardize), promotes the development of procedures for securing the improvements made during the first three steps. Post pictures of the original work area and pictures of how it looks after completing the first three steps to show employees how the space is to be maintained. Communicate to staff expectations for keeping the environment in an orderly and clean condition. People should be accountable for returning items to designated homes and following procedures for disposing of unnecessary items to prevent reappearance of clutter.

Imagine what would happen if no standard procedure existed for stocking materials in patient exam rooms. It would be unclear as to what items are routinely stocked in the room, where items are stored, and how often items need replenishing. Developing, communicating, and expecting standard work be followed by everyone (support staff, nurses, physicians, and so on) reduces the risk of unsafe surprises—such as needed supplies not being readily available in an emergency situation. Managers and supervisors assume an important role in promoting standard work. If people slip back into their own unique way of doing things, this behavior must be investigated immediately to determine the cause and formulate corrective actions.

Finally the fifth S, *shitsuki* (sustain), calls for maintaining over time the improvements gained from the 5S exercise. This is the most challenging phase of 5S as it requires a high level of commitment and discipline from all levels in the organization. Each individual must be responsible for working with others in the unit to keep the workplace uncluttered and follow standard work practices. It is recommended that managers periodically schedule time for a quick 5S exercise to help sustain and further improve workflow and the workspace. Over time, maintaining an organized and clean environment will become part of the work culture.

The 5S methodology is not simply a housekeeping function. The health care work environment is shared by multiple professionals who are constantly challenged to provide safe and efficient patient care in cluttered, complex, and disorganized work areas. The 5S process is a systematic method for sorting, straightening, scrubbing, standardizing, and sustaining a better working environment for everyone. An organized and visually presentable workspace improves efficiency, reduces errors, boosts staff morale, and presents a positive image to patients.

Visual Controls

A **visual control** is a simple and direct nonverbal method for relaying information to others. Visual controls are often developed as part of 5S events to organize workflow. Visual controls allow staff to understand the current situation, understand the process, or recognize when something is out of place. Examples of visual controls in hospitals include signs in patient rooms that convey information such as the patient's dietary status (nothing-by-mouth or liquid-only diet), digital control boards in emergency rooms indicating tests and medications ordered for patients, and colored patient wrist bands that alert staff to the patient's fall risk or allergies. These controls create a visual environment that helps reduce the chance for workplace errors. When developed, visual controls should be:

- Self-explaining: provide visual understanding of the current situation

- Self-ordering: provide visual understanding of the work process

- Self-regulating: provide information on the pace of work

- Self-improving: provide information when there is an abnormality

An example of a visual control is shown in Figure 12.2. This form was developed at Natchaug Hospital, Mansfield Center, Connecticut, to provide a visual aid for clinical staff managing patients in a behavioral health hospital. Patient care in this environment involves a multidisciplinary approach that includes specific standard tasks to be done by each discipline for all patients. Prior to the lean improvement project, a version of this form was used by the unit clerk to audit whether required tasks had been completed by the appropriate staff member. The audit process was time-consuming and there was no clearly defined process for alerting clinical staff to missing documentation or interventions.

FIGURE 12.2   Visual Aid for Clinical Staff Managing Behavioral Health Patient

Natchaug Hospital
HARTFORD HEALTHCARE

Required Documentation Sign-off

Name: _____
ID#: _____

Initial and Date in box when completed

	ALL DOCUMENTATION REQUIRES AUTHENTICATION WITH DATE AND TIME TO BE COMPLETE										
MD	Admitting Psychiatric Evaluation completed & signed										
	Attending Psychiatric Evaluation completed & signed										
	Admission Labs reviewed and initialed										
	Medication Consent form signed										
	AIMS form completed										
	MTP completed & signed-off within **72 hrs of admission**										
	TPU completed & signed-off **at least every 7 days**										
	Discharge summary dictated				Discharge summary signed						
RN	Initial Plan of Care completed & signed										
	Nursing Assessment completed & signed										
	Allergies identified & documented										
	MTP completed & signed-off within **72 hrs of admission**										
	TPU completed & signed-off **at least every 7 days**										
MHW	MHW Admission Checklist										
	Discharge checklist										
Therapist	Psychosocial Evaluation completed & signed										
	Discharge contact sheet started										
	MTP completed & signed-off within **72 hrs of admission**										
	TPU completed & signed-off **at least every 7 days**										
CRS	MTP completed & signed-off within **72 hrs of admission**										
	TPU completed & signed-off **at least every 7 days**										
Psych Testing	**Psychiatric Testing Sent for Scoring**										
	Received Scoring										

Natchaug Hospital, Mansfield Center, CT. Adapted with permission
Abbreviation key:
TPU: Treatment plan update
MHW: Mental health worker
MTP: Master Treatment plan
AIMs: Abnormal Involuntary Movement Scale Examination

During the improvement project (sometimes called a lean event), the team redesigned the audit form to become a worksheet for clinical staff to use in tracking completion of the patient care requirements. An initial worksheet was created by the improvement team and then pilot tested by frontline staff members, whose feedback helped to shape the final version.

This worksheet now serves as a real-time visual reminder of the specific care tasks that must be done prior to a patient's discharge. It is self-ordering in that each member of the clinical team understands what work needs to be completed at any given time. It is self-explaining in that it shows which tasks need to be completed and, for certain time-sensitive tasks, when the task needs to be completed. Finally, it is self-improving as the worksheet is used during group therapy sessions to discuss how best to ensure complete and timely patient care when there appears to be an issue with incomplete tasks. The form is located at the front of every patient record and provides the clinical staff with a visual control of the patient's progress during the hospital stay. With a quick glance at the worksheet, clinicians can immediately identify required tasks that have yet to be completed. Now missing documentation or interventions are addressed in real-time by clinical staff.

Kanbans

An additional tool utilized during 5S, and similar in nature to visual controls, are kanbans. **Kanban** is the Japanese word for sign board. A kanban is a special type of visual control used to indicate the need for movement of materials or patients through a specific process. For example, a sign outside of the x-ray room that indicates when the room is occupied or empty is a kanban. In addition, kanbans are often used for inventory management to point out when an item needs to be restocked. An example of a kanban used in inventory management is illustrated in Figure 12.3. The kanban card presented in the example would hang on the exterior of the appropriate bin in a supply bin. It provides visual and detailed information on the product to be ordered, the quantity needed and the time frame in which it will be required given the inventory amount kept on hand. For kanbans to be effective in the workplace they must be located in a visible space, readily understood by those involved in the process, and be part of the standard work.

Mistake-Proofing

Mistake-proofing is also known as **Poka-Yoke**, a term derived from two Japanese words: *yokeru* (to avoid) and *poka* (mistake). It is important to distinguish

FIGURE 12.3 Kanban Card for Inventory Control

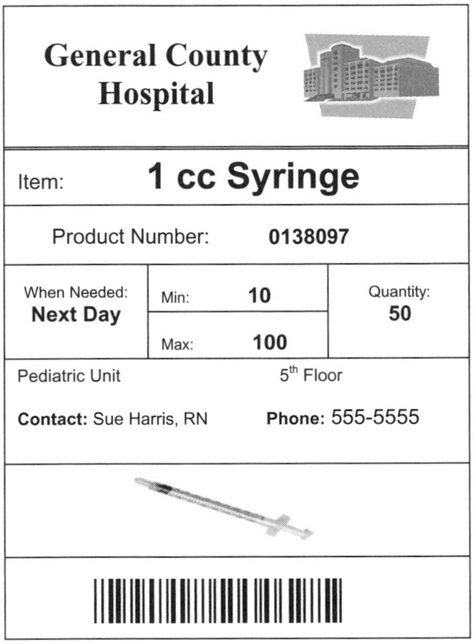

General County Hospital

| Item: | **1 cc Syringe** |

| Product Number: | **0138097** |

| When Needed: **Next Day** | Min: **10** | Quantity: **50** |
| | Max: **100** | |

Pediatric Unit   5th Floor

Contact: Sue Harris, RN   **Phone:** 555-5555

between mistakes and defects. Mistakes are defined by the Institute of Medicine as "failure of a planned action to be completed as intended or the use of a wrong plan to achieve an aim" (Institute of Medicine, 1999). Defects are the *outcome* of a mistake. For example, it is a mistake to allow a patient known to be at high risk of falling to walk without proper footwear. This mistake could cause a defect—a harmful fall.

Mistake-proofing is a method or device which prevents mistakes, allows for detection of mistakes so that they can be corrected, or reduces the harm that results from a mistake. Mistake-proofing exercises should be part of the organization's approach to improving process safety. The steps for mistake-proofing are as follows:

1. Define the mistake to be prevented

2. Identify red flags which may be present during the error

3. Determine the root cause of the mistake

4. Generate ideas to prevent the mistake from occurring

5. Develop a device or method to prevent the mistake from occurring in the future

In the first step the mistake to be prevented is clearly defined. During this step, the improvement team seeks to answer a series of questions: When does the mistake occur? How often has the mistake occurred? How is the mistake detected? What circumstances cause the mistake? Why did the mistake occur? Throughout this questioning, the team must keep an open mind and avoid making assumptions. Evidence to support the answers should be collected and evaluated in an unbiased manner.

The next step is to identify any **red flags** or warning signals that may be present when the mistake occurs. These situations heighten the risk of a mistake. If the same mistake has occurred more than once, the team can look for similarities between the events to see if common warning signal situations are evident. The following list includes several situations that often contribute to mistake-prone conditions (McClanahan, Goodwin, & Houser, 2000; Savary & Crawford-Mason, 2006; Zidel, 2006):

- Multiple process steps

- Similarity in product names or appearance

- High workload

- Insufficient staffing

- Infrequent performance of the tasks

- Unfamiliarity with practices or procedures

- Over-familiarity (complacency) from frequent task repetition

- Lack of or ineffective work standards

- Equipment changes

- Environmental conditions (for example, poor lighting, distractions, clutter)

In some circumstances, more than one red flag situation may exist. For example, during the summer months new physician residents begin practicing in the hospital. In the initial weeks on the job, residents are in a new and different environment. They are learning hospital procedures in addition to becoming comfortable with clinical responsibilities. When high patient volume occurs, residents are more likely to make mistakes due to the combination of inexperience and feeling overwhelmed with patient care duties. In this example, both unfamiliarity with procedures and high workload would be considered warning signals. All possible "red flags" should be identified and assessed during the mistake-proofing exercise.

The third step of mistake-proofing is to investigate the root cause of the mistake. Several techniques may be used to perform this investigation: root cause analysis, failure mode and effect analysis, 5-Whys, and cause and effect analysis. Some of these techniques are described in other chapters in this book. Regardless of the investigation model chosen by the team, it is imperative that information used to uncover the root cause of the mistake is current, complete, and accurate. The investigation results serve as the basis for the next step—identify how to prevent the mistake from occurring in the future.

The fourth step, generating ideas, is focused on identifying methods or devices that will prevent the mistake from happening. Often brainstorming sessions with improvement team members are the best way to generate lots of ideas. Once all mistake-proofing suggestions have been voiced, the team selects those ideas most likely to be successful at preventing the mistake or making it easier to detect and correct.

The fifth and final step in mistake-proofing is creation of the device or method that will detect or prevent the mistake from occurring. The solution does not need to be complex or expensive. A simple example of mistake-proofing is the surgeon's initial placed on the correct operative site of his patient. In Exhibit 12.1 is a case study illustrating a mistake-proofing exercise in perioperative services.

Applying Lean Tools

Lean improvement tools can be applied as needed during any patient safety improvement initiative. In addition some health care organizations sponsor lean or "kaizen" events. **_Kaizen_** is the Japanese word for continuous and incremental improvement. These improvement projects are traditionally conducted over a period of four to five days with the goal of achieving rapid change (Smith, 2003; Zidel, 2006). These initiatives provide an opportunity for people to intensely focus on a specific process needing redesign.

During a kaizen event, an interdisciplinary team is assembled to evaluate the targeted process, identify where improvements can be made, and initiate process redesign steps. Over the course of this short initiative, the team:

● Evaluates the current situation

● Identifies areas of opportunity

EXHIBIT 12.1

MISTAKE-PROOFING CASE STUDY IN PERIOPERATIVE SERVICES

The central decontamination department in a 500+ bed hospital noted an increase in damaged and dulled surgical instrumentation. Not only did this problem have cost implications, it also heightened the risk of damaged instruments being inadvertently included in sterilized surgical kits. If this occurred, the situation could be a safety concern for surgical patients. A team comprised of perioperative service clinicians and staff from the decontamination department came together to assess and improve the processing of surgical equipment.

First the team clearly defined the mistake that was to be prevented: damaged or dull surgical instrumentation. Next the team sought to determine the root cause and develop a solution to mistake-proof the instrumentation decontamination process. Steps in this process were identified as:

1. Surgical trays are received in decontamination following surgical procedures

2. Gross matter is removed from surgical instrumentation

3. Surgical instrumentation is stacked in trays and trays are sent through decontamination wash machines

4. Surgical trays are pulled from washers and stacked on shelving units

5. Surgical trays are counted and reassembled by decontamination staff

6. Surgical trays are wrapped and placed in sterilization machines

7. Surgical trays are removed from sterilization and allowed to cool

8. Sterilized trays are sent to surgical equipment room

Following direct observation of the process by team members and a cause-and-effect exercise, the root cause of damaged and dulled instrumentation was found to be: stacking of surgical trays directly on top of one another. Stacking of multiple trays caused the tips of towel clips and scissors to break and delicate surgical knives to bend and dull. Two red flag situations were found to increase the likelihood that multiple stacked trays would occur: high volumes in surgical cases and low staffing in the decontamination department (especially during night shift). The team discussed ideas to prevent stacking of surgical trays on shelving units. It was not possible to purchase additional shelves because of the cost and lack of space, although the team agreed that even with additional shelving units, trays might still be stacked.

To prevent stacking of trays on one another, the shelves were lowered to allow space for only one tray per shelf. This reconfiguration made it impossible for more than one tray to be placed on each shelf (no more tray stacking). It also freed up room for additional shelves to be added to the units; thereby increasing the usable space without taking away any floor space. The additional shelving cost approximately $1,500; however, the anticipated reduction in damage to the instrumentation was expected to save approximately $40,000 annually (cost avoidance for replacement and repair costs). Cost avoidance for prevention of a surgical mishap caused by damaged or dull instrumentation is incalculable.

- Uses lean tools (such as 5S, mistake-proofing, and visual controls) to improve the process

- Substantiates and enumerates improvements

- Implements training and standard work

Kaizen initiatives should be strategically important to the organization and processes chosen for improvement recognized by staff as areas in need of change. Team members consist of frontline staff intimately involved in the day-to-day processes. They map out current practices, identify areas for improvement, and initiate change. During the first day, team members walk through the entire process targeted for improvement. This hands-on observation allows team members to experience the process and make note of any constraints, areas of waste, or issues that may lead to unsafe or inefficient care.

The remaining project days involve creating a detailed map of the process (**value stream mapping**) to further highlight constraints and error-prone situations. Ideas for improving the process are generated by the team and prioritized for implementation. Once process improvements have been defined and agreed to, the team begins to make process changes. Within just a few short days, the team initiates improvements and assesses the impact of the changes on workflow and patient safety. This real-time evaluation allows the team to quickly make adjustments that might be necessary to ensure that the redesigned process is working well.

Exhibit 12.2 is an example of a kaizen event conducted in the emergency department (ED) in a small community hospital. Staff recognized that long waits for an inpatient bed after the ED physician's decision to admit a patient were causing delays in patient treatments. Furthermore, delays in transferring ED patients to inpatient beds caused longer waits for patients yet to be evaluated by the ED physician. Inefficiencies in the process had considerable impact on patient safety and timeliness of care.

EXHIBIT 12.2

KAIZEN EVENT SUMMARY: IMPROVING TIMELINESS OF INPATIENT ADMISSIONS FROM THE EMERGENCY DEPARTMENT

Goals/Objective

Delays of patient admissions to the inpatient unit from the emergency department (ED) compromises care by delaying necessary treatment. Opportunities exist to reduce the length of time patients spend in the ED once the decision to admit has been made. Patients who are to be admitted to the hospital have a significant delay in the ED from the time the admission is decided until transfer to the unit. On average, the wait time in the ED between admission and transfer is 54.6 minutes. Approximately seven patients per day presenting to the ED are admitted to inpatient status. Recognizing that this wait time delays care to patients, has a negative impact on customer satisfaction, and ties up valuable resources in the emergency room, the project focus was to reduce wait time by 50%. Secondary outcomes anticipated to come from this event include a decrease in the number of patients who leave the ED without being seen, and improvement in patient satisfaction scores.

Methods

A value stream mapping exercise was conducted to assess the current process to obtain consensus on specific steps adding value from the patient perspective. A flow chart was then utilized to map out the specific steps that take place once the ED physician has determined the necessity of patient admission to the hospital. The team identified constraints to the current process and countermeasures to improve the current process. Improvements were implemented in real-time and measured to assess the impact on patient wait times.

Results

Data obtained prior to the initiation of the event demonstrated an average patient wait time upon decision to admit to be 54.6 minutes (range 21–175 minutes). Constraints to the current process included:

- Delays in call time from ED physician to hospitalist to obtain orders for admission

- Variation in the process for nursing supervisor to obtain bed assignment for patients

- Variation in process (and time) for report from ED nurse to unit nurse for transferring patient care

- Delays in ED nurse charting required for patient transfer to unit

In addition, the team identified opportunities to maximize the ED white board to improve workflow with visual controls to staff regarding patient status of care and pending orders. To address the constraints and opportunities, the following changes were made:

- Implement a direct call from ED physician to hospitalist for admit orders

- Design and implement a preprinted admit order form for all patients

- Implement a standard process for specific nurse and bed assignment for anticipating first admission and nurse assignment for second and third patient admission

- Implement a standard process for nurse supervisor to obtain and communicate bed assignments for inpatient admissions

- Design and request changes to the ED white board to improve intradepartmental communication

The changes listed above resulted in a reduction in patient wait times to 30 minutes from time of completed orders for admission. Extrapolating this to the seven patients usually admitted every day to inpatient status, 2.5 hours of patient wait time will be eliminated each day. This reduction will significantly improve the timeliness of patient treatment on the inpatient units. In addition, 2.5 hours of staff resources spent on maintaining patients waiting for inpatient transfer will be eliminated. This frees up staff resources to care for more ED patients; thus reducing the wait time for newly arriving patients.

Conclusion

One of the guiding principles of the Toyota Motor Corporation is to "foster a corporate culture that enhances individual creativity and teamwork value, while honoring mutual trust and respect between labor and management" (Toyota Motor Corporation, 1997). Management's respect for people working in the organization is a key element of a lean organization. Successful adoption of the lean philosophy requires inspiring leaders willing to make a long-term commitment to continuous improvement. Frontline staff must feel empowered to recognize opportunities for building better and safer processes and be provided the training necessary to make this happen. In an organization that embraces lean core concepts, senior leaders openly acknowledge that frontline staff has the best understanding of day-to-day processes and the obstacles to safe patient care.

Becoming a lean organization is a journey in pursuit of patient care perfection. As such, it must be recognized that lean methods are not a one-time quick fix. Organizations must consistently strive to create standardized processes that are user-friendly for staff and allow for continuous flow of patients through the system of care. Factors that influence successful implementation of lean tools are:

- Maintaining the focus of creating value from the perspective of the patient

- Acquainting senior leaders administration with their supportive role

- Providing staff with lean tool training to ensure adequate knowledge of lean concepts

- Including frontline staff in making process changes

- Encouraging development of standard work and visual work environments

- Providing adequate staff training for any process changes and allow sufficient time for changes to be established as standard work

- Collecting data to evaluate the effectiveness of process redesigns

- Communicating to all staff members the safety improvements resulting from lean initiatives

The lean core concepts and process improvement tools provide a systems approach for continual evaluation and improvement of patient care for the purpose of creating more efficient and safer health care systems.

Discussion Questions

1. Discuss the benefits and challenges of adopting the lean philosophy for patient safety improvement initiatives.

2. Describe a personal health care experience in which you witnessed standard work practices. How can health services be made safer through the use of standard work practices?

3. What changes can be made in your place of employment to create a visual environment?

Key Terms

5S	Poka-yoke	User-friendly
Kaizen	Red flag	Value stream mapping
Kanban	Standard work	Visual control
Lean	Unobstructed throughput	

References

Feinstein, K. W., Grunden, N., & Harrison, E. I. (2002). A region addresses patient safety. *American Journal of Infection Control, 30*(4), 248–251.

Hirano, H. (1995). *5 pillars of the visual workplace.* New York: Productivity Press.

Institute of Medicine. (1999). *To err is human: Building a safer health system.* Washington, DC: National Academy Press.

Kenney, C. (2008). *The best practice: How the new quality movement is transforming medicine.* Jackson, TN: PublicAffairs.

McClanahan, S., Goodwin, S., & Houser, F. (2000). A formula for errors: Good people + bad systems. In P. Spath (Ed.), *Error reduction in health care* (pp. 1–14). San Francisco: Jossey-Bass.

McLaughlin, R. C. (2003). Redesigning the crash cart: Usability testing improves one facility's medication drawers. *American Journal of Nursing, 103*(4), 64A,64D, 64G–64H.

Nelson-Peterson, D., & Leppa, C. (2007). Creating an environment for caring using lean principles of the Virginia Mason production system. *Journal of Nursing Administration, 37*(6), 287–294.

Pape, T. (2006, February). Work around error. AHRQ WebM&M. Retrieved from http://webmm.ahrq.gov/casc.aspx?caseID=118#case.

Savary, L. M., & Crawford-Mason, C. (2006). *The nun and the bureaucrat.* Washington, DC: CC-M Productions.

Sirio, C., Segel, K., Keyser, D., Harrison, E., Lloyd, J., Weber, R., Muto, C., ... Feinstein, K. (2003). Pittsburgh regional healthcare initiative: A systems approach for achieving perfect patient care. *Health Affairs (Millwood), 22*(5), 157–165.

Smith, B. (2003). Lean and six sigma—a one-two punch. *Quality Progress, 36*(4), 37–41.

Toyota Motor Corporation. (1997, September). Guiding principles at Toyota. Retrieved from http://www2.toyota.co.jp/en/vision/philosophy/index.html.

Womack, J. P., Jones, D., & Roos, D. (2007). *The machine that changed the world.* New York: Free Press.

Zidel, T. (2006). *A lean guide to transforming healthcare.* Milwaukee, WI: Quality Press.

PART 5

FOCUSED PATIENT SAFETY INITIATIVES

CHAPTER 13

HOW INFORMATION TECHNOLOGY CAN IMPROVE PATIENT SAFETY

Donna J. Slovensky
Nir Menachemi

LEARNING OBJECTIVES

- Identify common challenges encountered in implementing information technology in health care organizations
- Describe ways that information technology can improve patient safety
- Recognize how to avoid frequently encountered information technology implementation problems

Information technology (IT) is pervasive in all aspects of our personal and work lives to the extent that we give technology-based tools little thought—until they malfunction or fail to meet our immediate needs. Broadly speaking, technology can be defined as any tool we use to complete a task. It may be "high-tech" or "low-tech" depending on the sophistication of the tool. For the purposes of this chapter, **health information technology (HIT)** refers to any tool used in a health care organization (HCO) to automate or mechanize clinical and administrative processes. Some common examples of automation in HCOs include:

- **Computerized Physician Order Entry/Clinical Provider Order Entry (CPOE):** Clinicians' drug or laboratory orders are entered into a computer system as free text or selected from menus, and transmitted electronically to other in-house or off-site locations.

- **Bar code scanning devices:** Items such as medical supplies and pharmaceuticals can be bar-coded and scanned to document administration to the patient and for charge transmission to the billing system and withdrawal from the inventory.

- Computer analysis of laboratory data: Specimens are affixed to computer-readable input media and evaluated against established analysis criteria for reporting.

- Picture archiving and communications system (PACS): X-rays and other images are stored in a computer database from which images can be accessed for viewing on a video display screen from multiple locations.

Automation has long been recognized as an important factor in reducing human errors in work processes, including those involving delivery of health care (Salvendy, 1997). Key components of automating a process typically include streamlining the work tasks into as few steps as possible and establishing a standard approach for performing each step. Ideally, when a process has been designed effectively and automated properly, the "right" work will be performed each time and the output of the work will be of consistent and acceptable quality.

A key benefit of work process automation is a decrease in the amount of time people spend on routine, repetitive processes. This time "saved" can be allocated to performing more complex work tasks that do not lend themselves to automation. In the context of patient safety, for example, reducing time spent in documenting patient vital sign information can result in more time for direct, hands-on patient care.

Not only can work processes be automated, but current technology resources allow automation of the data and information generated through or associated with work processes. This application of technology allows data and information to be more efficiently captured or recorded in real time. Computerized information processing provides data management capabilities that enable easy access to information in multiple formats to meet individual user needs. In short, HIT tools can deliver more, and more robust, information for decision making than could ever be achieved with manual approaches. In the context of patient safety, for example, an **electronic health record (EHR) system** can present all relevant patient data in a format that allows clinicians to rapidly synthesize information from multiple sources, diagnose patient problems, and initiate treatment efficiently.

Unfortunately, workflow and process changes often are difficult to implement in complex organizations such as HCOs. Additionally, technology "solutions" for inefficient work processes can sometimes introduce new difficulties that may inhibit achievement of desired improvements in patient safety. In this chapter, we discuss common HIT implementation challenges along with recommendations for more effective use of HIT for patient safety purposes.

What We Have Learned from Research and Practice

For many years, health service researchers have studied the potential benefits derived from the use of HIT and other technologies with regard to process efficiency and patient care effectiveness. Although HIT often is implemented to improve administrative efficiencies and lower operating costs, significant improvements in clinical quality and reductions in medical errors can also be realized.

The clinical and health care management literature includes many studies that demonstrate how various HIT applications can improve patient safety either directly or indirectly. A *direct effect* on patient safety occurs when the technology has a design feature that is specifically intended to perform or influence a patient care action. For example, HIT can directly influence patient safety when a system is designed to assist clinicians in decision making (for example, recommend a correct dosage of a drug or provide meaningful information about the patient's condition, such as a recent lab result). Improved decision making can prevent errors associated with the development of care plans and application of treatment protocols to diagnose illness, prescribe treatment and medications, or administer health services. An *indirect effect* on patient safety is achieved when technology designed for a purpose other than patient care support also improves a patient care process. In many cases, the indirect effect is improvement in access to clinical information or reduction in time spent on nonclinical tasks. Technologies designed to streamline work processes and reduce the amount of time needed for administrative tasks can afford clinicians more time for patient care activities. Fewer distractions from nonclinical activities can contribute to a safer patient care environment.

Direct Effects of HIT on Patient Safety

Some information systems are designed specifically to assist clinicians in decision making (for example, diagnosing a patient's condition, selecting appropriate treatment, and so on). In a widely cited early study, Bates and colleagues (1998) found that using a hospital-based CPOE application resulted in a 55% reduction in serious medication errors. Furthermore, when a clinical decision support system was used in conjunction with the CPOE system, an 83% reduction in overall medication error rates was achieved (Bates et al., 1998). Since the publication of this early study, similar studies in other settings have found that CPOE systems can prevent many medication errors. For example, 66% of medication-related errors were prevented with the use of a CPOE system in conjunction with a basic clinical decision support tool in a children's hospital setting (Fortescue, Kaushal, & Landrigan, 2003). Specialized software designed to improve the ordering of anti-infective agents resulted in a 59% decline in the rate of pharmacy interventions for erroneous drug doses among children (Mullett, Evans, Christenson, & Dean, 2000). Default dosing and order guidance alerts reduced the drug error of prescribing above the maximum dosage from 2.1% to 0.6% in an urban academic medical center (Teich et al., 2000). A review paper that summarized findings from studies of CPOE through May 2007 reported that 23 of 27 alert types showed benefit through improved prescribing behavior or a reduction in medical errors (Schedlbauer et al., 2008).

Handwritten documentation can be misinterpreted due to poor penmanship, a situation that can be greatly mitigated by implementing CPOE and other types of HIT systems. A significant number of patients are harmed every day when nurses or pharmacists have trouble interpreting poor penmanship, which results in dispensing of a wrong drug or a wrong drug dosage. In addition to eliminating poor handwriting, HIT systems can check for drug-drug, drug-allergy, or drug-food interactions which are other common adverse drug events (Bates & Gawande, 2003; Morimoto, Gandhi, Seger, Hsieh, & Bates, 2004). Manual approaches cannot compare with the scope of checks afforded by this type of automated system.

In addition to helping avert errors, HIT can also directly improve the use of preventive care. For example, two comprehensive literature reviews found that simple electronic reminders programmed into a computer system improved clinicians' use of blood pressure assessment, vaccinations, Papanicolaou tests, breast cancer screenings, colorectal cancer screenings, and other preventive care tests (Hunt, Haynes, Hanna, & Smith, 1998; Shea, DuMouchel, & Bahamonde, 1996).

HIT can also improve care when drug manufacturers are forced to recall a product due to safety reasons. Clinicians who use EHRs or other HIT systems can rapidly identify and notify individual patients about important changes to their drug therapy or provide information about unsafe devices. When a popular anti-inflammatory drug was pulled from the market, doctors with EHR systems were able to more quickly identify, contact, and then switch their patients over to safer FDA-approved medications (Jain et al., 2005).

Finally, certain features of HIT systems can help simplify and improve patient education. For example, EHR products can be used as tools for doctors to illustrate or explain procedures or conditions to patients. In addition, information handouts can be printed directly from the system and given to the patient during the clinic visit. Patients can enter key health monitoring information such as blood pressure or blood sugar readings in an electronic tracking file to record changes between doctor's visits. Presumably, more informed, better educated patients are able to better manage their conditions and avert errors that may be due to lack of relevant information or understanding of their condition or treatment.

Other direct patient safety benefits have been associated with the use of various technologies such as bar-coded medication management (Johnson, Carlson, Tucker, & Willette, 2002; Meyer et al., 1991), pharmacy information systems (Grams, Zhang, & Yue, 1996; Troiano, 1999), pharmacy dispensing systems (Kaushal, Barker, & Bates, 2001), clinical decision support systems (Berner, Maisiak, Cobbs, & Taunton, 1999), automated total parenteral nutrition ordering (Lehmann, Conner, & Cox, 2002), handheld personal digital assistants (Bates & Gawande, 2003), and computer-generated alerts to clinicians (Kuperman et al., 1999; Rind et al., 1994). In all of these studies, automation of some patient care activity resulted in improvements in quality of care. For example, when bar code medication management systems can interface with pharmacy information systems, the computer program can help assure that the right patient receives the correct dose of an intended medication at the right time and with the right route. Likewise, when clinicians are given access to real-time information about their patients via a handheld personal digital assistant or via a computer-generated alert, they are able to act more swiftly in managing a patient's clinical needs.

Indirect Effects of HIT on Patient Safety

As stated previously, an indirect effect occurs when a system designed for another purpose has a peripheral patient safety benefit. For example, HIT indirectly influences patient safety by reducing or eliminating tedious, repetitious, or administrative tasks that reduce the amount of time caregivers have available to spend with their patients. When doctors and nurses have fewer distractions and more time to focus on patients, outcomes can improve and errors can be averted. The use of an EHR system, for example, eliminates the need for health care staff to send hard copies of test results to physicians for review before adding the information to the patient's chart. Electronic data transfer can reduce lost or redundant information and assure test results are posted to the medical record and available to all caregivers as soon as they become available. In a study of a large outpatient clinic using an EHR system, Wang et al. (2003), reported that radiology results were significantly better utilized in a computerized format which also saved time and ultimately money for health care providers. Improving access to information that contributes to clinical decision making can effectively reduce delays in diagnosis and errors in treatment orders.

Along the same lines, using an EHR eliminates the need to retrieve, transport, and refile paper documents. Much time and effort are spent on creating, filing, searching for, and transporting paper records. The time lag between a clinician's request for a paper record and delivery of the record can compromise care if the information in the record is needed to avoid drug reactions or other patient risks. An EHR can provide ready access to complete and timely information for clinical decision support.

Another important benefit of HIT is improved communication among providers. When clinicians on the health care team all have access to the same electronic health record, an improvement in the coordination of care for patients occurs. Several studies have found that EHR systems allow all members of the health care team to document the care they provide and to access relevant and timely information about their patients generated by other caregivers. Additionally, the messaging feature built into many EHR systems allows clinicians to communicate in real time with each other. This feature has proved to be a great time saver (Cooper, 2004) and is particularly effective at improving chronic disease management (Epping-Jordan, Pruitt, Bengoa, & Wagner, 2004; Bodenheimer & Grumbach, 2003).

Lastly, a series of studies examining HIT adoption in Florida hospitals consistently found that hospitals with greater investments in HIT performed better in terms of quality of care and patient safety. Specifically, Menachemi, Chukmaitov, Saunders, and Brooks (2008) found that hospitals that adopted a greater number of HIT systems were significantly more likely to have desirable quality outcomes measured as mortality rates from various procedures and conditions treated in the acute-care setting. The same research team also found that hospitals with the most sophisticated and mature HIT infrastructures performed significantly better on a wide range of patient safety measures including iatrogenic infections, pressure ulcers, patient falls, and postoperative complications (Menachemi, Saunders, Chukmaitov, Matthews, & Brooks, 2007).

In a related cross-sectional study of 41 Texas hospitals, researchers used a previously validated assessment tool to measure physician interactions with information systems in providing care for patients with four selected medical conditions: myocardial infarction, congestive heart failure, coronary artery bypass surgery, and pneumonia (Amarasingham, Plantinga, Diener-West, Gaskin, & Powe, 2009). The extent of usage of the typical functions of order entry, test results, notes and records, and decision support was compared to inpatient mortality, complications, length of stay, and hospitalization costs. Significant relationships were found in several key areas:

- Greater usage of automated records and notes was associated with decreased mortality in all conditions.

- Greater usage of order entry was associated with decreased odds of death for myocardial infarction and coronary artery bypass graft patients.

- Greater usage of decision support tools was associated with decreased complications and decreased mortality from pneumonia.

- For most conditions, greater use of decision support, order entry, and test results were associated with lower costs.

Automating work processes enables clinicians to work more efficiently by improving access to information, improving communication among caregivers, reducing administrative tasks, and improving the decision-making process. These benefits can lead to less fragmented care, help identify errors more quickly, and facilitate correction of errors before patients are harmed. Significantly, these benefits and by-products also have a positive effect on clinician and patient satisfaction.

Nevertheless, it is important to note that merely the installation of HIT will not necessarily improve patient safety. Studies have returned mixed results about the presumed causal effects of technology on patient outcomes. One meta-analysis (Garg et al., 2005) concluded that the patient outcome effects of clinical decision support systems were "understudied and, when studied, inconsistent." David Bates (2009) suggests that the relationships identified may be circumstantial rather than causal. Additionally, limitations of using administrative data to measure patient safety indicators further confounds results in some studies (Parente & McCullough, 2009). At best, the role of HIT in patient care and its effect on patient safety are complex and highly contextual. Mistake-proofing features have obvious benefit, but to achieve the full potential of HIT, systems must be designed specifically for the work environment and culture of a given organization.

Unintended Consequences of Automation

Despite the positive impact of HIT on patient safety, several studies (Ash, Berg, & Coiera, 2004; Koppel et al., 2005; Han et al., 2005; Ash et al., 2007) and facility experiences have uncovered IT-related safety issues. A Joint Commission

Sentinel Event Alert (2008) refers to this phenomenon as a "technology-related adverse event," and suggests human-machine interface or system design as the likely problem sources. Announcement of this *Sentinel Event Alert* follows (and references) several previously published *Alerts* that addressed safety issues related to the following specific technologies.

- Infusion pumps (*Sentinel Event Alert,* Issue 15)

- Ventilators (*Sentinel Event Alert,* Issue 25)

- Patient-controlled analgesia (*Sentinel Event Alert,* Issue 33)

- Tubing misconnections (*Sentinel Event Alert,* Issue 36)

- Magnetic resonance imaging (*Sentinel Event Alert,* Issue 38)

In some instances, computer programming designed to make a task more efficient (for example, drop-down menus and default field entries) have made it *easier for people to make mistakes.* A quick click of the mouse when the cursor is not properly aligned on the menu item can cause the wrong test or treatment to be ordered. Besides subjecting a patient to an unnecessary test and any associated risk of injury, significant expenses can be incurred for equipment use, supplies, and employee time spent in processing a test that often cannot be billed for payment. Touch screen devices that do not make adequate surface contact can create similar problems, omitting or incorrectly reading information. These types of mistakes may actually result in *false documentation*, which constitutes fraud with regard to billing and may subject the organization to legal penalties. Clinical action taken as a result of the false information may be a cause of medical error. The potential for errors that result from system design has been cited by physicians as a significant point of concern in implementing HIT systems (McAlearney Chisolm, Schweikhart, Medow, & Kelleher, 2007).

A second unintended consequence is *efficiency loss instead of gain.* If insufficient information is available to the clinician or the format of the information is misleading, unnecessary time can be spent in correcting mistakes and rework. For example, a physician's office may use an electronic prescribing system that includes a database of local pharmacies. The physician selects the pharmacy from a drop-down menu that lists pharmacies by store name (first) and street name (second). Imagine how many CVS and Walgreen pharmacies might be located in a large metropolitan area! If the visible field for the pharmacy is truncated, the field entry might appear to be the same for two or more pharmacies. A physician viewing the truncated field on the display screen would need to spend extra time to expand the field to ensure choosing the correct pharmacy, or choices may be made that result in sending the prescription to the wrong pharmacy. Patients, pharmacists, and physicians all can lose valuable time in correcting such an error.

Automation also can result in *sending errors upstream*. This is an unintended consequence of system integration although integration is highly desirable, particularly in hospitals where multiple caregivers need quick access to current information. Patient birth date, age, weight, and gender usually are entered at the time of registration and transmitted among multiple systems. Unfortunately, numbers are easily transposed and wrong keys are struck frequently without being noticed. A transposed number in a birth date can result in a failure to integrate data files properly if the birth date is one of the linking fields. A drug that is calculated by body weight can be over- or underprescribed if the patient weight is wrongly documented. Though 10 pounds might not have a noticeable influence in drug dosing for a healthy adult, a one-pound error might impose significant risk to a neonate or toddler.

Some instances of IT implementation have actually *increased the workload* of caregivers without substantially improving patient safety. An assessment of centralized telemonitoring of intensive care unit patients (Berenson, Grossman, & November, 2009) found that lack of system interoperability required significant nursing time to connect the monitoring data with other clinical data. In this study some hospitals were investing additional funds to create interfaces with their EHR while others chose to continue using the inefficient disparate systems to avoid additional costs of integration. It is important to note that improvements in ICU quality of care were expected from decreased complications and lengths of stay, but a technology effect could not be isolated from concurrent process improvement activities.

Automation can induce *complacency about data quality and integrity*. Data existing in an automated system is assumed to be correct unless there is visual evidence to trigger user suspicion. End users of the data rarely question accuracy if the format is correct and the data appears reasonable. For example, an erroneously high blood pressure reading for an obstetric patient might go unchallenged if it is within a commonly encountered range. However, an apparent inconsistency between gender and diagnosis or procedure (such as a male with gynecologic information) would likely be investigated. In an integrated system a data error can be replicated in multiple applications and decisions based on the erroneous information can result in several medical errors. If a physician or other caregiver presumes that a process has been automated correctly when in fact errors have been automated and the system transmits erroneous information, their decisions based on the available information may well result in threats to patient safety.

As a final point, an attempted technology solution may *fail to achieve the intended goals*. We have learned from experience and through research that technology is "necessary but not sufficient" to reduce medical errors and improve patient safety. In fact, automating a poorly designed process will certainly highlight inefficiencies in the process and may actually increase the number of errors associated with the process. A CPOE implementation in a VA hospital improved adverse drug events associated with transcription but engendered more errors associated with drug ordering (Nebeker, Hoffman, Weir, Bennett, & Hurdle, 2005). A study of electronic medication administration in five nursing homes concluded that "technology could not solve chronic structure and process issues in isolation" (Scott-Cawiezell et al., 2009, p. 29). However, when technology was used in conjunction with focused process improvement efforts, positive results in late and missing medications were achieved. Again, the question might be posed whether the IT effect is circumstantial rather than causal (Bates, 2009).

An extensive three-year project using qualitative methods such as interviews and observations catalogued and described the following nine types of unintended adverse consequences of implementing a CPOE system (Ash et al., 2007):

- More or new work issues
- Workflow issues
- Never ending demands
- Paper persistence
- Communication issues
- Emotional reactions
- New kinds of errors
- Changes in power structure
- Overdependence on technology

HIT Implementation Challenges

As with any resource- and personnel-intensive organizational strategy, implementing HIT systems is fraught with barriers and challenges, not the least of which is the actual cost of system purchase and implementation. Costs associated with implementing technology solutions in HCOs are large and complex. The up-front purchase price can be staggering, but the ongoing maintenance and upgrade fees, user training costs, technical support expenses, and other "hidden" costs can exceed the purchase price over the life of the system. Health care, despite its classification as a service industry, is also a business. Like other businesses, HCOs make many decisions from a financial perspective. However, the service and patient care aspects of the organization's mission typically take precedence in strategic resource allocation decisions related to HIT. Thus, our discussion of implementation challenges will be focused on technological and sociological issues rather than financial barriers.

Technological Challenges

Though many computer products and applications may have specific issues associated with them, there are some challenges that are particularly problematic for health care system applications. Paramount among these challenges is the need for patient-specific clinical and administrative information to be transmitted or shared across a complex system of providers, payers, and oversight agencies. Data sharing must occur internally and between organizations. The level of industry standardization among HIT products needed to accomplish full interoperability and easy data exchange across systems has not yet been achieved. Just as consumers made choices between Betamax and VHS video tapes, 8-track and cassette audio tapes, and more recently between Blu-ray and High-Definition DVD, HCOs must choose among available HIT products with the hope that their choice becomes the industry standard or is at least compatible.

The lack of industry standards has been a significant impediment to HIT adoption in many HCOs. Standards are needed in five key categories to achieve full interoperability. Although progress has been made on standards in some categories, much work remains to be done in all categories.

Vocabulary Standards

Medical terminology and the broader language of health care are not precise vocabularies. Medical terms originate from ancient Greek and Latin, from more modern French and Spanish, and from other languages in addition to English, with new terms coming into use regularly. It is very common for two (or more) words with different origins to have the same meaning. For example, -*dynia* and -*algia* are both suffixes that mean pain. Although neurodynia and neuralgia both mean "nerve pain," a computer system may be programmed to recognize one but not the other. Further complexity arises from the plethora of abbreviations used in HCOs, including those that are created by individuals as personal "shorthand" for their own documentation.

Whereas spoken and written medical language may be readily understood due to context and opportunities for clarification, computer language is primarily one of "match" or recognition. A computer system will recognize only what it has been programmed to read. Thus, a medical term or data entry may be correct from a vocabulary perspective, but incorrect with regard to the programming of a specific computer application.

A universally agreed-upon medical vocabulary is needed to optimize the functionality of HIT and to ensure accuracy in data recording and information exchange. The vocabulary used for programming HIT products must be precise and unambiguous and must be validated within the medical community. Some of the widely recognized vocabularies, classifications, and nomenclatures currently used in designing clinical applications include:

- SNOMED (Systematized Nomenclature of Medicine)

- CPT (Current Procedural Terminology)

- DSM (Diagnostic and Statistical Manual of Mental Disorders)

- ICD (International Classification of Disease)

Although there are some commonalties among these and other vocabularies, they were designed to be used differently and none was designed specifically for automation of clinical data. The National Library of Medicine's Unified Medical Language System® (UMLS) project is a large-scale effort at industry standardization via a free resource for HIT system developers. The Metathesaurus®, a vocabulary database that incorporates dozens of classifications and code sets used in the health care industry in the United States and internationally, is one of the key elements of the UMLS (NLM, 2009).

Data Structure and Content Standards

Health care and clinical data are captured and documented in many formats, including text, numbers, graphics, sound, and images. The variations in how data can be documented are legion. Consider the simplistic example of the options for formatting a date in a Microsoft Excel file—more than 12 formats are given including:

- 3/14/2001

- March 14, 2001

- 3/14/01

- 14-Mar-01

- 14-Mar-2001

Imagine the complexity of designing data entry screens and reporting formats for laboratory values, patient history information, drug dosages, and other data elements with variable ranges and formatting options.

Standard formats designed on logical principles are needed to document clinical data as used in EHRs, decision support systems, and data archiving systems. Confusion can occur when one computer system codes a heart attack as "myocardial infarction" and another system refers to the same condition as "acute MI."

Security Standards

Capture, storage, use, and transmission of health data are governed by legal and ethical principles related to privacy and security of individually identifiable information. In general, use of individual health information is restricted to "need-to-know" for continuing provision of care without express permission of the individual for other uses. Putting a paper health record in a secure, locked room with restricted access is much easier than protecting an electronic record, elements of which may be stored in several systems with access by hundreds of users including those off-site.

Internal system access can be managed through a hierarchy of access privileges. The greater risk of security breaches comes from electronic data transfer, particular when using mobile or wireless networks. Though data encryption and additional security measures during transfer are standard practice, the type and extent of security may vary across organizations. A strong security measure used by one organization may prohibit data exchange with a business partner that does not employ the same security protocol.

The Health Insurance and Portability and Accountability Act (HIPAA) of 1996 included mandates for the Department of Health and Human Services (HHS) to develop national security standards for electronic health information (CMS, 2009). The HHS standards, published as a final rule in 2003, address physical security, technical issues and administrative requirements. However, the standards are intentionally flexible and allow HCOs to develop facility-specific security plans.

Electronic Patient Identification Standards

Accurate and reliable patient identification mechanisms are essential to avoiding medical errors. Small facilities may not experience the magnitude of duplicate patient names that occur in larger facilities; nonetheless the issue is universally important. Family names passed to children with a conventional addendum (such as Jr., II, or III) are less problematic than common names used repetitively in the general population, but still can cause errors if the addendum is not used in patient registration and other identifiers are not checked carefully. For instance, among the more than 5,000 people named Maria Gonzalez in Los Angeles, the odds are high there are some common birth dates, ages, and maybe common parental names.

The mobility of the population also creates a need for linking health data from geographically distant HCOs. Clearly, a robust system is needed to identify patients and their information during a single episode of care and to link a patient's health information from multiple episodes of care; however, a unique personal identifier remains elusive.

Several electronic identification techniques—both low-tech and high-tech products—have been developed for specific applications, but none are universally used and some remain cost prohibitive. Selected examples include:

- Bar coding—used to link documents in a patient record; used on patient bracelets for personal identification

- Electronic ID cards—used for personal identification of an individual

- Thumbprints—used for personal identification of an individual

- Retinal scans—used for personal identification of an individual

Sociological Challenges

Although financial and technological issues are important and require administrative attention, the most problematic HIT implementation challenges are sociological, or people issues. New technologies usually require workers to change their operational practices and learn new skills. Workflow is disrupted and perhaps even chaotic for some period of time. Worker productivity and job satisfaction may suffer. Few workers enthusiastically embrace a job change factor as complex as a new information system. The good news is that individuals newly entering the health care workforce are often more technology savvy than previous generations. One projection is that by 2012 more than 70% of physicians will have been trained using electronic information systems (Bierstock, 2008). However, even tech-savvy individuals may resist IT when it does not streamline work processes or is viewed as adversely affecting patient safety.

Resistance to Workflow Redesign

Much of the resistance to implementing new technologies is a reaction to the anticipated disruption to the existing workflow and the subsequent redesigns that will be needed. Stakeholder involvement is an essential success factor in the selection or design, planning, and implementation of a new system.

Whereas implementing any new system can be challenging, implementing IT products in clinical applications often engenders more resistance than business applications. Business applications typically are oriented toward transaction processing and have less textual and image data than clinical systems. Thus, they lend themselves to more straightforward programming and implementation.

Physicians and other clinical professionals are powerful stakeholders in HCOs, in large part due to their influence on patient preference for this HCO rather than a competitor organization. A single doctor can contribute a noticeable percentage of patient revenue. A productive group practice can wield significant power through their combined revenue-generating capacity. Thus, the acceptance of clinical technology by dominant physician groups can be an important success factor. Though some studies have shown that physician characteristics such as age and gender (Menachemi & Brooks, 2006; Kaushal et al., 2009) or practice specialty (Lindenauer et al., 2006; Corey, 2007) influence their technology adoption behaviors, recent examination of technology adoption within group practices suggests the importance of practice culture (Kralewski et al., 2008). Practices with autonomy cultures that involve physicians in the planning process have better IT adoption rates.

If clinicians perceive a technology application will cause them to be less productive or create new problems they may well boycott the application and thereby guarantee its failure. For example, transitioning from voice dictation or handwritten documentation to keyboard data entry can be especially challenging for older persons who did not begin their professional practice using this tool.

Few clinical professionals have formal keyboarding training; for most it is a self-taught skill and the skill level varies greatly among individuals. For those with less speed and dexterity this new approach to completing routine tasks can be quite time-consuming and frustrating, particularly if they had developed highly efficient personal approaches for using the existing system.

Being "told" to use a tool they did not choose, particularly one they find cumbersome to use, is frustrating at best and for some may be perceived as a challenge to their professional image and autonomy. Technology-related work process changes are often not well received if the existing manual system is perceived by clinicians as functional, particularly if the change disrupts patient care activities (Garrett et al., 2006; McAlearney et al., 2007). Additionally, few clinicians have "free" time in their workday to spend in training on new technology. A common "no time for training" scenario is described in Exhibit 13.1.

EXHIBIT 13.1

INFORMATION TECHNOLOGY IMPLEMENT SCENARIO

The hospital purchased a clinical documentation product for use in five critical care units. With awareness that the care units couldn't be shut down for nurses to attend classroom training as a group, the Health Information Systems (HIS) Department proposed a train-the-trainer model whereby much of the training and practice could occur at the patient care unit. Multiple HIS training sessions were scheduled to accommodate all shifts, and units were instructed to send one or more representatives for training at any of the scheduled sessions. On training dates several of the planned attendees were absent. Those who called to cancel their registration cited workload in the care unit as the reason for nonattendance. The training module was placed online for access in the care units for peer training and practice.

On the go-live date, the system install was successful and the program access icon appeared on monitor screens in the critical care units. As HIS personnel visited the care units to respond to any problems encountered with early use, it quickly became apparent that very few staff were able to use the system effectively. Some staff were unable to log in; others appeared to be searching for the correct data entry screen. HIS personnel attempted one-on-one training to aid the staff, but activity in the care unit did not allow adequate focus on immediate instruction.

Investigation by HIS staff and nursing supervisors revealed that less than one-third of the staff had participated in a training session.

Workflow Redesign Fears

People currently doing the job that will be redesigned by adopting HIT should be involved in the redesign efforts. These people are the best source of information about the various process steps and decisions that must be made throughout the process. A systems analyst or programmer has very little knowledge about the "person" steps of a process. The future HIT system users must be involved in planning for conversion from manual to automated processes. If IT implementation is left to "technocrats" simple things such as use of unfamiliar or nonstandard terminology can lead to errors that did not occur with the existing manual process.

Although user involvement is critical, changing a job process can be threatening to individuals doing the work or those affected by the work. Employees may fear they will not have the skills to perform the newly redesigned job or they may worry their position will be eliminated altogether. Though not often openly expressed, these concerns may cause some workers to withhold key information about process steps or performance factors or in some other manner prohibit accurate job analysis and redesign. In such cases the redesigned process may not be a significant improvement over the old process and may in fact be less efficient or subject to greater performance errors.

Fear of Performance Management

Automating the documentation associated with patient care can create anxiety about the performance surveillance aspect of the system. Most IT applications include an electronic date/time stamp when data are entered. Thus, an audit log can be created that shows when actions were performed. Tasks not completed at the prescribed time—such as medications administered late—are clearly evident. In some cases work-arounds such as the one described in Exhibit 13.2 are created. Nurses and other caregivers have many demands on their time during work shifts. They often make decisions about the priority of patient care tasks in real time and the documentation of their actions may necessarily be separated from the actual work task. A supervisor or manager who examines the timing of work without knowledge of the immediate care environment context when the work occurred may draw inappropriate conclusions about performance.

EXHIBIT 13.2

INFORMATION TECHNOLOGY WORK-AROUND SCENARIO

A newly installed medication administration system required nurses to scan a bar code affixed to the medication package when it was removed from the cart and administered to the patient. The system captured the time the bar code was scanned and documented it for the medication administration record (MAR). After a few weeks, review of the MARs showed that a large proportion of medications were given to patients well past the scheduled time. The supervisors stressed the importance of administering medications at the prescribed time to the nurses. Subsequently, the nurses adopted a personal practice of copying the bar codes and scanning them at the appropriate time as removed from the cart, but actually administering the medications when unit workflow permitted.

Solutions

The problems discussed in the previous section are not universal in all HCOs or with all HIT implementations. However, they do happen frequently and should be considered as potential barriers to successful implementation when planning any new HIT system. Many of the issues presented can be mitigated by using tactics that address more than one issue.

Solutions to Technological Challenges

As we have seen with numerous consumer products, technology standards usually begin as a proprietary product that performs exceptionally well. As competitors enter the market with similar products the battle for market share begins. Over time, one product becomes dominant and the associated technology becomes the "standard." Competitors wanting to stay in the market adopt the technology and adapt their products to it. A recent example is the wireless data protocol Bluetooth used in mobile telephone headsets. Mobile telephones made by various vendors (such as Nokia, Sony, Motorola) are compatible with the Bluetooth protocol.

The sheer size of the HIT industry and the scope of products available make it unlikely that technology standards will follow the consumer products model. A third party is needed to negotiate consolidation of standards for HIT products and devices. Potential third parties include the government, professional associations, and key stakeholder groups. HCOs should employ rigorous due diligence in selecting HIT vendors. In particular, the vendor's tenure in the industry, market share, and commitment to interoperability are important considerations.

In the absence of communication and data standards, system designers are advised to rely on industry best practices for maximizing the system functionality to achieve desired controls. A basic but highly reliable tool is the use of algorithms for safety checks. For example, when the CPOE is linked with the pharmacy system, standard dosing information can be compared with specific orders. Discrepancies can be communicated to the ordering physician using an "alert" function.

Establishing and documenting format specifications is a low-tech solution, but one that offers exceptional return in data accuracy and information reliability. The length of a data field, the order and visibility of fields in entry and viewing screens, and the formatting of printed and on-screen reports can be problematic if not designed specifically to support the ways in which the system will be used. A viewing screen that truncates a key field such as a drug name can contribute to prescribing errors that may range from an inconvenience to a catastrophic event.

There is a critical need for employment of clinical professionals, especially physicians and nurses, with expertise in HIT or medical informatics. Physicians and nurses have a far more intimate understanding of the processes of care than HIT system engineers. As more doctors and nurses receive HIT training or express an interest in working closely with HIT developers, systems designed with the needs of clinical end users will become readily available.

Solutions to Sociological Challenges

Implementing a new HIT system can be an occasion of change management at its most complex. A broad range of personnel and management skills is required to facilitate the process of re-visioning how an individual's job tasks will be performed in an automated environment, including:

- Communicating and obtaining buy-in for the vision

- Interviewing about current job requirements

- Coaching and encouragement during the change process

- Training in new processes and IT skills

- Performance evaluation pre- and post-implementation

- Scheduling and workload management

- Motivating employees through change process

Strong leadership involvement is crucial. Failure to sufficiently engage both administrative and clinical leaders in the planning phase can have devastating effects on system acceptance and usability. Both types of leaders must be actively involved in establishing the organization's HIT strategy and in communicating the vision for the technology infrastructure—how "wired" the HCO will be. The leadership team should articulate the criteria by which a system will be evaluated when integrated into the HCO's operating environment. It is important to remember that "success" can have more than one definition, including the following:

- The application or system was installed as planned (on time, within budget)

- The application or system is used as intended (functional)

- The application or system makes a difference (improving performance or outcomes)

Being clear about which (or which ones) of these options is necessary to guide decision making throughout the system development cycle. Aligning the incentives for designers and staff to achieve the desired system goals is essential.

Experience has shown that early involvement of employees in system design or selection processes is a key success factor in HIT implementation. Employees performing the work processes are most knowledgeable about the processes and often have information that is not documented in policies and procedures. Understanding the nuances of the current processes is essential. Getting employee buy-in for the system change early in the process creates a positive environment in which to initiate major changes. Staff members and clinicians who wield significant informal power in their work units can be strong assets in the planning and selection processes. If these individuals "sell" the system and any work-related changes to their colleagues, broad-based user support can be achieved early in the process.

Among the most important approaches to managing the "people" issues in implementing HIT are conducting comprehensive workflow analyses and ensuring thoughtful redesign of work processes *prior to* selecting an HIT product. Automating a poorly designed or dysfunctional process will highlight process problems and usually will result in expensive system redesign post-implementation. Not only will this prolong the implementation process and expand the costs, employees can become frustrated and demotivated to use the system.

Another important approach is to plan for and manage extensive training and user technical support during implementation and for a reasonable length of time post-implementation. People learn new skills at differing speeds and with different performance outcomes from the same training. Training should be user specific to ensure that workers achieve a desired level of skill and confidence. Faster learners can be partnered with those who learn more slowly for just-in-time training and reinforcement. Teaching a skill to someone else can be a learning process that further extends the skills of both the student and the teacher.

A key point illustrated by Exhibit 13.1 is that staff member workload must include time to access necessary training on new systems. In a cost-constrained environment, staffing is necessarily lean. If a clinician leaves a care unit for training, other staff must increase their workload; patient care duties cannot be delayed until the clinician returns from training. Staffing modifications such as flex-pool coverage during the training phase must be included in planning and budgeting models.

Staged implementation that provides system redundancy during the immediate transition period can further ease the difficulty of changes in process and workflow. Just-in-time training and necessary adjustments to control unintended consequences of the system can be made without loss of data integrity or undue risk to patients.

As noted previously, problems encountered in technology implementation are not universal. A solution to an identified problem is not one-size-fits-all either, as organizational context and culture are important factors. The solutions presented here address leverage points where organizations can tailor their approach to technology implementation to avoid some of the frequently encountered problems reported in the research and practice literature. These leverage points include:

- Applying due diligence in selecting vendors and vendor products

- Using the design features of the technology to maximum advantage for safety checks

- Using industry best practices to select design features and data protocols

- Involving line staff and clinical professionals in system selection or design

- Plan for the right type and amount of user training

- Design or redesign processes for work efficiency prior to system selection

Specific suggestions for solutions to technological and sociological problems are:

- Apply due diligence in selecting HIT vendors

- Use algorithms and other technology features for safety checks

- Establish and document data format specifications

- Involve frontline workers and clinical professionals in systems analysis and design

- Involve clinical and administrative leaders in "selling" IT solutions

- Provide extensive user training before, during, and for a reasonable period after implementation of new technologies

- Create training partnerships for peer teaching

- Make training user specific

- Conduct workflow analysis and process improvement activities prior to system redesign or HIT selection

- Modify work schedules or employ additional staff to cover patient care activities while staff are in training

- Stage implementation for system redundancy during transition

Conclusion

HIT is not intended to replace people. Rather, it is a highly sophisticated tool used by people to:

- Do more work

- Work faster and more efficiently

- Improve work outcomes

- Achieve consistent outcomes

HIT has achieved a level of robust functionality that enables clinicians and administrators to view it as a member of the health care team. Well-designed HIT applications can collect and analyze data, compare data to standards, suggest appropriate actions, and perform error checks and a myriad of other processes. A primary function of HIT is to facilitate communication among members of the caregiving team. Enabling data sharing in real time among the team is a strong contributor to reducing medical errors.

Though the acknowledged benefits of automation and technology adoption for health care processes are numerous, the challenges to achieving an optimal return on technology investments in HCOs are plentiful as well. The evolution of information technology resources from transaction processing devices to decision support systems has occurred relatively rapidly, with the technology availability and capability increasing much more rapidly than organizational systems can adopt (financial and technical constraints) or adapt (sociological constraints). Organizational learning to inform technology decisions is further constrained by insufficiently generalizable research findings and practice literature.

Despite these and other challenges, IT is a ubiquitous and necessary tool in the delivery of health care, one that continues to evolve toward the goal of full integration and interoperability across the health care system. Although many tactics for achieving measureable improvements in patient safety and error reduction in a specific context have been reported, a few key strategies are evident in most successful HIT implementations.

First, leadership involvement—both administrative and clinical—is pivotal to successful implementation. Members of the organization's "C-suite,"—the chief executive officer, the chief operating officer, the chief financial officer, the chief information officer, and the chief medical officer—have the organizational clout to sell the vision and benefits of major process changes. They also are the individuals responsible for establishing criteria for evaluating the system implementation and ensuring that incentives are appropriate to secure the desired outcome.

Second, stakeholders must be involved in the design and selection of applications and systems. Frontline workers, in particular, have the most to gain (or lose) from implementing HIT products to automate work processes. Harnessing workers' knowledge about job processes and workflow early in the design process can result in a smoother transition and significant savings in time, money, and energy.

Third, major technology implementations should be staged, that is, the old system should remain functional during the "go live" for the new system. This approach provides opportunities to fix problems and system inefficiencies that arise during implementation without compromising the quality of the system output. Additionally, this approach allows time for users to become familiar with the system, to experience the range of activities the system must accommodate, to identify needed improvements, and to establish new habits or routines required by process changes. If the new system does not satisfy users' needs it will not achieve the desired level of acceptance and utilization.

Fourth, user training must be comprehensive, extensive, and ongoing. Workers need training in a simulated environment prior to implementation and just-in-time training during the "go live." When pre-implementation training is inadequate, workers often revert to the previous system for convenience, thus delaying the acceptance period. Typically users will not experience the full range of system functionality for some time after installation. Therefore, ongoing training and rapid user support and troubleshooting are important to build user skills and confidence in the system's functionality.

Fifth, the HIT tool must be viewed as a member of the health care team. HIT does not replace people; it replaces repetitive tasks that people do. As with all team members, HIT has several communication responsibilities, including the responsibility to:

- Make important information readily available
- Suggest alternatives when decisions must be made

- Point out redundancies

- Correlate links between pieces of information

Despite rigorous workflow and job analyses, thoughtful system selection and careful implementation, some HIT installations will be rated as "unsuccessful" according to one or more of the criteria previously stated. These events should be pursued as learning opportunities not only for the sponsoring HCO, but also for the larger health care community. Problems encountered, responses to those problems, and sequential decisions should be documented and shared as contributions to the growing body of knowledge related to HIT implementation and use. In the absence of robust and generalizable research findings, experiential learning may offer important guidance to HCOs pursuing similar HIT goals.

Discussion Questions

1. What are the major patient safety advantages of HIT? What are the potential disadvantages?

2. What key "people skills" are required in successful HIT implementation in HCOs?

3. What are some benefits to be gained from involving stakeholders in HIT design and selection?

4. What is meant by HIT being considered as a "member of the health care team?"

Key Terms

Bar code scanning devices

Computerized physician/ provider order entry (CPOE)

Electronic health record (EHR) system

Health information technology (HIT)

References

Amarasingham, R., Plantinga, L., Diener-West, M., Gaskin, D. J., & Powe, N. R. (2009). Clinical information technologies and inpatient outcomes: A multiple hospital study. *Archives of Internal Medicine, 169*(2), 108–114.

Ash, J. S., Berg, M., & Coiera E. (2004). Some unintended consequences of information technology in health care: The nature of patient care information system-related errors. *Journal of the American Medical Informatics Association, 11*(2), 104–112.

Ash, J. S., Sittig, S. F., Poon, E. G., Guappone, K., Campbell, E., & Dykstra, R. H. (2007). The extent and importance of unintended consequences related to computerized provider order entry. *Journal of the American Medical Informatics Association, 14*(4), 415–423.

Bates, D. W. (2009). The effects of health information technology on inpatient care. *Archives of Internal Medicine, 169*(2), 105–107.

Bates, D. W., Leape, L. L., Cullen, D. J., Laird, N. M., Petersen, L. A., Teich, J. M., et al. (1998). Effect of computerized physician order entry and a team intervention on prevention of serious medication errors. *JAMA, 280*(15), 1311–1316.

Bates, D. W., & Gawande, A. A. (2003). Improving safety with information technology. *New England Journal of Medicine, 348*(25), 2526–2534.

Berenson R. A., Grossman, J. M., & November, E. A. (2009). Does telemonitoring of patients—The eICU—Improve intensive care? *Health Affairs, 28*(5), w937–w947.

Berner, E. S., Maisiak, R. S., Cobbs, C. G., & Taunton, O. D. (1999). Effects of a decision support system on physicians' diagnostic performance. *Journal of the American Medical Informatics Association, 6*(5), 420–427.

Bierstock, S. (2008). Adoption in its own time. *Healthcare Informatics, 25*(3), 58.

Bodenheimer, T., & Grumbach, K. (2003). Electronic technology: A spark to revitalize primary care? *JAMA, 290*(2), 259–264.

Centers for Medicare and Medicaid Services. (June, 2009). Security standard overview. Available from http://www.cms.hhs.gov/SecurityStandard/.

Cooper, J. (2004). Organization, management, implementation and value of EHR implementation in a solo pediatric practice. *Journal of Healthcare Information Management, 18*(3), 51–55.

Corey, C. C. (2007). Clinical information technology adoption varies across physician specialties. *Data Bulletin (Center for Studying Health System Change), 34*, 1.

Epping-Jordan, J. E., Pruitt, S. D., Bengoa, R., & Wagner, E. H. (2004). Improving the quality of health care for chronic conditions. *Quality and Safety in Health Care, 13*(4), 299–305.

Fortescue, E., Kaushal, R., & Landrigan, C. (2003). Prioritizing strategies for preventing medication errors and adverse drug events in pediatric inpatients. *Pediatrics, 111*(4 Pt. 1), 722–729.

Garg, A. X., Adhikari, N. K. J., McDonald, H., Rosas-Arellano, M. P., Devereaux, P. J., Beyene, J., Sam, J., & Haynes, R. B. (2005). Effects of computerized clinical decision support systems on practitioner performance and patient outcomes: A systematic review. *JAMA, 293*(10), 1223–1238.

Garrett, P., Brown, A., Hart-Hester, S., Hamadain, E., Dixon, C., Pierce, W., & Rudman, W. J. (2006). Identifying barriers to the adoption of new technology in rural hospitals: A case report. *Perspectives in Health Information Management, 3*(9), 1–11.

Grams, R., Zhang, D., & Yue, B. (1996). A primary care application of an integrated computer-based pharmacy system. *Journal of Medical Systems, 20*(6), 413–422.

Han, Y. Y., Carcillo, J. A., Venkataraman, S. T., et al. (2005). Unexpected increased mortality after implementation of a commercially sold computerized physician order entry system. *Pediatrics, 116*(6), 1506–1512.

Hunt, D. L., Haynes, R. B., Hanna, S. E., & Smith, K. (1998). Effects of computer-based clinical decision support systems on performance and patient outcomes. *JAMA, 280*(15), 1339–1345.

Jain, A., Atreja, A., Harris, C. M., Lehmann, M., Burns, J., & Young, J. (2005). Responding to the Rofecoxib withdrawal crisis: A new model for notifying patients at risk and their health care providers. *Annals of Internal Medicine, 142*(3), 182–186.

Johnson, C. L., Carlson, R. A., Tucker, C. L., & Willette, C. (2002). Using BCMA software to improve patient safety in Veterans Administration medical centers. *Journal of Healthcare Information Management, 16*(1), 46–51.

Kaushal, R., Barker, K. N., & Bates, D. W. (2001). How can information technology improve patient safety and reduce medication errors in children's health care? *Archives of Pediatric and Adolescent Medicine, 155*(9), 1002–1007.

Kaushal, R., Bates, D. W., Jenter, C. A., Mills, S. A., Volk, L. A., Burdick, E., Tripathi, M., & Simon, S. R. (2009). Imminent adopters of electronic health records in ambulatory care. *Informatics in Primary Care, 17*(1), 7–15.

Koppel, R., Metlay, J. P., Cohen, A., Abaluck, B., Localio, A. R., Kimmel, S. E., & Strom, B. L. (2005). Role of computerized physician order entry systems in facilitating medication errors. *Journal of the American Medical Association, 293*(10), 1197–1203.

Kralewski, J. E., Dowd, B. E., Cole-Adeniyi, T., Gans, D., Malakar, L., and Elson, B. (2008). Factors influencing physician use of clinical electronic information technologies after adoption by their medical group practices. *Health Care Management Review, 33*(4), 361–367.

Kuperman, G. J., Teich, J. M., Tanasijevic, M. J., Rittenberg, E., Jha, A., Fiskio, J., et al. (1999). Improving response to critical laboratory results with automation. *Journal of the American Medical Informatics Association, 6*(6), 512–522.

Lehmann, C. U., Conner, K. G., & Cox, J. M. (2002). Provider error prevention: Online total parenteral nutrition calculator. *Proceedings of the AMIA Symposium*, 435–439.

Lindenauer, P. K., Ling, D., Pekow, P. S., Crawford, A., Naglieri-Prescod, D., Hoople, N., Fitzgerald, J., & Benjamin, E. M. (2006). Physician characteristics, attitudes, and use of computerized order entry. *Journal of Hospital Medicine, 1*(4), 221–230.

McAlearney, A. S., Chisolm, D. J., Schweikhart, S., Medow, M. A., & Kelleher, K. (2007). The story behind the story: Physician skepticism about relying on clinical information technologies to reduce medical errors. *International Journal of Medical Informatics, 76*(11–12), 836–842.

Menachemi, N., & Brooks, R. G. (2006). EHR and other IT adoption among physicians: Results of a large-scale statewide analysis. *Journal of Healthcare Information Management, 20*(3), 79–87.

Menachemi, N., Chukmaitov, A., Saunders, C., & Brooks, R. G. (2008). Hospital quality of care: Does information technology matter? The relationship between information technology adoption and quality of care. *Health Care Management Review, 33*(1), 51–59.

Menachemi, N., Saunders, C., Chukmaitov, A., Matthews, M. C., & Brooks, R. G. (2007). Hospital adoption of information technologies and improved patient safety: A study of 98 hospitals in Florida. *Journal of Healthcare Management, 52*(6), 398–409.

Meyer, G. E., Brandell, R., Smith, J. E., Milewski, F. J., Jr., Brucker, P., Jr., & Coniglio, M. (1991). Use of bar codes in inpatient drug distribution. *American Journal of Hospital Pharmacies, 48*(5), 953–966.

Morimoto, T., Gandhi, T. K., Seger, A. C., Hsieh, T. C., & Bates, D. W. (2004). Adverse drug events and medication errors: Detection and classification methods. *Quality and Safety in Health Care, 13*(4), 306–314.

Mullett, C., Evans, R., Christenson, J., & Dean, M. (2000). The impact of a pediatric antiinfective decision support tool [Abstract]. Proceedings of the AMIA Annual Fall Symposium 2000, 1096.

National Library of Medicine. (May, 2009). Unified Medical Language System. Available from http://www.nlm.nih.gov/research/umls/.

Nebeker, J. R., Hoffman, J. M., Weir, C. R., Bennett, C. L., and Hurdle, J. G. (2005). High rates of adverse drug events in a highly computerized hospital. *Archives of Internal Medicine, 165*(10), 1111–1116.

Parente, S. T., & McCullough, J. S. (2009). Health Information Technology and patient safety: Evidence from panel data. *Health Affairs, 28*(2), 357–360.

Rind, D. M., Safran, C., Phillips, R. S., Wang, Q., Calkins, D. R., Delbanco, T. L., Bleich, H. L., & Slack, W. V. (1994). Effect of computer-based alerts on the treatment and outcomes of hospitalized patients. *Archives of Internal Medicine, 154*(13), 1511–1517.

Salvendy, G. (1997). *Handbook of human factors and ergonomics*. New York: Wiley.

Schedlbauer, A., Prasad, V., Mulvaney, C., Phansalkar, S., Stanton, W., Lib, D., Bates, D. W., & Avery, A. (2008). What evidence supports the use of computerized alerts and prompts to improve clinicians' prescribing behavior? *Journal of the American Medical Informatics Association, 16*(4), 531–538.

Scott-Cawiezell, J., Madsen, R. W., Pepper, G. A., Vogelsmeier, A., Petroski, G., & Zellmer, D. (2009). Medication safety teams' guided implementation of electronic medication administration records in five nursing homes. *Joint Commission Journal of Quality and Patient Safety, 35*(1), 29–35.

Shea, S., DuMouchel, W., & Bahamonde, L. (1996). A meta-analysis of 16 randomized controlled trials to evaluate computer-based clinical reminder systems for preventive care in the ambulatory setting. *Journal of the American Medical Informatics Association, 3*(6), 399–409.

Teich, J. M., Merchia, B. S., Schmiz, J. L., Kuperman, G. J., Spurr, C. D., & Bates, D. W. (2000). Effects of computerized physician order entry on prescribing practices. *Archives of Internal Medicine, 160*(18), 2741–2747.

The Joint Commission. (December 11, 2008). Safely implementing health information and converging technologies. *Sentinel Event Alert, 42.*

Troiano, D. (1999). A primer on pharmacy information systems. *Journal of Healthcare Information Management, 13*(3), 41–52.

Wang, S. J., Middleton, B., Prosser, L. A., et al. (2003). A cost-benefit analysis of electronic medical records in primary care. *American Journal of Medicine, 114*(5), 397–403.

CHAPTER 14

A STRUCTURED TEAMWORK SYSTEM TO REDUCE CLINICAL ERRORS

Daniel T. Risser
Robert Simon
Matthew M. Rice
Mary L. Salisbury
John C. Morey

LEARNING OBJECTIVES

- Discuss the role of teamwork training as a patient safety solution
- Identify the five dimensions of teamwork behaviors
- Describe how to identify teamwork failures that contributed to an adverse event
- Recognize what teams must do to effectively coordinate and communicate with each other to solve problems.

The first decade of the twenty-first century has been productive for exploring teamwork training as a systems solution to reduce medical errors and promote patient safety. This period witnessed the publication of the Institute of Medicine report that identified teamwork training as a potential patient safety intervention (Kohn, Corrigan, & Donaldson, 2000), major publications reviewing the contribution of crew resource management (CRM) training to aviation safety and its potential to improve patient safety (Baker, Salas, & Barach, 2003; Musson & Helmreich, 2004; Salas, Burke, Bowers, & Wilson, 2001; Salas, Wilson, & Burke, 2006; Wilson-Donnelly, Burke, & Salas, 2004), adoption of CRM-based crisis resource management training in anesthesia practice (Gaba, Howard, Fish, Smith, & Sowb, 2001), and the recognition that systems-level solutions are the most fruitful and enduring avenues for improvements in patient safety (Leape, 1994, 2004; McClanahan, Goodwin, & Houser, 2000).

Because health care is delivered as an interdisciplinary and team-level enterprise, practitioners and patient safety advocates have looked for models of teamwork training to adapt to the health care environment. The twenty-year evolution of teamwork training from changing attitudes to changing behaviors in commercial and military aviation provided CRM as a mature model for the translation of teamwork training into the health care community (Helmreich, Merritt, & Wilhelm, 1999; Leedom & Simon, 1995). As these developments were taking place, the MedTeams® program of research, funded through the U.S. Army, completed its field evaluation of the first CRM-based training program developed for hospital emergency departments (ED) (Morey et al., 2002). MedTeams training has been commercially available since 1999 and versions of the program for the ED, OR, and hospital-wide clinical staffs were offered to military hospitals until 2004. Major components of the MedTeams curriculum appear in the Team Strategies and Tools to Enhance Performance and Patient Safety (TeamSTEPPS®) program that became available in 2006 from the Agency for Healthcare Research and Quality (King et al., 2008).

The development of the MedTeams team training curriculum began with a needs analysis that included a review of closed risk management cases at a major medical center. As this chapter will describe, the interdependent teamwork behaviors taught in MedTeams training provide a means to recognize and avoid, or to mitigate, the impact of clinical errors. Should an adverse event occur, the MedTeams system provides a framework for conducting a systematic analysis to identify the teamwork failures contributing to that event.

We are deeply indebted to the vision of Dr. Dennis Leedom, formerly of the Army Research Laboratory, who initiated this project and his outstanding successor, Mr. Mike Golden, who chaperoned it through all phases. We also wish to thank the visionary leaders of the participating hospitals who recognized that improving teamwork was important even before The Joint Commission raised the visibility of the issue. But most important, we wish to thank the exceptional doctors and nurses they sent us, the members of the MedTeams Consortium for their dedication, diligence, insight, perseverance, sense of humor, and willingness to step into the breach to make this sea change occur. We also owe a great debt to Roland Loranger, Joseph Melino, and Joan Flynn of Lifespan Risk Management for their willingness to educate us about incidents, claims, and the world of risk management. And finally we wish to thank Dr. Lucian Leape of the Harvard School of Public Health for his encouragement and support when we were just a small group initiating the project and for his long perseverance in surfacing and framing the problem of error in medicine.

The MedTeams research reported in this chapter was supported by contract DAAL01–96-C-0091 from the Army Research Laboratory. The views, opinions, and findings expressed are those of the authors and should not be construed as an official position of the U.S. Department of Defense or its agencies. MedTeams® is a registered trademark of Dynamics Research Corporation.

Teamwork Training Addresses Safety Challenges

Teamwork is defined as a "distinguishable set of two or more people who interact, dynamically, interdependently, and adaptively toward a common and valued goal" (Salas, Dickenson, Converse, & Tannenbaum, 1992, p. 4). More than two decades of research in aviation has shown that effective teamwork is critical to flight safety (Leedom & Simon, 1995; Prince & Salas, 1999). Both the armed services and commercial aviation organizations have standardized training systems in place for teamwork. What the aviation industry has found is that teamwork training reduces the risk that crews will make a fatal error or permit a fatal string of errors to unfold because the crew failed to communicate, coordinate, and check with each other. The training has significantly improved teamwork, resulting in saved aircraft and lives. For Army aviation, teamwork training has meant over 20% improvement in mission performance, over 40% reduction in safety-related task errors, and an estimated annual savings of 15 lives and $30 million (Gayman, Gentner, Canbaras, & Crissey, 1996; Grubb, Simon, & Zeller, 2001).

There is an increasing awareness in the health care community that teamwork training can have similar patient safety benefits. Shifts in caregivers' attitudes and beliefs, such as those listed below, have prompted the health care community to examine the various accident reduction methods used in industries such as aviation.

- The realization that all humans are fallible and that even the most diligent and conscientious clinicians will make mistakes frequently simply because they are human (Bartlett, 1998; Bogner, 1994; Koss, 1993; Leape, 1994, 1996; Leape et al., 1991; Reason, 1990; Reason & Mycielska, 1982; Weiler et al., 1993). The willingness to face such human limitations and seek solutions that are attentive to these limitations has historically been missing in health care (Bogner, 1994; Leape, 1994, 1996).

- The realization that one caregiver's error can often be anticipated and prevented or corrected by another caregiver if the clinical work environment can accept and actively embrace the idea of mutual real-time monitoring for errors by peers. Peer monitoring is beginning to be seen positively as a safety net that protects both the patient and the caregiver. Permitting, perhaps even asking, other caregivers to regularly check one's actions is a dramatic attitude change for the health care community (Simon et al., 1997).

- The realization that the health care delivery system is complex and poorly designed for safety. This poor design, in combination with medicine's complexity, dramatically increases the risk of error (Chassin, Galvin, & the National Roundtable on Health Care Quality, 1998; Dorner, 1996). The medical community recognizes that problems exist in the ways caregivers coordinate services (Joint Commission on Accreditation of Healthcare Organizations, 1998; Schmidt & Moore, 1993). Better solutions will only come from a better understanding and better design of the care processes (Binder & Chapman, 1995; Leape, 1994; Millenson, 1997; Xiao et al., 1996).

- The realization that caregiver training is too narrow. Although health care professional education does an excellent job of teaching clinical skills, attention to coordination skills has been missing (Chassin, Galvin, & the National Roundtable on Health Care Quality, 1998; Vincent, Taylor-Adams, & Stanhope, 1998). The teaching of teamwork skills and team concepts to improve care delivery has been dramatically absent (Joint Commission on Accreditation of Healthcare Organizations, 1998).

There is a strong potential that teamwork training for health care providers, and emergency care providers in particular, will have benefits that are comparable to aviation. Functionally, the emergency care world has much in common with aviation. It requires effective and often rapid coordination of groups of technical professionals to execute critical technical tasks, demands appropriate sequencing and timely execution of tasks, often demands quick decision making using incomplete information, and imposes high standards of performance and high levels of responsibility and stress on the professionals involved. Just as crews, passengers, and aircraft are placed in danger when aircrew teamwork fails, patients suffer when emergency caregivers improperly coordinate care or fail to help each other prevent clinical errors. Such errors, in the most extreme forms, permanently injure patients and lead to deaths. In a less extreme form, errors uselessly consume time and resources and slow patient recovery (Leape et al., 1991). Both forms of error provide good reasons to pursue solutions.

This chapter describes a structured teamwork system that was tested and shown to increase the performance of teamwork behaviors and reduce the incidence of clinical errors (Morey et al., 2002). It is now used in emergency departments around the country. Small teams of caregivers with different sets of clinical skills have learned to work closely and in a coordinated fashion to define, execute, and monitor the delivery of care to patients assigned to the **team**. The goal of such teamwork is to provide the highest standard of care to all patients belonging to the team.

Patients in other acute care units of the hospital are also likely to benefit significantly from this type of teamwork system. The application of this structured teamwork approach possibly could reduce clinical errors in other high-stress, high-performance environments where caregivers are often forced to deliver care to patients under conditions of incomplete information. These units include the following:

- Labor and delivery units
- Special care units (including intensive care, critical care, neonatal intensive care, and so on)
- Operating rooms
- Postanesthesia care units
- Emergency medical departments or units

Caregivers in these units often manage care delivery for several unstable patients simultaneously. Communication conditions are often less than ideal, and patients can face grave and immediate consequences if mistreatment occurs. The stresses on caregivers for high standards of performance are great. Tight coordination is essential and caregivers must respond quickly to changing situations. It seems likely that the MedTeams teamwork system could help in each of these environments.

The adaptation of MedTeams for the unique staffing patterns and operational features of labor and delivery units was evaluated in a research study at a cohort of fifteen major medical centers (Nielsen et al., 2007). The focus of this study was the clinical outcomes that resulted from teamwork training. While the researchers' interest in patient outcomes was timely and necessary, their failure to find significant impacts on patients from teamwork training was attributed to issues of management oversight, promotion of staff acceptance of the program, and details of program implementation (Harris, Treanor, & Salisbury, 2006). Successfully introducing a teamwork program like MedTeams requires careful assessment of site readiness to adopt team-based care, attention to changing culture and management practices, and follow-through with organizational reinforcement of teamwork practices once the training is completed (Morey & Salisbury, 2002; Salas et al., 2009).

Readers are also introduced to one of the tools of the MedTeams system, the Teamwork Failure Checklist. This checklist can be used by caregivers during an incident or accident investigation to identify teamwork failures that contributed to the event. This tool, originally designed by Dynamics Research Corporation for an analysis of ED closed claims, can help organizations recognize the teamwork breakdowns that contributed to the undesirable patient care event. The checklist can also be used prospectively to identify and correct inadequate teamwork performance that could lead to a sentinel event.

Teamwork Challenges in Emergency Care

Although individual clinical errors can, and sometimes do, precipitate dramatic adverse events, it is often a sequence of errors (an "error chain") that precipitates such events (Leape, 1994; Gaba, 1994). The only positive aspect to such error chains is that they commonly unfold over a period of time and consequently provide significant opportunities for caregivers to recognize the emerging problem and intervene to break the chain. The following is a summary of an actual closed malpractice case where the chain was never broken. This case reveals several common teamwork failures and demonstrates the potentially dramatic consequences.

A female in her late thirties came to the emergency department reporting an increased incidence of her normal angina chest pains over the preceding two weeks. She denied any current chest pain when the triage nurse inquired, but did report some mild shortness of breath. The patient had a long history of heart disease, including documented coronary artery disease. She was on multiple medications. She was triaged as "urgent," the second highest triage category in a four-tier triage system, even though she had abnormal vital signs and a significant history that should have placed her in the highest category, "emergent patient." The ED was extremely busy and the patient was in the department for almost one hour before being evaluated by a medical student. The patient complained of mild (3 on a scale of 1 to 10) chest pain and was found to have virtually no pulse in her limbs. One-and-a-half hours after presentation to the ED, repeat vital signs by the nurse showed very low blood pressure (61/32). This was not communicated to the medical student or the physician. To relieve the patient's chest pain, the physician ordered nitroglycerin (NTG) to be given under the tongue. During the investigation following this incident, the nurse reported on a written statement that she was uncomfortable giving NTG, a drug that will lower blood pressure, to a patient with very low blood pressure (hypotension); however, she indicated that she thought the physician "knew what he was doing."

The patient continued to complain of chest pain and shortness of breath so another drug (morphine sulfate) and an NTG intravenous drip were instituted. Almost one-half hour after the initial hypotensive episode, the patient's low blood pressure was noted by the physician and the NTG infusion was discontinued. At this time a consult with the internal medicine resident was called, and the resident arrived in the ED one-half hour later. The patient remained hypotensive, and her chest pain and extreme breathing difficulties (dyspnea) worsened. The patient became extremely hypotensive, her heart rate dropped far below normal, and the "code team" was activated. Cardiac resuscitation, including epinephrine, atropine, defibrillation, external pacing, and pericardiocentesis was unsuccessful. The patient was pronounced dead three hours and ten minutes after entering the ED (Simon, Morey, Locke, Risser, & Langford, 1997, p. 16).

FIGURE 14.1   Most Frequent Teamwork Errors

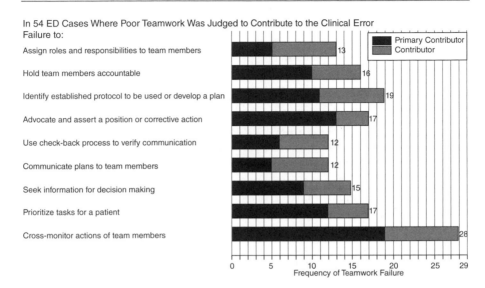

In 54 ED Cases Where Poor Teamwork Was Judged to Contribute to the Clinical Error

This case demonstrates a chain of errors in which poor climate, lack of team structure, poor task priority setting, poor communication, and lack of cross-monitoring and assertiveness within the ED contributed to a catastrophic patient outcome that sadly rippled into the lives of many people. The consequences of this team failure were dramatic: the patient died, the family was devastated, the staff was distressed and demoralized, the hospital's reputation was harmed, and over $2 million was paid in settlement (Simon et al., 1997).

Teamwork failures like these are more common than most clinicians or patients want to believe. For example, Dynamics Research Corporation found in a 1997 retrospective review of ED closed claims arising from 4.7 million patient visits that consequential teamwork failures occurred in 43% of the ED closed claims (Risser et al., 1999; Simon et al., 1999). For this 43%, the average number of teamwork failures per case was 8.8 (ranging from 1 to 32). The teamwork failures most frequently cited in the study as contributing to clinical errors are shown in Figure 14.1. Note that the single teamwork failure most frequently cited as contributing to the occurrence of clinical error was "cross-monitoring." A cross-monitoring failure refers to a failure to recognize a clinical error created by one caregiver that was readily visible and could have been caught by another caregiver. Such failures occur all too frequently in the current culture because it is generally unacceptable behavior for one caregiver to check another caregiver's actions. The care community has done little to cultivate such monitoring habits and much to inhibit them.

Perhaps the most alarming fact was that 8 of the 12 deaths reviewed were judged to be preventable if appropriate teamwork action had been taken. Moreover, 5 of the 8 major permanent impairments (for example, significant heart damage, loss of a limb, loss of ability to manage daily living activities) were judged to be preventable if appropriate teamwork actions had been taken.

In addition, it was estimated that better ED teamwork, on average, would save $560,479 (in 1999 dollars) per closed case where teamwork can influence the outcome (that is, prevent or mitigate the error). Examined from another perspective, this turns out to be $345,460 in savings per 100,000 ED patients, or nearly $3.50 for every patient seen by the ED. This is believed to be a conservative estimate of true costs that could be avoided by better teamwork (Risser et al., 1999; Simon et al., 1999).

The Teamwork System

The summary presented here is an overview of the teamwork system created by the MedTeams Project, a large applied research project that developed an emergency care teamwork system that was evaluated in nine hospitals across the country (Morey et al., 2002). This teamwork system is designed to improve care delivery performance and reduce the occurrence of clinical errors. It teaches team members to actively coordinate and support each other in the course of clinical task execution using the structure of work teams. Teams and teamwork behaviors do not replace clinical skills but rather serve to ensure that clinical activities are properly integrated and executed to deliver effective emergency care. Teamwork is a management tool to expedite care delivery to patients, a mechanism to give caregivers increased control over their constantly changing environment, and a safety net to help protect both patients and caregivers from inevitable human failings and their consequences. The basic concepts and behaviors of teamwork are taught to staff in a half-day course. The behaviors taught become habits and skills through daily practice.

Team Definition and Composition

Early on in the MedTeams Project it was found that ED caregivers often had an expanded, varied, and abstract concept of a "team" that lacked the precision necessary to create practical, manageable work teams. They tended to include within the team boundary not only the many members of the ED staff but also members of other departments, such as laboratory, housekeeping, and administration. This was "team" in the big-group, loose sense of the word. For the teamwork system to be effective, a tighter, narrower definition of "team" had to be introduced (Morey, Simon, Jay, & Rice, 2003). The ED needed to create small, mission-focused, technically skilled teams similar to those of the cockpit crews in aviation.

In the MedTeams System an ED core team consists of a set of three to as many as ten clinically skilled caregivers who have been trained to use specific teamwork behaviors to tightly coordinate and manage their clinical actions. (Average core team size in the research project was six.) Each core team consists of at least one physician and one nurse. The most experienced physician on the team is usually the team leader. The team leader only serves as leader to one team during a specific work shift. Team members always know who is on their team and who is the team leader. To make coordination easier, individuals who are members of the same team may wear a unique, readily visible identifier (such as a colored patch, an armband, or badge, a type or color of clothing, and so on) that denotes an individual as belonging to a specific team.

Team Responsibilities

The goal of each ED core team is to deliver high-quality clinical care to the set of ED patients assigned to it. To achieve this goal, team members coordinate directly and repeatedly with each other to ensure proper and timely clinical task execution and to detect and help overloaded teammates. Each team member works to maintain a clear understanding (a common situation awareness) of the care status and care plan for each patient assigned to the team and the workload status of each team member. Teams hold brief meetings to make team decisions, assign or reassign responsibilities and tasks, establish or reestablish situation awareness, and exchange lessons learned.

The team oversees and directly manages the use of all care resources needed by the patients assigned to the team. Figure 14.2 shows the range of care resources commonly used by the team to support patient care.

The team oversees all care actions involving the team's patients. The team must always be provided with a clear explanation of any patient care action taken by a non–team member because the team is ultimately responsible for the patient. Team members may not leave the team without first notifying their team leader and making appropriate hand-offs of responsibilities to the remaining team members. Table 14.1 shows basic team characteristics associated with the team's mission and goals, performance, and membership.]

FIGURE 14.2   Care Resources Managed by the ED Core Team

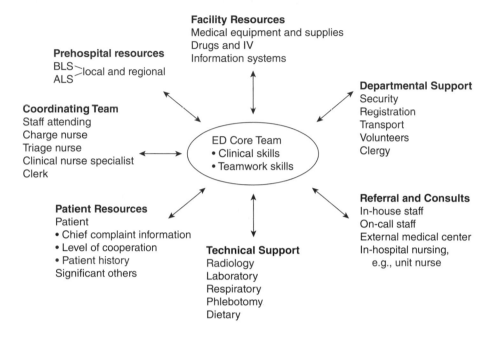

Facility Resources
Medical equipment and supplies
Drugs and IV
Information systems

Prehospital resources
BLS
ALS ⟩ local and regional

Departmental Support
Security
Registration
Transport
Volunteers
Clergy

Coordinating Team
Staff attending
Charge nurse
Triage nurse
Clinical nurse specialist
Clerk

ED Core Team
• Clinical skills
• Teamwork skills

Patient Resources
Patient
• Chief complaint information
• Level of cooperation
• Patient history
Significant others

Technical Support
Radiology
Laboratory
Respiratory
Phlebotomy
Dietary

Referral and Consults
In-house staff
On-call staff
External medical center
In-hospital nursing,
    e.g., unit nurse

Teamwork Dimensions and Behaviors

Teamwork behaviors can be organized into a framework composed of five **team dimensions** or objectives:

1. Maintain team structure and climate

2. Plan and problem solve

3. Communicate with the team

4. Manage workload

5. Improve team skills

The basic interrelationship of the five team dimensions is shown in Figure 14.3. The first objective—*maintain team structure and climate*—seeks to establish and maintain appropriate team structures and an organizational climate conducive to teamwork. The teamwork behaviors focus on the daily formation and preparation of the core team for the work shift and expectations regarding professional interactions. Success in meeting the other four objectives presupposes success in

Table 14.1 Team Characteristics

Factor	Characteristics
Mission and goals	Teams are oriented to accomplishing a well-defined, time-bound objective. There is a definable standard of performance
Performance	Teams have a time orientation to their work. The team has an identifiable start and stop time for its tasks and duties. There is real-time communication by team members. Members operate in parallel and their actions must be coordinated. Certain team tasks are routine and can be choreographed or scripted. Other aspects of working together are ad hoc coordination and can only be guided by teamwork rules and principles. Decision making takes place (planned or on the fly) that immediately affects the team's care delivery actions. Members coordinate to develop and execute plans. Teams actively intervene to eliminate task overloads on individual team members whenever possible. A team can improve its performance through practice and after-action review.
Membership	Individuals can identify themselves as members of the team. Team membership is structured. The roles of leader and follower are understood by the team members, but there are opportunities to emergent leadership and followership roles depending on the demands of patient care and the skills of the team member. Team membership is driven by the skill mix the team mission requires. Partial overlap of skills permits a degree of flexibility in task assignment within the team. During the temporary life of the team, the team's duties are superordinate to the personal goals of the individual team members.

meeting this first objective; Team Dimension 1 provides the foundation upon which the others rest.

Team Dimensions 2, 3, and 4 address daily operational teamwork objectives. These objectives are not addressed in any particular sequence. Each comes into focus many times in the course of a clinical shift, and they are often intertwined. Moreover, teams and team members rapidly and frequently change their focus between clinical task execution and team coordination issues. A team member's focus at any given point in time is driven by the need to balance (1) the demands of the immediate patient care requirements against (2) the need to monitor and maintain situation awareness in order to prevent errors and ensure the quality of impending care.

Team Dimension 2—*plan and problem solve*—brings caregivers face to face with their human fallibility as it relates to the decision-making process and error

FIGURE 14.3 Interrelationships of the Five Team Dimensions

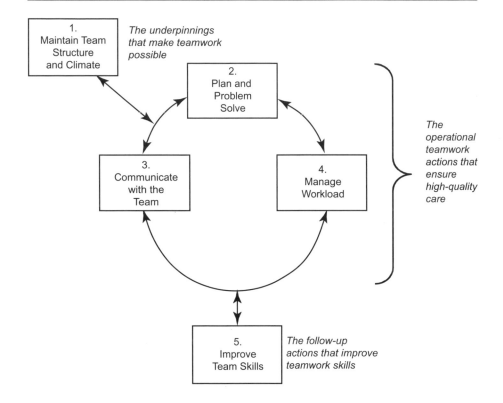

management. This objective addresses actions that can be taken to minimize the occurrence of errors within the team. Success in applying many of the error-avoidance actions identified in this dimension is dependent on team members holding a common understanding of the care plan and the status of care plan execution for each patient.

Team Dimension 3—*communicate with the team*—focuses on communication activities that help team members establish and maintain a common understanding of patient and operational issues affecting the team and team situation awareness. This objective is generally focused on timely and accurate information transfer and on maintaining a common situation awareness so team members can effectively coordinate actions and recognize pending errors. By "situation awareness" we mean one's level of awareness of important mission-related information and events that are occurring in the immediate operational environment (Endsley, 1995). This means an awareness of the patient status and care plan for patients assigned to the team and awareness of the workload levels of fellow team members. This dimension addresses specific teamwork actions taken to ensure timely and accurate clinical communication. Team members cannot deliver proper care or effectively coordinate actions without an accurate awareness of the current state of affairs.

The fourth team objective or dimension—*manage workload*—focuses on eliminating immediate work overload on individual team members by having team members help each other with tasks. Task assistance is a risk-avoidance activity that reduces the potential for clinical errors that stem from stress, fatigue, lack of the necessary skills, or individual overload. The concept is simple—help others and ask others for help.

The last teamwork objective—*improve team skills*—focuses on improving teamwork skills through team review meetings, one-on-one coaching, and situation-specific teaching conducted during real-time patient care activities. In this dimension, shift reviews enable the team to examine the experiences during the shift, discuss the teamwork and care performance, and provide immediate lessons and feedback to team members. The coaching and teaching actions provide similar insights and feedback. This dimension is important because it provides a feedback mechanism to revise and improve the team's performance. Establishing new habits and skills requires regular practice. Absorbing new concepts takes time.

Primary descriptors for each team dimension or objective are found in Table 14.2, the Teamwork Behavior Matrix. Primary descriptors help organize course training materials. The practical daily actions actually taken by team members for each team dimension are found in the last column in the matrix.

Team Activities

There are two basic categories of teamwork activity: teamwork conferences and individual teamwork. Teamwork conferences refer to those few times during the shift when the full team comes together for a meeting. There are usually only a few of these meetings each shift unless the team is very small (two or three caregivers), because it is simply too difficult to convene the full group. Most commonly there is one meeting at the beginning of the shift and one near the end of the shift. Each meeting typically lasts two to three minutes. These meetings are most often used to assign duties, establish situation awareness, gather information, discuss problems, or exchange lessons learned.

The bulk of the teamwork activities are done by caregivers operating as individual team members observing or briefly connecting with one other team member. Common individual team members' teamwork actions could include the following:

Table 14.2 Teamwork Behavior Matrix

TD#	Team Dimension	Primary Descriptors	Teamwork Actions by Core Team
1	Maintain Team Structure and Climate	Organize the team	a) Establish the leader b) Assemble the team c) Designate roles and responsibilities d) Communicate essential team information
		Cultivate team climate	e) Acknowledge the contributions of team members to team performance f) Demonstrate mutual respect in all communication g) Hold each other accountable for team outcomes
		Resolve conflicts	h) Address professional concerns directly i) Achieve acceptable resolution with follow-up discussions if needed
2	Plan and Problem Solve	Conduct situational planning	a) Engage team members in planning process b) Establish a shared mental model c) Communicate the plan to teammates
		Engage in error-management actions	d) Cross-monitor actions of team members e) Advocate and assert a position or corrective action f) Apply the two-challenge rule when necessary
3	Communicate with the Team	Maintain situation awareness (SA)	a) Request situation awareness updates b) Provide situation awareness updates
		Use standards of effective communication	c) Use common terminology in all communications d) Call out critical information during emergent events e) Use check-backs to verify information transfer f) Systematically hand off responsibilities during team transitions g) Communicate decisions and actions to team members
4	Manage Workload	Prioritize	a) Integrate individual assessments of patient needs b) Reprioritize patients in response to overall caseload of team c) Prioritize tasks for individual patients
		Manage team resources	d) Balance workload within the team e) Request assistance for task overload f) Offer assistance for task overload g) Constructively use periods of low workload
5	Improve Team Skills	Engage in informal team improvement strategies	a) Engage in situational learning and teaching with the team b) Engage in coaching with team members c) Conduct event reviews d) Conduct shift reviews
		Engage in formal team improvement strategies	e) Participate in educational forums addressing teamwork f) Participate in performance appraisals addressing individual's contributions to teamwork

- Caregiver A helps B with a clinical task. (A and B could be any two members of the team.)

- Caregiver A observes B's actions and notes nothing unusual so no direct interaction occurs.

- Caregiver A corrects B's situation awareness when she notes an unexpected care action by B.

- Caregiver A alerts B to the fact that he is about to make an error so B alters his action.

- Caregiver A informs B that he has made an error and they initiate corrective actions.

- Caregiver A discovers an error by B, initiates corrective actions, and alerts B and the team to the error and the actions taken.

- Caregiver A has her own situation awareness corrected by B when she asks a question about a presumed error.

These are examples of actions that give teamwork its operational power. Teamwork at the operational level involves an integration of these actions into a recurring intermittent process of monitoring, intervening, and correcting errors or deviations in situation awareness. These actions are known as "**check actions**." Such actions are just another part of the common daily work activities of team members. Each team member readily moves between clinical tasks and check tasks as a part of the normal process of caring for patients and monitoring for errors. A model of the basic teamwork check cycle employed by caregivers is shown in Figure 14.4.

The teamwork check cycle begins with each team member monitoring his or her own situation awareness (1) and cross-monitoring (2) the actions of his or her teammates. Occasionally when monitoring a teammate, the caregiver in a monitoring mode will observe what he or she believes is an error or see a team-mate behavior that suggests an error is about to occur or sense that the team-mate's situation awareness is incorrect (3). At this point, the individual will intervene with a simple direct question or an offer of information (4) to correct what he or she believes is a simple error; (5) that is, a slip, lapse, mistake, or loss of situation awareness. Most of the time, the error will be a simple one and the erring teammate will quickly recognize it, acknowledge it, correct it, and move on (6). Note that sometimes it may actually be the monitoring teammate who has lost situation awareness. In such a case, the monitored party's feedback allows the monitoring teammate to correct his or her situation awareness and continue. Either way, the action has served to keep the team on track. If,

FIGURE 14.4 The Teamwork Check Cycle

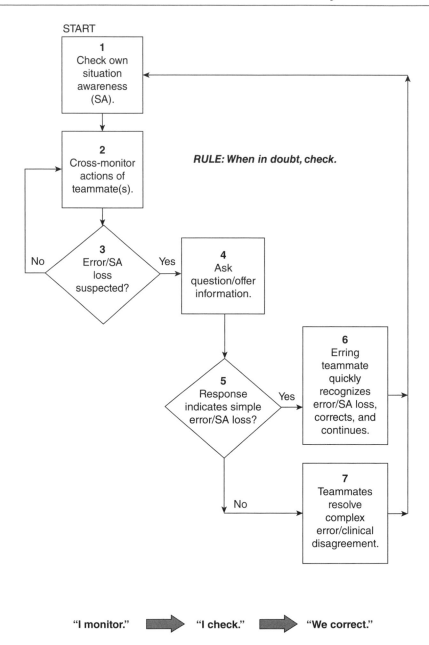

START

1
Check own situation awareness (SA).

2
Cross-monitor actions of teammate(s).

RULE: When in doubt, check.

3
Error/SA loss suspected?

No

Yes

4
Ask question/offer information.

5
Response indicates simple error/SA loss?

Yes

No

6
Erring teammate quickly recognizes error/SA loss, corrects, and continues.

7
Teammates resolve complex error/clinical disagreement.

"I monitor." ➡ "I check." ➡ "We correct."

on the other hand, a more complex error has occurred, or team members are in strong disagreement about how patient care should proceed, then (7) advocacy, assertion, and occasionally third-party involvement may be needed to reach resolution. Ultimately, however, the individuals resolve their disagreement and each returns (back to 1) to check and adjust his or her own situation awareness.

Each team member executes this check cycle as often as possible during a shift, given the demands of the clinical actions for which he or she is also responsible. Once these cross-monitoring habits have been firmly established and the staff has become receptive to the idea that checking is helpful, caregivers accomplish much of this monitoring with little or no conscious attention required until a potential error is sensed. Monitoring becomes second nature, with little or no active attention required until there is a perceived deviation.

The value of this recurring cycle is that the individual team member, by independently executing this monitoring process, can significantly contribute to the following:

- Maintaining his or her own situation awareness

- Maintaining the situation awareness of teammates questioned

- Catching simple errors made by teammates monitored

- Occasionally initiating true best-practice conflicts

Note that although in reality there are few actual conflicts in teams over what is the best practice for a particular patient, it is extremely important for the effective functioning of the teamwork system that staff know they will not have "their heads cut off" for challenging an action that they believe may harm the patient. Doctors and nurses in this teamwork system learn to explain their actions in a calm, civil manner. This openness is imperative because if the senior members of the team intimidate the junior members with sharp rebukes, the junior members will not be willing to inquire about apparently simple errors for fear that they will inadvertently stumble into best-practice disagreements. If open communication is suppressed, simple slips and lapses will not get caught.

Over time the recurring monitoring actions of the check cycle become part of the ingrained habits of each caregiver. The aggregate impact of multiple team members simultaneously and continuously conducting the check cycle as a normal part of their daily work routine is dramatic: hundreds of checks on the team each day. Conscientious use of the teamwork check cycle breaks error

FIGURE 14.5 Teamwork Failure Checklist

Case or Claim Case # _____

Reviewer Codes _____

Description of Error/Incident _____

(Describe the error in a short, brief sentence)

Part A – Assessment of Teamwork Failures That Contributed to the Error

Instructions: Thoroughly review the available facts of the case before beginning. For each teamwork behavior answer each question by marking "Yes" or "No" with an X. Answer each of the four assessment questions in order from left to right until you make a "No" response or complete Question 4. Then move to Question 1 for the next teamwork behavior and repeat the assessment process. Continue until all the teamwork behaviors have been reviewed.

TD Code	Teamwork Behavior	1. Was the behavior appropriate for the situation?		2. Was there a teamwork behavior failure?		3. Did the failure contribute to the error?		4. Was the failure a primary contributor to the error?	
		No	Yes	No	Yes	No	Yes	No	Yes
1	a) Establish the leader		X→		→		→		
	b) Assemble the team		X→		→		→		
	c) Designate roles and responsibilities		X→		→		→		
	d) Communicate essential team information		X→		→		→		
	e) Acknowledge the contributions of team members to team performance		→		→		→		
	f) Demonstrate mutual respect in all communication		X→		→		→		
	g) Hold each other accountable for team outcomes		X→		→		→		
	h) Address professional concerns directly		→		→		→		
	i) Achieve acceptable resolution with follow-up discussions if needed		→		→		→		
2	a) Engage team members in planning process		X→		→		→		
	b) Establish a shared mental model		X→		→		→		
	c) Communicate the plan to teammates		X→		→		→		
	d) Cross-monitor actions of team members		X→		→		→		
	e) Advocate and assert a position or corrective action		→		→		→		
	f) Apply the Two-challenge Rule when necessary		→		→		→		

FIGURE 14.5 *Continued*

TD Code	Teamwork Behavior	1. Was the behavior appropriate for the situation?		2. Was there a teamwork behavior failure?		3. Did the failure contribute to the error?		4. Was the failure a primary contributor to the error?	
		No	Yes	No	Yes	No	Yes	No	Yes
3	a) Request situation awareness updates		X→		→		→		
	b) Provide situation awareness updates		X→		→		→		
	c) Use common terminology in all communications		X→		→		→		
	d) Call out critical information during emergent events		→		→		→		
	e) Use check-backs to verify information transfer		X→		→		→		
	f) Systematically hand off responsibilities during team transitions		X→		→		→		
	g) Communicate decisions and actions to team members		X→		→		→		
4	a) Integrate individual assessments of patient needs		→		→		→		
	b) Re-prioritize patients in response to overall caseload of team		X→		→		→		
	c) Prioritize tasks for individual patients		X→		→		→		
	d) Balance workload within the team		X→		→		→		
	e) Request assistance for task overload		→		→		→		
	f) Offer assistance for task overload		→		→		→		
	g) Constructively use periods of low workload		→		→		→		
5	a) Engage in situational learning and teaching with the team		→		→		→		
	b) Engage in coaching with team members		→		→		→		
	c) Conduct event reviews		→		→		→		
	d) Conduct shift reviews		X→		→		→		
	e) Participate in educational forums addressing teamwork		→		−)		→		
	f) Participate in performance appraisals addressing individual's contributions to teamwork		→		→		→		

Part B
Assessing the Impact of Effective Teamwork

Question 5. What impact would effective teamwork have had on this case?
(circle one answer)

    a. Would <u>have prevented</u> the error(s) from occurring.

    b. Would <u>have mitigated </u>the impact of the error(s) but not have prevented it.

    c. Would <u>not have prevented</u> the error(s) or mitigated the impact of the errors.

Source: Dynamics Research Corporation. Copyright © 2009. All rights reserved.

chains. (Additional details on the MedTeams Teamwork System are available at http://teams.drc.com.)

Identifying Teamwork Failures in Incidents

There is recognition in the health care world that organizations must learn from the incidents that occur. The Joint Commission has made this recognition explicit in its sentinel event guidance (Croteau, 2010). In addition, individual hospitals and facilities recognize the need to learn about their system weaknesses from less dramatic incidents that are also symptoms of system failure. The Teamwork Failure Checklist (Figure 14.5) is a tool to help organizations gain insight into system weaknesses as they relate to teamwork. It allows the organization to identify teamwork failures that contributed to an error. The insight gained from the assessment permits the organization to consider teamwork improvement options (for example, revise work structures to establish teams, provide staff training in teamwork, or alter reward structures) and make appropriate plans for system improvement. And where a sentinel event has occurred, the checklist can provide an assessment of teamwork breakdowns and aid in determining if they contributed to the error occurrence. Completion of the checklist becomes a component of the formal root cause analysis (RCA).

Completion of the Checklist

For any one incident, the completion of the Teamwork Failure Checklist is a three-stage process (Figure 14.6): (1) collect the facts, (2) review the facts, and (3) complete the checklist. The main objective in the fact collection phase is to bring all the facts together into one file so that the data can be easily reviewed. When the incident has been brought to the attention of the risk manager shortly after its occurrence and the risk manager has initiated a claim file to capture the relevant facts, significant amounts of reliable data will be available. If a claim file is not initiated until a suit is filed (often months or years after the incident), the quality and completeness of the data will be dramatically reduced, making completion of the Teamwork Failure Checklist difficult, if not impossible.

Unless the parties conducting the formal interviews of the caregivers involved in the incident specifically ask questions regarding the interactions between the caregivers, interview reports typically are silent on the coordination actions between caregivers. Caregiver coordination information was often missing in the retrospective review of incidents conducted by Dynamics Research Corporation. If you intend to evaluate team performance in future incidents, it is strongly recommended that you ask the risk manager to ensure that all future caregiver

FIGURE 14.6   Individual Claim Assessment Process

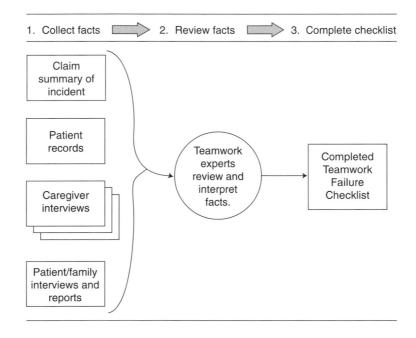

1. Collect facts ➡ 2. Review facts ➡ 3. Complete checklist

Claim summary of incident

Patient records

Caregiver interviews

Patient/family interviews and reports

Teamwork experts review and interpret facts.

Completed Teamwork Failure Checklist

interviews include detailed questions about the communication and coordination actions. Direct questions about these actions provide the best facts and insights for assessing teamwork. However, recognize that where no claim file exists it will be very difficult, and in many cases impossible, to acquire the incident data after the fact.

In the second phase of completing the checklist, the collected facts are reviewed and interpreted to understand the incident story. This interpretation is most effectively accomplished by using a physician-nurse pair (p-n pair), in particular a pair who are seasoned caregivers and have had formal training in teamwork. It is better still if they have had experience working in a team-based care system or another team-structured unit. The pairing is needed because physicians and nurses often have very different views of the world. Both perspectives tend to be necessary to fully understand the story, and it is often the discussions between the two reviewers that reveal the story and the teamwork breakdowns that occurred. Moreover, because objectivity is important, the physician and nurse used in this integration and evaluation role should have no connection to the incident being examined. If all the caregivers in the department are too close to the incident, it is best that the pair be drawn from another unit or outside organization with the previously mentioned background and training. A particular caution is placed against conducting a review and inter-pretation using only a physician or only a nurse; the risk of bias occurring will be high and the risk of the perception of bias will be even higher. Incident analysis by a lone reviewer will raise questions of assessment validity and trigger resistance to any proposed solutions stemming from it. The selection of the reviewers is an important issue for assessment credibility.

Once the physician and nurse have reviewed the file (caregiver interviews, depositions, patient records, and/or case summaries) and understand the incident chronology and the story, the Teamwork Failure Checklist (Figure 14.5) is used to formally assess the quality of the teamwork during the event chain. The case file is reviewed in detail and the p-n pair decides if there were teamwork failures and whether those failures contributed to the error that occurred. The individual teamwork behaviors, shown in column two of the checklist, are grouped according to the relevant team dimensions (see column two of the matrix in Table 14.2). Each teamwork behavior shown in the checklist is assessed by answering a sequence of four contingent questions:

1. Was the behavior appropriate for the situation?

2. Was there a teamwork behavior failure?

3. Did the failure contribute to the error?

4. Was the failure a primary contributor to the error?

For each teamwork behavior the two reviewers move horizontally through the series of four questions shown in columns three through six on the checklist. Question asking continues until either one of the four questions is answered "no" or all four questions have been answered. The reviewers then move to the next teamwork behavior and repeat the four-question sequence. This process is repeated until all teamwork behaviors have been reviewed.

The Teamwork Failure Checklist comes preprinted with an "X" in the "yes" column for the first question for some teamwork behaviors. These teamwork behaviors are considered to be applicable for all situations. For example, the teamwork behavior "Establish the leader" (1a) is always an applicable behavior. The team should never be in doubt regarding who is the leader. If any one of the caregivers involved in the incident indicates in an interview uncertainty about who the leader was, then there was a teamwork failure with respect to this behavior and an "X" would be placed in the "yes" column for Question 2. And, continuing with this example, if the caregiver's focus on trying to discover who the leader was contributed to his forgetting to give a medication to a patient, and that patient later went into convulsions because he had not received the needed drug, then the teamwork failure would be a contributor to the incident. In this instance, an "X" would be placed in the "yes" column for Question 3. The failure to designate a leader could even become a primary contributor (Question 4) if a conflict erupted between two caregivers over who was leader during a code and the conflict delayed delivery of time-critical care and the patient died. Recognize that the judgment of the extent to which the teamwork failure contributed to the clinical error occurrence requires an understanding of the clinical situation, the clinical options available, and the teamwork actions possible.

Note that there are also teamwork behaviors where the first question has not been pre-answered with a "yes" in the first question. These teamwork behaviors are only appropriate under particular situations. For example, if the staff were under conditions of high workload during the incident and the entire shift, then obviously the teamwork behavior "constructively use periods of low workload" (4g) is not relevant to the situation surrounding the incident. Similarly, if there is neither perceived nor real caregiver disagreement in an incident, then "Advocate and assert a position or corrective action" (2e) is not a relevant teamwork behavior given the case situation. One would not expect a caregiver to display this behavior. "Advocating a position" would be an irrelevant behavior in the absence of a perceived or real disagreement.

The last question on the form (after the individual behaviors have all been reviewed) asks the p-n pair to decide what impact they believe sound teamwork would have had on the error associated with the incident. It asks the pair to decide if proper teamwork would have prevented the error, mitigated the impact of the error, or had no impact on the error. To answer this question the pair should first review the checklist and the decisions they made regarding the individual teamwork behaviors and then decide whether they believe better teamwork could have prevented or mitigated the error. The pair might also wish to prepare a summary statement explaining their position on the impact of the teamwork failures on the clinical error.

Figure 14.7 shows a completed Teamwork Failure Checklist for the analysis that was conducted for the incident described earlier that involved the young woman presenting with chest pain who died as a result of poor care. This incident occurred in an ED environment with no formal team structure and a poor organizational climate. During the woman's stay in the ED there were multiple caregiver communication failures and there was a dramatic lack of caregiver assertiveness on behalf of the patient. The patient should have been triaged as "emergent" at arrival and should have immediately received medical attention and a thorough workup. Cross-monitoring by any caregiver with even basic clinical training should have surfaced this triage error and the high risk involved

FIGURE 14.7 Example of a Completed Teamwork Failure Checklist

Case or Claim Code # 2372

Reviewer Codes Dr. J and Nurse Z.

Description of Error/Incident   Failure to recognize and treat hypotensive crisis
(Describe the error in a short, brief sentence)

Part A – Assessment of Teamwork Failures That Contributed to the Error

Instructions: Thoroughly review the available facts of the case before beginning. For each teamwork behavior answer each question by marking "Yes" or "No" with an X. Answer each of the four assessment questions in order from left to right until you make a "No" response or complete Question 4. Then move to Question 1 for the next teamwork behavior and repeat the assessment process. Continue until all the teamwork behaviors have been reviewed. *(Note that for this example we used a check (✓) to show the evaluator entry more clearly.)*

TD Code	Teamwork Behavior	1. Was the behavior appropriate for the situation?		2. Was there a teamwork behavior failure?		3. Did the failure contribute to the error?		4. Was the failure a primary contributor to the error?	
		No	Yes	No	Yes	No	Yes	No	Yes
1	a) Establish the leader		X→		✓→		✓→		✓
	b) Assemble the team		X→		✓→		✓→	✓	
	c) Designate roles and responsibilities		X→	✓	→		→		
	d) Communicate essential team information		X→	✓	→		→		
	e) Acknowledge the contributions of team members to team performance	✓	→		→		→		
	f) Demonstrate mutual respect in all communication		X→	✓	→		→		
	g) Hold each other accountable for team outcomes		X→		✓→		✓→	✓	
	h) Address professional concerns directly		✓→		✓→		✓→		✓
	i) Achieve acceptable resolution with follow-up discussions if needed		✓→		✓→		✓→	✓	
2	a) Engage team members in planning process		X→		✓→		✓→	✓	
	b) Establish a shared mental model		X→		✓→		✓→		✓
	c) Communicate the plan to teammates		X→		✓→		✓→	✓	
	d) Cross-monitor actions of team members		X→		✓→		✓→		✓
	e) Advocate and assert a position or corrective action		✓→		✓→		✓→		✓
	f) Apply the Two-challenge Rule when necessary	✓	→		→		→		

FIGURE 14.7 *Continued*

TD Code	Teamwork Behavior	1. Was the behavior appropriate for the situation?		2. Was there a teamwork behavior failure?		3. Did the failure contribute to the error?		4. Was the failure a primary contributor to the error?	
		No	Yes	No	Yes	No	Yes	No	Yes
3	a) Request situation awareness updates		X→		✓→		✓→	✓	
	b) Provide situation awareness updates		X→		✓→		✓→	✓	
	c) Use common terminology in all communications		X→	✓	→		→		
	d) Call out critical information during emergent events	✓	→		→		→		
	e) Use check-backs to verify information transfer		X→	✓	→		→		
	f) Systematically hand off responsibilities during team transitions		X→	✓	→		→		
	g) Communicate decisions and actions to team members		X→		✓→		✓→	✓	
4	a) Integrate individual assessments of patient needs		✓→		✓→		✓→	✓	
	b) Re-prioritize patients in response to overall caseload of team		X→	✓	→		→		
	c) Prioritize tasks for individual patients		X→		✓→		✓→	✓	
	d) Balance workload within the team		X→	✓	→		→		
	e) Request assistance for task overload	✓	→		→		→		
	f) Offer assistance for task overload	✓	→		→		→		
	g) Constructively use periods of low workload	✓	→		→		→		
5	a) Engage in situational learning and teaching with the team	✓	→		→		→		
	b) Engage in coaching with team members	✓	→		→		→		
	c) Conduct event reviews		✓→		✓→	✓	→		
	d) Conduct shift reviews		X→	✓	→		→		
	e) Participate in educational forums addressing teamwork	✓	)		→		→		
	f) Participate in performance appraisals addressing individual's contributions to teamwork	✓	→		→		→		

Part B
Assessing the Impact of Effective Teamwork

Question 5. What impact would effective teamwork have had on this case?
(circle one answer)

    (a.) Would <u>have prevented</u> the error(s) from occurring.

    b. Would <u>have mitigated</u> the impact of the error(s) but not have prevented it.

    c. Would <u>not have prevented</u> the error(s) or mitigated the impact of the errors.

Source: Dynamics Research Corporation. Copyright © 2009. All rights reserved.

in giving nitroglycerin to a patient with low blood pressure. None of the needed teamwork actions that could have broken this error chain occurred.

Several of the team behaviors are checked as "not appropriate" in this situation. These behaviors involve teaching and coaching and work environment. It was determined by the p-n pair reviewing this event that although the ED was busy at the time the woman presented, this was not a situation of task overload triggering the errors. Poor organizational climate appears to have been the chief culprit because it significantly undermined communication among caregivers. Both the climate and the busy pace of the ED probably precluded real-time situation teaching and coaching and may have sabotaged opportunities for team reviews during the shift.

Furthermore, note that team reviews and case reviews or forums addressing teamwork concerns almost never help break the error chain while an event is still unfolding. These education actions more commonly have a delayed impact; that is, they make the caregivers smarter and more capable of recognizing and breaking error chains in future incidents. Only when an error chain unfolds very slowly over a period of many hours or perhaps days can team reviews and case reviews or forums possibly contribute to the breaking of a specific unfolding chain. In general, Team Dimension 5 actions are not primary contributors to the breaking of error chains.

As shown in part B of the Teamwork Failure Checklist (Figure 14.7), the p-n pair reviewing the incident felt that effective teamwork would have prevented the error from occurring. In the 1997 retrospective analysis of ED closed claims, Dynamics Research Corporation found that the participating p-n pairs generally thought that in cases with two or more "primary contributor" teamwork failures, proper teamwork would have prevented the error. In this case you will find five "yes" answers to Question 4 on the checklist.

Finally, as part of the retrospective analysis, a check of rater pair reliability was conducted using 16 cases. Two different p-n pairs each independently rated the 16 cases using the Teamwork Failure Checklist. The results demonstrated good instrument reliability. There was a strong correspondence between the pairs with respect to total teamwork failure count ($r = +.85, p < .001$). Correspondence of judgments between the pairs for the global impact question (the three-level Prevent/Mitigate/No Impact scale) was good ($t_b = +.61, p = .006$).

Use of Teamwork Failure Assessments

The Teamwork Failure Checklist can be used in a number of ways. It can help explain how an incident occurred and provide talking points for meeting with an upset family. Meeting in an honest, open fashion may help diffuse the anger and frustration and may actually reduce the risk of litigation. It can also allow periodic checks by management on the quality of the teamwork being provided. Reviewing a case's failures in various team dimensions provides management with a sense of where the problems lie. For example, a manager might discover that although the team structures are in place and the climate is supportive, the staff still demonstrates weak team communication habits. This finding would alert the clinical leaders as to where they need to focus teamwork sustainment training.

The checklist can also be used to assess and prepare cases for mortality and morbidity (M&M) conference presentations to the staff. It can also serve as the teamwork subanalysis in a root cause analysis conducted in response to a sentinel event. Recall that the Joint Commission guidance on sentinel events has identified weak teamwork as one of the Achilles heels in the health care system that is in need of repair (The Joint Commission on Accreditation of Healthcare Organizations, 1998). Moreover, if multiple claims files exist, analysis of a set of checklists completed for five or ten other incidents would help an organization confirm the presence of teamwork failure trends that might be discovered in an RCA. Such trend data would reassure leadership that the action plan they had proposed in response to the sentinel event is on a sound footing. These potential uses of the Teamwork Failure Checklist findings are described in more detail in Table 14.3.

Because reviewing of incidents almost always introduces legal concerns, any consideration of a review action should begin with a meeting with the risk manager. The risk manager must be involved in establishing rules for the control of the documents and any interactions with staff. The fact files needed to assess the teamwork performance must be handled with care so that legal privileges of the organization are not damaged (Barton, 1997; Davis & McConnell, 1997). To control legal risks, the risk manager should also be involved in any decisions regarding the release and use of the information (Sassano & Dronsfeld, 1991).

The p-n pair involved in incident review should be briefed by the risk manager on restrictions and protocols for accessing and using the claim fact files. Reviewers may be asked to sign nondisclosure agreements in order to gain access to files. Likewise, reviewers must adhere to any rules established regarding the distribution and protection of any notes and documents created.

Organizations must act aggressively to learn lessons and improve the care system, but they must do so in ways that avoid unreasonable legal risks. The actions and reactions of risk managers to a request for access to case facts may vary dramatically from one hospital to another. Their willingness or reluctance to help will be driven by the attitudes of the organization's senior leaders and the legal risks that are imposed by the laws of the particular state. If the senior leaders are not proactive and committed to preventive measures, then gaining access to case files will be difficult.

Table 14.3 Potential Uses of Teamwork Failure Checklist Findings

Use ID#	Use of Teamwork Failure Checklist Findings	Findings Derived from	Value of Findings to Organization/ Health Care Community	Risk Management Considerations in Use of Findings
1	Identify incident talking points for meeting with patient and family to explain incident.	Single case in own organization	Acknowledgment of a simple human failing may help diffuse anger and avoid litigation action; many patients and families are most concerned that the problem not happen again.	Consider establishing nondisclosure agreements with parties involved; consider access to and distribution of any acknowledgments with senior management and organization attorneys before meeting.
2	Limited in-house management review of teamwork weaknesses	Single case in own organization	• Flag possible teamwork problem areas and alert management to the possible need for training and management actions; may trigger training requirement or need for further trend analysis • Feedback to teamwork sustainment training efforts to improve performance	Restrict access to such a review; only show to senior management and managers directly involved in creating and implementing practical solutions; coordinate with risk manager to determine if a more in-depth analysis is appropriate and possible given the claim files available.
3	Case for morbidity/ mortality review: example of teamwork failure with serious consequences	Single case in own organization	Educate caregivers on specific teamwork failures that occurred and discuss important teamwork follow-through in future care management.	Provided to both physician and nursing staff as a normal part of the peer review process; parties appropriately cautioned not to discuss after M&M meeting has adjourned.

4	Root cause analysis (RCA) for a sentinel event: teamwork subanalysis	Single case in own organization	Addresses teamwork failures that contributed to the sentinel event and generates potential inputs to action plan.	Carefully consider access to, and distribution of, any such analysis; only reveal results to senior management unless otherwise authorized.
5	In-house trend analysis to identify recurring teamwork problems unique to the organization	Multiple cases from own organization	Flag recurring teamwork problems and risks that exist in your own particular organizations.	Restrict distribution of findings to senior management; reports that contain only statements of the problem should have a very limited distribution; reports that state problems and planned solutions may be more widely distributed.
6	Corroborate RCA findings regarding teamwork.	Multiple cases from own organization	Check that teamwork failures that have been identified in the RCA action plan are true recurring problems.	Attach as additional analysis action supporting the RCA; restrict access to those individuals authorized to see the RCA.
7	Research common teamwork failures that regularly occur in many health care organizations.	Multiple cases from own organization	• Pooled data from sentinel events and/or closed cases allow identification of common recurring teamwork failures associated with major errors and significant indemnity costs (reactive research). • Pooled data from recent risk cases can allow early identification of emerging types of clinical error and associated teamwork breakdowns before they develop into major litigation areas (proactive research).	Only release data to research efforts where (1) data from multiple organizations are pooled and (2) only aggregate results will be reported; de-identify any cases released; restrict access to individual cases to a very small set of researchers and their assistants. Have all parties with access to individual interviews and completed checklist sign nondisclosure agreements.

It is also imperative that the managers and researchers conducting these assessments coordinate closely with the risk managers on use of the information generated. Senior leaders must consider carefully what information is to be released, to whom, in what form, and when it will be released. Some suggestions regarding risk management issues are shown in the last column of Table 14.3. Recognize that these suggestions may require adjustments based on the tort laws of the particular state in which the organization resides.

Implementing a Teamwork System

Implementation of the MedTeams teamwork system involves a significant climate change for most departments and units. Only a sustained commitment from senior leaders will make it happen (Salas et al., 2009; Phillips, 1997). They must ensure a supportive department climate, work to change attitudes, and ensure that caregivers receive significant training and practice until the new teamwork behaviors become habits. Senior leaders must support and work closely with the line-level implementers who oversee the daily teamwork training and practice in the department.

Recognizing that the official titles may be different from one facility to another, the senior leaders who should be involved and the roles they should play are listed below:

- The *chief executive officer* is responsible for promoting the project vision at executive leadership levels, including board of director presentations.

- The *vice president of clinical services* is responsible for ensuring that the strategic plan envisions teamwork implementation and makes fiscal accommodations to ensure that this occurs.

- The *human resource director* is responsible for ensuring integration of teamwork factors into performance review process.

- The *department physician director* is responsible for ensuring that the strategic plan is integrated into the physician practice plan.

- The *department nurse director* is responsible for ensuring the strategic plan has the fiscal or operational support necessary to initiate and sustain teamwork implementation.

- *Department clinical leadership* is responsible for ensuring that staff accountability for daily implementation of the teamwork system.

The basic types of support actions these senior leaders need to take are shown in Exhibit 14.1. The particular attitudes and beliefs that must be encouraged for effective teamwork to emerge were discussed at the beginning of this chapter.

EXHIBIT 14.1

SENIOR LEADER ACTIONS NECESSARY TO SUPPORT TEAMWORK IMPLEMENTATION

1. Endorse the teamwork implementation initiative to board members, management, and staff as an important contributor to the control of clinical errors.

2. Select a strong physician-nurse pair (p-n pair) to lead implementation and send them to a teamwork training course.

3. Ensure that core care delivery teams (composed of physicians, nurses, and technicians) are established as part of the unit's standard daily work structure.

4. Revise policies to include procedures and protocols related to teamwork.

5. Include teamwork performance criteria in the personnel evaluation system.

6. Meet with the p-n pair on a regular basis to understand implementation difficulties and discuss possible solutions.

7. Include adequate implementation planning time in p-n pair work schedule.

8. Encourage staff to serve as program facilitators to aid implementation through support to the p-n pair

9. Make a brief statement of organizational commitment to teamwork at the beginning of each training class.

10. Provide visible support and encouragement to the implementation leaders in the presence of the staff.

11. Hold teamwork implementation progress reviews.

12. Include teamwork failure analyses in root cause analyses of sentinel events.

13. Develop a sustainment strategy, including a plan for the replacement of teamwork implementation leaders as they move on.

FIGURE 14.8   Teamwork System Implementation

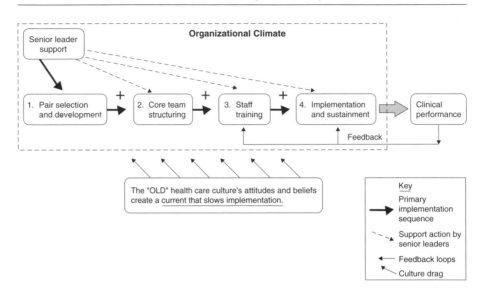

A simplified conceptualization of the teamwork implementation process is shown in Figure 14.8. Although senior leadership commitment and support (shown at the top left) is clearly the driving force in implementation success, the sound execution of the four operational actions (shown in the middle) is the practical key to successful implementation. Action 1, selection and development of a physician-nurse pair, defines who will provide teamwork training for the staff and lead or facilitate the daily actions involved in implementation. This must be a seasoned physician-nurse pair that has the respect of the staff. They must have respect for each other and work well together. They may or may not be managers in the department but they must have the respect and support of the managers and senior leaders. This support must be provided as both protected time for planning, teaching, implementation, and evaluation and time for coordination with department leadership to address the broad range of implementation issues that arise.

Use of a p-n pair in the teamwork implementation process is important because a critical part of the initiative is improving communication and coordination between physicians and nurses. These two individuals will come with their respective professional community's view of the clinical unit or department and how it works. This pairing also symbolically demonstrates the core team structure on which the teamwork system is built. Ultimately, however, success will rest on the ability of the p-n pair to coordinate with each other, effectively communicate with the staff, and solve problems. They must be able to do the following:

- Lead actions that revise staff structure and create core teams.

- Adjust management procedures to ensure maintenance of team structures over shift changes.

- Establish schedules for staff teamwork training.

- Deliver training to staff.

- Determine fiscal support requirements.

- Acquire and distribute implementation support materials (for example, core team identification devices such as scrubs, armbands, badges, training materials, and so on).

- Oversee team system start-up on the appointed day.

- Establish teamwork coaching procedures and protocols to ensure that proper teamwork skills and habits are formed based on daily feedback.

- Find, develop, and enlist the support of additional teamwork facilitators (current clinical preceptors).

- Put feedback mechanisms in place (such as short three-to-five-minute self-review team meetings near the end of the shift, and teamwork failure reviews in morbidity and mortality conferences) so that system corrections and improvements will occur as a normal part of the implementation process.

The teamwork-trained physician-nurse pair must manage and oversee the remaining operational actions involved in implementation: structure core teams (Action 2 in Figure 14.8), train the staff (Action 3), and implement and sustain the system (Action 4). The formal training required to prepare a physician-nurse pair to oversee the implementation of this teamwork system in their department takes less than one week. Their in-house preparation time before start-up is three to six weeks, depending on the size of the organization.

Again, as suggested by the box at the bottom of Figure 14.8, the ease with which teamwork is embraced by a department is influenced by the attitudes and beliefs of the caregivers. The caregiver culture either facilitates or impedes the implementation depending on where the particular caregiver community stands. For resistant staffs, implementing the team structures and employing the teamwork behaviors will eventually begin to move resistant attitudes to friendlier ground—but the movement will occur slowly. The time commitment and direct involvement of leadership are imperative to a successful and long-lived teamwork system. Dynamics Research Corporation believes effective teamwork system implementation ultimately occurs only when there is the following:

- A positive attitude on the part of senior leaders

- A practical commitment to implementation by the senior leaders

- A capable p-n pair to manage the transition and oversee the daily actions of training and implementation

Conclusion

Shifts in the attitudes of the health care community are allowing changes in emergency care and other services that will ultimately improve care delivery and reduce the error rates associated with care. Movement toward these newer attitudes and beliefs significantly improves the opportunities for teamwork system implementation. In particular, changes in caregiver beliefs and attitudes regarding personal fallibility, work approach, care system complexity, primary source of clinical error, peer checks of one's actions, and caregiver skills required will make teamwork implementation easier.

Finally, existing research suggests that improved teamwork can have a profound impact on patient care (Gaba, 1994). The teamwork concepts discussed here, the teamwork system that was tested, and the Teamwork Failure Checklist tool for assessing teamwork performance in incidents are devices that will improve the teamwork component of health care. The ultimate key to implementation lies in the willingness of the organization's senior leaders to commit to the initiative. With senior leadership commitment and a little patience and perseverance, caregivers will learn coordination skills and communication habits that will enable them to better integrate their clinical actions and implement a team-based, patient-focused cultural change. And, at least as important, caregivers will learn to more openly accept help from others to avoid the inevitable errors that are part of being human.

Discussion Questions

1. The MedTeams System emphasizes that a physician-nurse pair deliver teamwork training, share the responsibility of coaching teamwork behaviors in the

workplace, and collaborate in conducting a teamwork failures analysis. Discuss the strengths and weaknesses of this pairing of professionals to perform these tasks.

2. When specific teamwork errors are found to have contributed to an adverse event, what organizational responses and remedial actions might be needed to correct these errors?

3. List some of the actions that need to occur at the organizational level to ensure that a teamwork training system like MedTeams is effectively implemented.

Key Terms

Check actions   Team dimensions   Teamwork

Team

References

Baker, D. P., Salas, E., & Barach, P. (2003). *Medical teamwork and patient safety: The evidence-based relation.* Washington, DC: The American Institutes of Research.

Bartlett, E. (1998). Physicians, cognitive errors, and their liability consequences. *Journal of Healthcare Risk Management, 18*(4), 62–69.

Barton, E. (1997). Claims and litigation management. In R. Carroll (Ed.), *Risk management handbook for healthcare organizations* (2nd ed.). Chicago: American Hospital Publishing.

Binder, L. S., & Chapman, D. M. (1995). Qualitative research methodologies in emergency medicine. *Academic Emergency Medicine, 2*(12), 1098–1102.

Bogner, S. (Ed.). (1994). *Human error in medicine.* Hillsdale, NJ: Erlbaum.

Chassin, M., Galvin, R., & National Roundtable on Health Care Quality. (1998). The urgent need to improve health care quality. *Journal of the American Medical Association, 280*(11), 1000–1005.

Croteau, R. J. (Ed.). (2010). *Root cause analysis in health care: Tools and techniques* (4th ed.). Oakbrook Terrace, IL: Joint Commission Resources.

Davis, K., & McConnell, J. (1997). Data management. In R. Carroll (Ed.), *Risk management handbook for healthcare organizations* (2nd ed.). Chicago: American Hospital Publishing.

Dorner, D. (1996). *The logic of failure: Recognizing and avoiding error in complex situations.* New York: Metropolitan Books.

Endsley, M. (1995). Toward a theory of situation awareness in dynamic systems. *Human Factors, 37*(1), 32–64.

Gaba, D. M. (1994). Human error in dynamic medical domains. In S. Bogner, (Ed.), *Human error in medicine.* Hillsdale, NJ: Erlbaum.

Gaba, D., Howard, S., Fish, K., Smith, B., & Sowb, Y. (2001). Simulation-based training in anesthesia crisis resource management (ACRM): A decade of experience. *Simulation and Gaming, 32*(2), 175–193.

Gayman, A. J., Gentner, F. C., Canbaras, S. A., & Crissey, M. J. (1996, December). *Implications of crew resource management training for tank crews.* Paper presented at the Interservice/Industry Training Systems and Education Conference, Orlando, FL.

Grubb, G., Simon, R., & Zeller, J. L. (2001). *Effects of crew coordination training and evaluation methods on AH-64 attack helicopter battalion crew performance* (ARI Contractor Report 2002–10, ADA 398770). Alexandria, VA: U.S. Army Research Institute for the Behavioral and Social Sciences, pp. 14–17.

Harris, K. T., Treanor, C. M., & Salisbury, M. L. (2006). Improving patient safety with team coordination: Challenges and strategies of implementation. *Journal of Obstetric, Gynecologic, and Neonatal Nursing, 35*(4), 557–566.

Helmreich, R. L., Merritt, A. C., & Wilhelm, J. A. (1999). The evolution of crew resource management training in commercial aviation. *International Journal of Aviation Psychology, 9*(1), 19–32.

Joint Commission on Accreditation of Healthcare Organizations. (1998). *Sentinel events: Evaluating cause and planning improvement.* Oakbrook Terrace, IL: Author.

King, H., Battles, J., Baker, D., Alonso, A., Sales, E., Webster, J., Toomey, L., & Salisbury, M. (2008, August). *TeamSTEPPS®: Team Strategies and Tools to Enhance Performance and Patient Safety.* Retrieved from http://www.ahrq.gov/downloads/pub/advances2/vol3/Advances-King_1.pdf.

Kohn, L. T., Corrigan, J. M., & Donaldson, M. S. (Eds.). (2000). *To err is human: Building a safer health system.* Washington, DC: National Academy Press.

Koss, L. (1993). Cervical (PAP) smear: New directions. *Cancer Supplement, 71*(4), 1406–1412.

Leape, L. (1994). Error in medicine. *Journal of the American Medical Association, 272*(23), 1851–1857.

Leape, L. (1996, October 13). Errors in health care: Problems and challenges. Paper presented at Examining Errors in Health Care: Developing a Prevention, Education, and Research Agenda, Rancho Mirage, CA.

Leape, L. (2004). Human factors meets health care: The ultimate challenge. *Ergonomics in Design, 12*(3), 6–12.

Leape, L., Brennan, T., Laird, N., Lawthers, A., Localio, A., Barnes, B., Hebert, L., … Hiatt, H. (1991). The nature of adverse events in hospitalized patients: Results of the Harvard Medical Practice Study II. *New England Journal of Medicine, 324*(6), 377–384.

Leedom, D., & Simon R. (1995). Improving team coordination: A case for behavior-based training. *Military Psychology, 7*(2), 109–122.

McClanahan, S., Goodwin, S., & Houser, F. (2000). A formula for errors: Good people + bad systems. In P. Spath (Ed.), *Error reduction in health care* (pp. 1–14). San Francisco: Jossey-Bass.

Millenson, M. L. (1997). *Demanding medical excellence: Doctors and accountability in the information age*. Chicago: University of Chicago Press.

Morey, J., Simon, R., Jay, G., Wears, R., Salisbury, M., Dukes, K., & Berns, S. (2002). Error reduction and performance improvement in the emergency department through formal teamwork training: Evaluation results of the MedTeams project. *Health Services Research, 37*(6), 1553–1581.

Morey, J. C., & Salisbury, M. (2002). Introducing teamwork training into healthcare organizations: Implementation issues and solutions. *Proceedings of the Human Factors and Ergonomics Society 46th Annual Meeting*. Santa Monica, CA: Human Factors and Ergonomics Society, 2069–2073.

Morey, J. C., Simon, R., Jay, G. D., & Rice, M. M. (2003). A transition from aviation crew resource management to hospital emergency departments: The MedTeams story. *Proceedings of the Twelfth International Symposium on Aviation Psychology*. Columbus: The Aviation Psychology Laboratory of The Ohio State University, pp. 826–832.

Musson, D. M., & Helmreich, R. L. (2004). Team training and resource management in health care: Current issues and future directions. *Harvard Health Policy Review, 5*(1), 25–35.

Nielsen, P., Goldman, M., Mann, S., Shapiro, D., Marcus, R., Pratt, S., Greenberg, P., & Sachs, B. (2007). Effects of teamwork training on adverse outcomes and process of care in labor and delivery. *Obstetrics & Gynecology, 109*(1), 48–55.

Phillips, K. (1997). *The power of health care teams: Strategies for success*. Oakbrook Terrace, IL: Joint Commission on Accreditation of Healthcare Organizations, p. 105.

Prince, C., & Salas, E. (1999). Team processes and their training in aviation. In D. J. Garland, J. A. Wise, & V. D. Hopkin (Eds.), *Handbook of aviation human factors*. Mahwah, NJ: Erlbaum.

Reason, J. (1990). *Human error*. New York: Cambridge University Press.

Reason, J., & Mycielska, K. (1982). *Absent-minded? The psychology of mental lapses and everyday errors*. Englewood Cliffs, NJ: Prentice Hall.

Risser, D., Rice, M., Salisbury, M., Simon, R., Jay G., & Berns, S. (1999). The potential for improved teamwork to reduce medical errors in the emergency department. *Annals of Emergency Medicine, 34*(3), 373–383.

Salas, E., Almeida, S., Salisbury, M., King, H., Lazzara, E., Lyons, R., Wilson, K., McQuillan, R., (2009). What are the critical success factors for team training in health care? *The Joint Commission Journal on Quality and Patient Safety, 35*(8), 398–405.

Salas, E., Burke, C., Bowers, C., & Wilson, K. (2001). Team training in the skies: Does crew resource management (CRM) work? *Human Factors, 43*(4), 641–674.

Salas, E., Dickinson, T., Converse, S., & Tannenbaum, S. (1992). Toward an understanding of team performance and training. In R. W. Swezey & E. Salas (Eds.). *Teams: Their training and performance*. Norwood, NJ: Ablex.

Salas, E., Wilson, K., & Burke, C. (2006). Does crew resource management work? An update, an extension, and some critical needs. *Human Factors, 48*(2), 392–412.

Sassano, M., & Dronsfeld, J. (1991). Securing risk management information from discovery. In G. Henry (Ed.), *Emergency medicine risk management: A comprehensive review.* Dallas: American College of Emergency Physicians.

Schmidt, J., & Moore, G. P. (1993). Management of multiple trauma. *Emergency Medicine Clinics of North America, 11*(1), 29–51.

Simon, R., Morey, J., Rice, M., et al. (1999). Reducing errors in emergency medicine through team performance: The MedTeams project. *Proceedings of Enhancing Patient Safety and Reducing Errors in Health Care.* Chicago: National Patient Safety Foundation.

Simon, R., Morey, J., Locke, A., Risser, D., & Langford, V. (1997). *Full scale development of the Emergency Team Coordination Course® and evaluation measures.* Andover, MA: Dynamics Research Corporation.

Vincent, C., Taylor-Adams, S., & Stanhope, N. (1998). Framework for analyzing risk and safety in clinical medicine. *British Medical Journal, 316*(7138), 1154–1157.

Weiler, P., Hiatt, H., Newhouse, J., Johnson, W., Brennan, T., & Leape, L. (1993). *A measure of malpractice: Medical injury, malpractice litigation, & patient compensation.* Cambridge, MA: Harvard University Press.

Wilson-Donnelly, K., Burke, C., & Salas, E. (2004). Does crew resource management (CRM) training work in health care? *Proceedings of the Human Factors and Ergonomics Society 48th Annual Meeting.* Santa Monica, CA: Human Factors and Ergonomics Society, pp. 2587–2591.

Xiao, Y., Hunter, W., Mackenzie, C., Jefferies, N., & Horst, R., (1996). Task complexity in emergency medical care and its implications for team coordination. *Human Factors, 38*(4), 636–645.

CHAPTER 15

MEDICATION SAFETY IMPROVEMENT

Yosef D. Dlugacz

LEARNING OBJECTIVES

- Describe various national efforts to reduce medication errors
- Understand the impact of organizational culture on medication safety
- Describe risk points in the medication delivery process
- Identify medication error reduction strategies
- Explain the role of patients in promoting medication safety

Medication safety has been a growing national concern since the Institute of Medicine (IOM) report focused the nation's attention on the number of preventable errors that injure hospitalized patients (IOM, 1999). A more recent IOM report found that medication errors injure approximately 1.5 million people in the United States and cost billions annually. Conservative estimates are that between 380,000 and 450,000 **adverse drug events** occur in U.S. hospitals every year. The medication error rate for outpatients is even worse, with 530,000 adverse events occurring annually in the Medicare population alone (IOM, 2006). In response to these reports most health care organizations have stepped up their medication error reduction strategies. Throughout the country, issues associated with medication delivery processes are being evaluated, redesigned, and improved. Yet, medication errors continue to occur.

The National Coordinating Council for Medication Error Reporting and Prevention (NCC MERP), an independent conglomerate of health care organizations, including the American Medical Association, The Joint Commission, the American Hospital Association and others, defines a medication error as "any preventable event that may cause or lead to inappropriate medication use or patient harm while the medication is in the control of the health care professional, patients, or consumer" (NCC MERP, 2005, p. 4).

This chapter describes the safety risks that contribute to medication errors and what health care professionals and organizations can do to reduce these risks. Many improvement recommendations originate from the work of national groups involved in medication safety. Some process changes aimed at eliminating medication errors are derived from error-proofing practices found in high-reliability organizations (HROs) and from lean process improvement techniques. Quite likely you will find a number of concepts and practices described herein also discussed in other chapters in this book. This chapter is intended as a central point of reference for readers particularly interested in reducing medication errors.

National Efforts to Improve Medication Safety

Governmental, advisory, and accreditation organizations have prioritized medication error reduction and are suggesting solutions. National groups are exerting pressure on health care organizations to adopt defined medication safety practices through the use of financial incentives, threat of negative publicity, and accreditation requirements. In addition to encouraging health care organizations to adopt safer medication delivery practices, many groups offer consumer education, tools, and forums on the topic of medication safety. Several (of the many) influential national groups involved in promoting medication safety are described in the next section.

Government Agencies

Federal regulations and government-sponsored research are helping to support ever safer medication safety in all health care environments. These activities have a major influence on safe medication practices.

Agency for Healthcare Research and Quality (AHRQ)
The AHRQ (http://www.ahrq.gov), part of the U.S. Department of Health and Human Services, has as its mission to improve the quality, safety, efficiency, and effectiveness of health care for all Americans. The organization provides quality and patient safety information and resources to clinicians and consumers of health care services. Through an online peer-reviewed journal on patient safety, WebM&M (Morbidity and Mortality Rounds on the Web) (http://www.webmm.ahrq.gov), experts analyze medical errors that have been anonymously reported to the organization. Included among the several guides published by the AHRQ to help consumers navigate safely through medical care is

Your Medicine: Play It Safe, which addresses common questions about medication safety. Another guide, *Twenty Tips to Help Prevent Medical Errors in Children,* provides facts to help parents help their children avoid errors involving medicines and hospital stays.

Centers for Medicare and Medicaid Services (CMS)

The CMS works collaboratively with public and private organizations to improve medication safety. These partnerships encourage public reporting of preventable errors and defining measures of care. The CMS has developed several initiatives to respond to the crisis of medication errors. For example, they support electronic prescribing to improve the efficiency of providing prescription drugs, and also electronic messaging that would ensure that pharmacists and physicians have accurate and complete information about their patient's medical history. They advocate data collection and analysis to identify safety problems and adverse events, with the hope of improving understanding of problems related to pre-scribing practices and other errors. To highlight performance improvements, the CMS collects and publishes data on performance measures related to the effec-tive use of medications. Their Web site (http://www.HospitalCompare.hhs.gov) provides consumers with comparative measures of hospital performance, includ-ing some measures of medication safety practices.

Federal Drug Administration (FDA)

The FDA is responsible for drug safety in the United States through error track-ing and education. The FDA receives medication error reports from its adverse event reporting program, MedWatch (http://www.fda.gov/safety/MedWatch/). They also receive medication error information from the Institute for Safe Medication Practices (ISMP) and the U.S. Pharmacopeia (USP), a nongovern-mental medication standard-setting organization. The FDA distributes informa-tion to consumers and health professionals on new drug warnings and other safety information, drug label changes, and shortages of medically necessary drug products.

Advisory Groups

Medication safety is the primary focus of many advisory groups who represent or interact with health care professionals in various settings. The efforts of these advisory groups are contributing to ever improving medication safety.

American Society of Health-System Pharmacists (ASHP)

The ASHP (http://www.ashp.org) is a professional association of pharmacists dedicated to helping people use medications safely and effectively. They provide advice on medication use and safe practices to health care professionals working in hospitals, ambulatory care clinics, long-term facilities, and home care services. On the ASHP safe medication Web site (http://www.safemedication.com) consumers can learn about appropriate use of medications and medication safety tips.

Institute of Medicine (IOM)

The IOM (http://www.iom.edu) is a not-for-profit, nongovernmental agency that is part of the National Academy of Sciences, whose purpose is to provide independent, scientific, expert information and advice on medicine and health to professionals and the public. In addition to conducting studies for the U.S. Congress and other federal and independent organizations, the IOM offers informational forums, roundtables, and discussion opportunities to educate and promote improved safety in health care.

The IOM is committed to educating the public about medication risks and advising the public on ways to reduce those risks. For example, in 2006, the IOM published a fact sheet, "What You Can Do to Avoid Medication Errors," designed to inform the public about common dangers involving the medication process and offering advice about how to ensure improved safety. When the U.S. Congress urged the CMS to sponsor a study on medication safety, the IOM addressed this issue. Their report, *Preventing Medication Errors* (IOM, 2006) concluded that medication errors are common and costly. The report contains various recommended medication error reduction and prevention strategies to decrease mistakes. For example, the IOM recommends that physicians routinely reconcile medication changes with the patient's pharmacy record (for both hospital patients and outpatients), and at transition points, such as admission, transfer, and discharge. The IOM suggests that at every office visit, patients bring along all their medications so the physician can see what drugs the patient is actually taking.

Institute for Safe Medication Practices (ISMP)

The ISMP (http://www.ismp.org) is a nongovernmental, nonprofit group of health care professionals dedicated to understanding and reducing medication errors and promoting safe medication use. The organization works closely with health care practitioners and institutions, regulatory agencies, professional organizations, and the pharmaceutical industry. The ISMP offers tools, resources, educational programs, teleconferences, and online newsletters, such as "ISMP Medication Safety Alert," which provides health care professionals and consumers with up-to-date information and advice about medication safety. It also sponsors an informative consumer-oriented medication safety Web site (http://www.consumermedsafety.org).

National Coordinating Council for Medication Error Reporting and Prevention (NCC MERP)

The NCC MERP (http://www.nccmerp.org) is an independent group of health care organizations that collaborate to discuss causes of medication errors and promote increased safety in medication delivery. By reviewing over 500 narrative reports of errors, the NCC MERP has identified common at-risk professional behaviors and determined what is needed to reduce the effect of these behaviors on safe delivery of medication (for example, do not take shortcuts). Several process change recommendations have been disseminated by the NCC MERP. For example, to reduce errors associated with prescription writing, the NCC MERP advises that, when appropriate, the prescription includes information about the purpose of the medication (for example, to treat a cough) to help ensure that the proper medication is being dispensed. The addition of information about the medication's purpose adds an extra safety check to the prescription and dispensing process.

U.S. Pharmacopeia (USP)

The USP (http://www.usp.org) is a nongovernmental, not-for-profit public health organization that sets standards for all prescription and over-the-counter medicines and other health care products manufactured or sold in the United States. Under federal law, these standards must be met. USP provides continuing education for physicians, pharmacists, and nurses and distributes evidence-based drug information to health care providers through their Web site and at conferences.

The Leapfrog Group

The Leapfrog Group, a conglomeration of big business and industry, is attempting to reduce medical errors by using their purchasing power to influence hospital care. They reward hospitals for outstanding quality and safety by recommending that their employees frequent hospitals that meet their criteria. On the group's Web site (http://www.leapfroggroup.org) are ratings for hospitals on quality and safety measures, including use of specific safety practices such as use of computerized physician order entry (CPOE) technology.

Accreditation Groups

Many hospitals seek voluntary accreditation and the standards of these groups include requirements related to medication safety. The two primary groups that accredit hospitals are listed here.

The Joint Commission (TJC)

TJC is a not-for-profit accrediting agency that certifies health care organizations for adhering to stringent performance and quality standards. To maintain accreditation, organizations, including office-based surgery practices, have to comply with standards for medication management. In a 2007 national survey of hospitals, TJC targeted three issues that seriously compromised patient safety with regard to medication: medication storage (secure, safe), medication orders (written clearly, transcribed correctly), and pharmacist review of orders (for appropriateness) (Kienle & Uselton, 2008). Hospitals are expected to address these issues and develop processes to eliminate medication safety dangers. National Patient Safety Goals, developed and promulgated by TJC, include several directly related to improving medication safety. For example, health care organizations are expected to standardize and limit the number of drug concentrations used and disseminate a list of look-alike or sound-alike drugs to alert caregivers to the potential for misidentifications. The current National Patient Safety Goals can be found on the TJC Web site (http://www.jointcommission.org).

The 2010 standards for office-based surgery practices include medication management requirements. These requirements address management of high-alert and hazardous medications, storing the medications safely, preparing, labeling, dispensing, and so on. The standards also require effective response to real or **potential adverse drug events** and medication errors.

DNV Healthcare

Another agency that accredits hospitals, and is recognized as an authority for Medicare and Medicaid programs, is DNV Healthcare, Inc. (http://www.dnv .com/industry/healthcare). This accreditation group is part of a Norway-based foundation that evaluates compliance with standards in several industries. The medication related standards found in the National Integrated Accreditation for Healthcare Organizations (NIAHO) issued by DNV are similar to those of The Joint Commission. For instance, to meet the NIAHO standards organizations must have a formal and systematic approach for reconciling patient medications across the continuum of care, including unit-to-unit and provider-to-provider (DNV Healthcare, 2009).

Medication Safety Improvement Barriers

With so many groups working to improve medication safety and with so much public attention focused on reducing errors, it is remarkable that more progress has not been made. The hospital medication delivery process is still riddled with problems, with over 400,000 preventable medication-related injuries occurring in hospitals annually (IOM, 2006). In long-term care facilities, Gurwitz et al. (2005) found the overall rate of adverse drug events was 9.8 per 100 resident-months, with a rate of 4.1 preventable adverse drug events per 100 resident-months.

Health care providers have access to recommendations from various groups regarding safer medication practices, yet these recommendations are often not implemented. Why? The organizational and social culture of health care does not readily embrace change. A cultural change is necessary, one where each member of the organization is committed to safety. If principles of high-reliability organizations (see Chapter Three) were adopted, the necessary cultural mind-set to improve would be in place. Cultural barriers include lack of sensitivity to the inherent risks of medication delivery and lack of understanding of the dangers involved (IOM, 2003). Unclear organizational values have also been cited as contributing to risks to patient safety, such as not addressing medication delivery problems with pharmacy in a timely way and fear of punishment (Kalisch & Aebersold, 2006).

Health care professionals often have a justifiable fear of censure or reprisal if they report errors. In spite of Joint Commission standards that encourage health care organizations to create a blame-free environment for error reporting, individuals may still be blamed for errors that are caused by flawed systems. In some organizations, if a nurse makes an error—such as administering an incorrect medication or an incorrect dose of medication—the nurse is subject to reprimand. Professionals working in these organizations are reluctant to disclose errors or near misses (an event which did not cause patient injury but might have if not caught and corrected). Without such reports, the organization cannot identify safety and reliability gaps in the medication system. The organization loses opportunities to fix error-prone processes and systems. Even when errors and near misses are reported, the information may not be uniformly tracked and analyzed in a systematic way. The resources necessary for accomplishing these analyses may be lacking if the organization is not truly committed to medication safety improvement.

Traditional work patterns and staff organization can also pose barriers to medication safety. For example, a 2006 study by the Emergency Nurses Association investigated why the medication-related National Patient Safety Goals were poorly adhered to by emergency department (ED) nurses. Poor compliance with the goals was found to be related to complexity of the work environment, the nurses' involvement in education of residents-in-training, and mixed-shift nursing hours (Juarez et al., 2009).

Technology improvements, such as point-of-care access to pharmaceutical decision support resources, can reduce medication errors; however, many health care organizations have yet to adopt these technologies. In particular, many primary care physician offices do not have the infrastructure, commitment, or resources to introduce new technology and processes into their offices (Galt, 2003). Introducing, implementing, and financing new technologies in health care facilities, in addition to incorporating new systems into current information systems, is not easy (see Chapter Thirteen). Staff members must be trained in the new technology and psychological barriers to changing current practices must be overcome. Other technological barriers, such as drug manufacturers not placing bar codes on each unit dose package of medication, also contribute to medication errors.

Impact of Organizational Culture

Until leadership adopts HRO principles, medication safety improvements will come slowly. HRO principles—sensitivity to operations, preoccupation with failure, deference to expertise, resilience, and reluctance to simplify—focus on establishing an organizational state of mind in which reliability and safety are central. In an organization committed to high reliability, risks are identified in a blame-free environment, lines of accountability and responsibility are clearly defined, clinicians are empowered to make changes, and communication is effective. Attention to and focus on risk is considered everyone's job, not only the specialists. The goal for everyone must be reliability, that is, to deliver medication safely, accurately, and appropriately and do it consistently every single time (Weick & Sutcliffe, 2007).

Leaders have a significant impact on creating a **just culture** that supports a reliable and safe medication delivery system. Cultural assumptions generally reflect leadership values, as described by Dr. Lucian Leape, a longtime patient safety advocate (Schyve, 2004, p. 656):

> The secret of culture change is, I believe, quite simple: leadership and champions. Putting it in the negative, culture change cannot happen without strong leadership from the top and active leaders, physician champions, at the front line. Leaders must articulate the goals, demonstrate their commitment in everyday life, and persuade others to make the changes needed. In those institutions and systems where the leaders have truly made safety the top priority, dramatic changes have occurred. The challenge is how to get more of them aboard.

EXHIBIT 15.1

MEDICATION ERROR CASE STUDY

A woman with a cardiac condition was admitted to the ICU of a large teaching hospital during the night shift. A first-year resident ordered a new medication, with which he was unfamiliar, for the patient. The pharmacist who dispensed the drug labeled the medication with a "red flag," a warning that the medication had to be diluted before being administered to the patient. The nurses on the unit were inexperienced, having very recently completed their orientation and they too were unfamiliar with the new medication.

Inexperienced and unfamiliar as they were, however, they did not seek the information necessary to safely administer the drug. Because they did not want to appear to be inexperienced, neither the resident nor the nurse checked with their supervisors or with the pharmacy. Remarkably, they did not notice the prominently displayed red warning flag. The new nurse was reluctant to question the resident about the medication, and did not follow policy to explicitly articulate for the physician the name of the medication and the dosage when she handed the syringe to the resident for administration. Likewise the resident did not confirm the medication with the nurse, as policy required. He simply took the medication as it was handed to him and injected the patient with the undiluted drug. The patient had a cardiac arrest and died.

Note: This example is compiled from several actual events.

Exhibit 15.1 is a case study illustrating how the culture in an organization can affect compliance with safe practices. In this instance, a harmful medication error occurred.

The case study highlights how issues of education and culture can prevent professional staff from using available resources. The clinicians seemed to avoid open communication. Because the resident was unfamiliar with the drug and its effects, he could have discussed the medication order with the chief resident or the attending physician. The nurses could have sought information about the medication from the nurse educator who was available or called the pharmacist for administration instructions. The pharmacist might have alerted the clinicians about the medication and its delivery. Certainly the nurse and the resident should have communicated with each other about the medication before it was injected.

Cultural and hierarchical barriers prevented the nurse from admitting that she did not know about the medication. If she had questioned others about the medication or discussed her reservations with peers or with the resident, her inexperience would have become evident. The resident wanted to demonstrate his authority and so also did not ask for confirmation, advice, or information from peers or superiors. This tragic event could have been prevented.

In an HRO, the nurses' preoccupation with failure would cause them to focus attention on their lack of information and inexperience with a new medication. The red flag warning of the pharmacist would have been noticed. If the nurses were sensitive to operations, they would be alert to potential dangers in this high-risk situation, especially during the night shift when staffing is low. In an HRO, inexperienced clinicians know the importance of deferring to expertise when necessary and they ask for assistance.

Understanding Medication Errors

Administration of medication is the most frequent intervention in medical care, with patients often prescribed multiple medications. To understand the issues involved in medication safety it is necessary to understand the complexity of the medication delivery system. This section focuses on medication delivery in a hospital or similar institutional setting. However, many of the principles and error prevention strategies are applicable to outpatient settings as well. Medication delivery in a hospital involves many steps and many people—which increases the safety risks (see Figure 15.1).

The process is not continuous but rather fragmented by disciplines. Adding to potential risk, no single authority is **accountable** for oversight of the entire process. Therefore transitions from one task to the next may not be effectively or safely managed.

Consider the number of steps involved in delivering the right medication to the right patient at the right time. The physician has to correctly diagnose the

FIGURE 15.1　Hospital Medication Administration Process

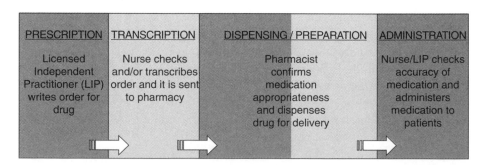

PRESCRIPTION	TRANSCRIPTION	DISPENSING / PREPARATION	ADMINISTRATION
Licensed Independent Practitioner (LIP) writes order for drug	Nurse checks and/or transcribes order and it is sent to pharmacy	Pharmacist confirms medication appropriateness and dispenses drug for delivery	Nurse/LIP checks accuracy of medication and administers medication to patients

patient's condition and prescribe the correct medication at the correct dosage and delivery mode. The prescription has to be written legibly and accurately. Next, the prescription has to be transcribed accurately by the nurse and communicated correctly to pharmacy. If the hospital has a CPOE system, the medication order has to be properly entered into the computer by the physician and accurately transmitted to the pharmacy. The pharmacist has to fill the prescription with the correct medication and affix the right label for the right patient. Then the correctly labeled medication has to be delivered to the right unit in a timely way. The route for giving the medication needs to be accurately communicated to the administering nurse as well. The nurse then has to confirm the accuracy of the medication and give the medication correctly to the right patient at the right time.

To create a safe medication delivery system, the process complexity and risk potential at each step must be taken into account. A preoccupation with risk, errors, and safety gaps is necessary to ensure reliable performance.

Risk Points in Medication Delivery

Errors can occur at any point in the medication delivery process. Adding to the error risk are issues such as competence of the professionals involved and effectiveness of communication among the different disciplines at each step. Understanding **risk points**, where errors occur, helps focus attention on the system problems that cause mistakes.

Prescription Errors

Physicians can prescribe the wrong medication or the wrong dosage. This can occur for any number of reasons. For instance, the physician may have incomplete or incorrect information about the patient's clinical condition. The physician may not be aware of the patient's allergies or herbal supplements that the patient is taking. The physician may not be aware of the latest drug warnings or contraindications that need to be considered before prescribing the medication. Once choosing a medication for the patient, the physician needs to write a prescription or order the medication with the correct dosage and timing of administration. Even when physicians choose the correct medication, their orders may contain dangerous abbreviations or other communication shortcuts that are easily misinterpreted by nurses or pharmacists.

Transcription Errors

Issues of legibility and completeness can affect safety when nurses manually transcribe medication orders. The medication can be written incorrectly in the patient's record or information regarding type of medication, timing, dosage, frequency, duration, administrative route can be incorrect or incomplete. This same information can be incorrectly entered into a computer system by the physician or nurse. Errors also occur as medication information is transferred between providers when patients move to different levels of care. Incorrect or incomplete information is particularly dangerous when patients are discharged from a hospital or long-term care facility (Davis, Toombs Smith, & Tyler, 2005; Callen, McIntosh, & Li, 2009).

Dispensing and Preparation Errors

Pharmacists are important safeguards in the medication delivery system as they are responsible for reviewing all medication orders for accuracy and completeness. Unfortunately, because of the way information flows within a hospital, pharmacists are not always aware of patients' current diagnoses and chronic conditions, if any. Pharmacists may not have access to essential laboratory information about patients. These shortcomings weaken the ability of pharmacists to be effective safeguards in the medication delivery process (Cina et al., 2006). The pharmacist can prepare and dispense the wrong drug, or the right drug at the wrong dose, or the wrong amount. Labeling of medications can be inaccurate, incomplete, or misinterpreted. Concentrated forms of medication can be improperly diluted for intravenous administration. These errors often occur when pharmacy staff are interrupted or inadequately staffed (Desselle, 2005).

Medication packaging by suppliers can also lead to pharmacist errors. For example, similarly packaged medications can provoke errors, especially if the pharmacist is distracted. Medications that have passed their expiration date or not stored properly can lead to safety problems as well.

Administration Errors

An administration error occurs when the patient does not receive the intended medication at the right time in the right way. Errors of omission (the drug is not given at all or not given at the correct time) are as common in hospitals as errors of commission (wrong drug given, drug given by wrong route, or expired drug given). Excluding wrong-time errors, omission of an ordered medication is generally the most common type of drug administration error in nursing homes (IOM, 2006).

Administration of intravenous (IV) medications is complex and particularly susceptible to errors (Taxis & Barber, 2003). Adverse events relating to the speed of IV medication delivery can occur. For example, "red man syndrome," so-called because the patient becomes flushed, experiences burning, itching, and other discomfort such as chest pain, can occur when IV Vancomycin (an anti-biotic) is given too quickly. In addition, mistakes occur when caregivers are unfamiliar with the medication to be given, the administration process, or the medication delivery equipment.

Similar medications stored next to one another in the same area can cause nurses to give the wrong drug to a patient (Bates, 2002). This same mistake can occur when medication containers are not properly labeled or when caregivers are interrupted or distracted during medication delivery.

Locate Your Risk Points

Although the medical literature is filled with information on the causes of medication errors, organizational leaders should identify the actual risk points in their particular system. This information can be derived from incident and near-miss reports generated by caregivers. Pharmacists and nurses, frontline safeguards in the medication delivery process, are best positioned to recognize and report actual and potential mistakes. To create a culture where reporting of errors is encouraged, the organization must encourage a blame-free environment where reports can be made without fear of personal reprisals.

Allowing staff to anonymously report mistakes (not sign their name to the report) is one way health care organizations have been able to gather more information about medication system risk points. Pharmacists, nurses, and quality management staff in one health care system collaborated in establishing an anonymous near-miss reporting form (see Figure 15.2).

Frequency of reporting increased with the use of the form in Figure 15.2. Analysis of the reported near misses data revealed that over 11% of near misses were related to anti-hypertensive agents, primarily mistakes involving medication dosing. By establishing an effective near-miss reporting program and by analyzing the reporting results, leadership was able to locate the risk points in their medication delivery system and target improvement efforts to reduce the likelihood of an actual harmful mistake.

Using data from medication-related incident reports, quality professionals and pharmacists in an 800-bed teaching hospital, identified where errors were occurring in the delivery process (see Figure 15.3).

Analysis of medication-related incidents revealed that 62% of errors were related to the way the orders were written (prescription errors). Problems of legibility, transcription, use of abbreviations, and incorrect medication accounted for these errors. Thirty-four percent of errors were related to the administration of medication. Using this information, the hospital targeted improvement efforts to improve risky processes.

FIGURE 15.2 Anonymous Medication Error Report

Unit: _____   DATE OF OCCURRENCE: ___/___/___   TIME OF OCCURRENCE: _____

PERSON INVOLVED IN OCCURRENCE:
☐ RN   ☐ MD   ☐ PA/NP   ☐ CSA   ☐ PHARMACIST   ☐ OTHER _____

PERSON REPORTING OCCURRENCE:
☐ RN   ☐ MD   ☐ PA/NP   ☐ CSA   ☐ PHARMACIST   ☐ OTHER _____

NAME OF MEDICATION: _____   CATEGORY OF MEDICATION: _____

Proscription	Transcription	Dispensing	Time of Calculation/Preparation
☐ Wrong Patient	☐ Wrong Patient	☐ Wrong Patient	☐ Wrong Patient
☐ Wrong Medication	☐ Wrong Medication	☐ Wrong Medication	☐ Wrong Medication
☐ Wrong Dose	☐ Wrong Dose	☐ Wrong Dose	☐ Incorrect Calculation
☐ Wrong Route	☐ Wrong Route	☐ Wrong Route	☐ Wrong Route
☐ Wrong Frequency	☐ Wrong Frequency	☐ Wrong Frequency	☐ Missing Dose
☐ Wrong Diluent	☐ Wrong Diluent	☐ Wrong Diluent	☐ Wrong Frequency
☐ Wrong Rate	☐ Wrong Rate	☐ Wrong Rate	☐ Duplication of Dose
☐ Illegible Order	☐ Illegible Order	☐ Excess Dose	☐ Allergy to Medication
☐ Allergy to Medication	☐ Allergy	☐ Allergy to Medication	☐ Wrong Diluent
☐ Drug – Drug Interaction	Allergy to Medication	☐ Drug – Drug Interaction	☐ Wrong Rate
☐ Drug – Food Interaction	Not Written on MAR	☐ Drug – Food Interaction	☐ Drug – Drug Interaction
☐ No Renewal	☐ Drug – Drug Interaction	☐ Wrong Dosage Form	☐ Drug – Food Interaction
☐ Unclear telephone order	☐ Drug – Food Interaction	☐ Delay in Dispensing	☐ Wrong Dosage Form
☐ Incomplete Order	☐ Delay in Transcription		
	☐ MAR not recopied properly		
	☐ Computer mis-entry		

Brief description of near miss and action taken: _____

Legend:

MAR = Medication administration record

PA/NP = Physician assistant/nurse practitioner

CSA = Clerical Support Associate

FIGURE 15.3 Medication System Error Analysis

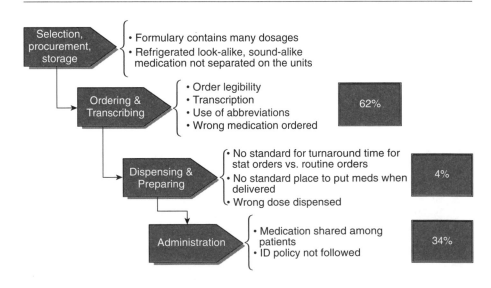

Medication Error Prevention Strategies and Practices

Medication errors occur because people are fallible and the delivery process is complex, involving many people and processes. Because errors are inevitable, processes must be designed to reduce the possibility of error and, when errors do occur, the process must allow for rapid error detection and correction.

National groups, including those mentioned earlier in this chapter, have proposed many solutions for reducing and preventing medication errors. For example, a strategic plan for medication safety was developed by a partnership of the American Hospital Association, Health Research and Educational Trust and the ISMP (2003). The plan proposed seven tactics to address system and process issues related to medication safety:

- Demonstrate a leadership-driven culture of safety
- Improve medication error detection and reporting
- Evaluate the role of technology in reducing medication errors
- Focus on the prescription and administration of high-alert medications
- Establish a blame-free environment
- Involve the community in safety programs
- Control the formulary to select medications based on safety rather than cost

Some of these recommendations relate to the organizational culture that supports medication safety improvement, some address the human factors related to medication delivery, and some speak to process redesign priorities.

Supportive Culture

When organizations embrace the HRO principles described in Chapter Three, improving the safety of medication delivery is less challenging. If every health care worker is preoccupied with the risk of failure and has a mind-set focused on reliability, there will be fewer errors. For example, in organizations sensitive to operations, high-alert drugs—such as chemotherapy medications, narcotics, and anticoagulants—would be recognized by caregivers as especially dangerous and handled more cautiously. During prescribing, transcribing, dispensing, preparation, and administration of these medications people would pay careful attention to preventing mistakes.

In an organization reluctant to simplify, the medication process is analyzed using failure mode and effect analysis (or another proactive risk assessment method) to strengthen process reliability before an adverse event occurs. In organizations committed to safety and reliability staff report a high percentage of near misses and errors. This information is regularly analyzed to identify safety concerns. Less risky processes are designed, tested, implemented, and sustained. HRO principles support the creation of a preventive culture rather than one that only reacts to adverse events when they occur.

Medication safety is largely dependent on the knowledge and competence of physicians, pharmacists, and nurses. These professionals must be constantly mindful of the risks involved in medication delivery and the potential and actual harm that results from gaps in safety. In an HRO, if a physician incorrectly prescribes a medication, the pharmacist or the nurse feels free to challenge and correct the error. Not only is the pharmacist or nurse empowered to speak up, they are also compelled to do so because of the organization's commitment to error prevention and patient safety.

The traditional hierarchical culture of the hospital has to be addressed so that residents, nurses, respiratory therapists, and others feel comfortable questioning physicians when they suspect that a medication error might occur. Typically a physician heads the hierarchy and does not elicit confirmation for decisions from others. The organizational culture of medication delivery has to change from a silo model—one where different disciplines and specialties work independently often without interdisciplinary communication—to one where the patient's safety is protected through the collaborative effort of everyone on the caregiving team. The Joint Commission cites ineffective communication among caregivers as the most frequent root cause of sentinel events (Jackson, 2005).

Human Factors

A factor that clearly causes people to make mistakes is poorly designed systems. However, a well-designed system does not eliminate the risk of human error. Mistakes can be caused by the way people interact with the system or by human conditions such as stress, tension, and mental distractions that adversely affect performance. Interventions to improve medication safety are most successful when both the system factors and the human factors are addressed (Grasha, 2000).

The NCC MERP (2005) has identified common professional at-risk behaviors that contribute to medication errors. These behaviors include:

- Using medication without complete knowledge of the medication

- Failing to double-check high-alert medications before dispensing or administering

- Failing to effectively communicate information

- Feeling reluctant to ask for clarification when unsure of proper medication use

According to NCC MERP, these at-risk behaviors occur because of system-level flaws, such as an organizational culture that tolerates at-risk behaviors and the complexity of the medication process. It is recommended that organizations question whether they tolerate risky behavior and also question why people are engaging in this behavior. The goal is to uncover and correct the culture or process flaws that contribute to at-risk behaviors.

Dr. Anthony Grasha, professor of psychology at the University of Cincinnati, created an annotated human factors checklist that details culture and system changes intended to reduce errors during medication delivery (Grasha, 2002). His recommendations include modifications to the physical environment, task analysis and design, building better human-equipment interfaces, selecting the right people for the job, and providing appropriate training for individuals in the workplace. The checklist is available from Pharmsafety.org (http://www.pharmsafety.org).

Protocols, standard order sets, checklists, and other care management tools can be employed to improve communication among clinicians along the continuum of care. One such tool is a clinical pathway. This is a description of daily interventions (including medications) and outcome targets for patients with specific conditions. Many of the recommended treatments found on a pathway are grounded in **evidence-based medicine** (policies and practices derived from scientifically studying the effectiveness of various treatments). Clinical pathways standardize care and provide a means of communicating patient treatment and outcome expectations among various disciplines. Communication and standardization of treatment, via clinical pathways, especially as the patient moves through various levels of care, can reduce medication errors and improve safety.

Figure 15.4 shows Day 1 of a clinical pathway for the treatment of heart failure. The medication intervention is highlighted, as are the related outcomes. If the standard medications are not given, the clinician is required to provide the reason. This tool ensures that medication is not forgotten or overlooked and that every member of the caregiving team has access to the same information regarding the clinical treatment.

FIGURE 15.4   Heart Failure Clinical Pathway

HEART FAILURE
CLINICAL PATHWAY

DAY 1   DATE: ____/____/____

		Intervention		Outcomes	
ASSESSMENT	CONSULTS	Nutrition screen		Nutrition consult ordered ☐	
		1. Physical Therapy screening			
	TESTS	2. Echocardiogram ordered if EF		Echocardiogram performed: ☐	
		not known		EF documented in the medical record as _____ %	
				or mild, moderate or severe dysfunction	
		Cholesterol profile, BNP level			
		Electrocardiogram		Electrocardiogram performed ☐	
		Pulse Oximetry		Oxygen level greater than 90% ☐	
	MONITORS & TEAM PROCESS	Admission history and assessment		Admission history and assessment completed ☐	
		Vital signs every _____ hours		Patient initial weight: _____	
		3. Daily weight performed		1. Initial weight on nursing admission form	
				Met: ☐ Unmet: ☐ Initials:	
		Patient smoked in last year: Yes ☐ No ☐		2. If smoker, smoking cessation counseling given	
				Met: ☐ Unmet: ☐ Initials:	
		Pain management assessed ☐		Patient is pain free ☐	
		Skin assessment ☐		Patient's skin is intact ☐	
		Telemetry ordered ☐			
	PROBLEMS/	1.	3.		5.

PLAN	MEDICATIONS	If EF is below 40% use:	Patient on ACE-1 ☐ or ARB ☐ Or is intolerant ☐
		ACE inhibitors (ACEI) ☐ or angiotensin	Reason _____
		II receptor blocker (ARB) ☐ unless	ACE-I/ARB held: Hypotension ☐ Renal failure ☐
		Contraindicated	Other ☐ Specify_____
		Diuretic prescribed: Yes ☐ No ☐	If diuretic yes, intravenous ☐ or oral administration ☐

	ACTIVITY	Out of bed as tolerated ☐ Bedrest ☐		Activity guidelines discussed ☐	
	TEACHING	4. Patient Friendly CareMap@ given		Patient verbalizes understanding of Heart Failure plan of care ☐	
		initial: _____		Patient verbalizes understanding of medications and	
		Orient to unit, review plan of care.		pain scale ☐	
		teach disease process, diet, fluid restriction.			
		medications, signs and symptoms to report.			
		daily weights, safety precautions.			
		smoking cessation, pain scale ☐			
	DISCHARGE PLANNING	CMS guidelines for smoking		Guidelines for smoking cessation and EF entered on Heart	
		cessation and EF assessed ☐		Failure Specific Supplemental Discharge Instruction Sheet ☐	
		Assess support network ☐			
		Assess discharge planning needs ☐			
	TEAM SIGNATURES AND TITLE	1.	3.		5.
		2.	4.		6.

CMS11-D (0.07)   3

Process Redesigns

The system factors affecting medication safety are dealt with through redesign of various steps in the medication delivery system. Common process redesign strategies known to improve the reliability of any process will also improve medication safety. These strategies include (Agency for Healthcare Research and Quality, 2008):

- Standardize the process

- Build decision and memory aids into the system

- Make the desired action the default choice

Table 15.1 Process Redesign Tactics Applied to
Medication Delivery

Tactic	Examples
Standardize	Physicians use standard order sets for high-risk medications such as chemotherapy and anticoagulant therapy.
Decision and memory aids	Pop-up screens in CPOE system reminds ordering physician of common drug interactions and other important information that may influence their choice of medication.
Desired action is default	Physician has to actively choose not to prescribe the agreed-on prophylactic antibiotics for particular types of surgery.
Habits, work patterns, and scheduling	Pharmacists use morning patient rounds as an opportunity to educate caregivers about unusual medications, formulary changes, and other patient-specific medication safety issues.
Process risks and risk-reduction actions known	Caregivers informed about dangerous abbreviations and use of these abbreviations is prohibited when ordering medications.
Redundancies	Medication reconciliation is done prior to a patient's discharge to double check appropriateness and accuracy of discharge medication prescriptions.
Independent backups	Prior to administering IV medications, two nurses separately check infusion pump rate and medication concentration and then compare findings.

- Take advantage of people's usual habits, work patterns, and scheduling

- Make process risks and actions to reduce risk known to caregivers

- Create redundant processes

- Make use of independent backups

Table 15.1 summarizes examples of medication system improvements in the above categories.

Standardize the Process
Researchers found standard order sets resulted in higher rate of venous thromboembolism prophylaxis in patients admitted to the hospital through the ED (Levine, Hergenroeder, Miller, & Davies, 2007). Standard order sets for particular diseases should be developed by multidisciplinary task forces and vetted by the relevant professionals, from the Pharmacy and Therapeutics (P&T) committee to the medical departments. Well-developed order sets clearly (and legibly)

communicate all process steps, allowing caregivers access to the same information about what is expected and in what order. Medication errors can occur if a step in the process is overlooked or eliminated. For example, often a patient requires hydration with saline before administration of medication or requires anti-nausea medication prior to chemotherapy.

The Indianapolis Coalition for Patient Safety (http://www.indypatient safety.org) chartered a task force to standardize intravenous medication concentrations and dosage units across adult hospitals for safer and more consistent practices in administering high-risk intravenous medications to patients. A single concentration and dosage unit standard was developed for 25 high-risk medications using manufacturers' recommendations, reference materials, and a consensus-driven approach. This standardization decreased the potential for medication errors within hospitals and on patient transfer between hospitals in the seven Indianapolis health systems.

Build Decision and Memory Aids into the System

Hospitals with CPOE systems should use the technology to reduce the likelihood of medication errors. The system can be configured to alert physicians of potential drug–drug interactions, allergic responses, or drug–food interactions. Flags in the CPOE system can automatically alert physicians to correct medication dosage, frequency, strength, and duration. In addition, the system can provide useful information about drugs that are not commonly prescribed.

The clinical pathway in Figure 15.4 is an example of a paper-based memory aid. It helps physicians remember to order medications commonly prescribed for patients with heart failure. Color coding is another example of a memory aid that can reduce medication-related errors. Researchers in Florida found a color-coded medication safety (CCMS) system that provides nurses with immediate access to necessary pediatric medication information reduced medication calculation errors and made it easier to recognize physician ordering errors (Feleke et al., 2009).

Environmental changes can help people choose the correct medication during the ordering, dispensing, preparation, and administration steps. Products with similar names are particularly prone to mistakes (Institute for Safe Medication Practices, 2009). These types of mistakes can be reduced by highlighting the appearance of look-alike medication names on computer screens, pharmacy and nursing unit shelf labels and bins (including automated dispensing cabinets), pharmacy product labels, and medication administration records. This highlighting can be done through the use of bold face, color, and/or tall man letters on the parts of the names that are different (for example, hydr**OXY**zine, hydr**ALA**zine).

Make the Desired Action the Default Choice

When the accepted evidence-based medication prescription is the default choice (such as on a clinical pathway or in the CPOE system), physicians have to document their reason for choosing a different medication. For example, in our health system, if a physician orders a different medication from the one recommended, the CPOE system alerts the pharmacist who then checks the reason for the variance. One orthopedic surgeon objected to using a particular surgical prophylactic antibiotic, indicating that the antibiotic he had always used resulted in good outcomes and he saw no reason to change. Because his choice of medication did not conform to the default choice, he had to document in the patient's chart why evidence-based treatment was not being ordered.

Take Advantage of People's Usual Habits, Work Patterns, and Scheduling

Evaluate how to incorporate medication safety improvements into the way patient care is now carried out. For instance, every patient taken to surgery enters through the OR door. If that patient needs a dose of antibiotics prior to the start of surgery, it may be easier for staff to remember to start the dose if it is done when they "hit the button" to open the OR door. Do nurses conduct regular bed rounds on hospitalized patients? Add medication safety checks, such as verification of correct IV flow and rate, to their bed rounding routine. Change-of-shift reports are another opportune time to double check medication safety issues. Hicks, Becker, and Chuo (2007) recommend change-of-shift reporting in NICU settings include additional systems and safety checks to prevent mistakes involving intralipid therapy. These checks should include inspection of the infusion pump and validation of infusion rates.

Make Process Risks and Actions to Reduce Risk Known to Caregivers

Everyone involved in medication administration needs to be trained on risky behaviors—some of these behaviors are just natural, inherently human behaviors, but in medication administration they become high-risk behaviors. An example is the natural human behavior to use abbreviations, acronyms, and symbols in written communications. However, if used when writing a medication prescription, these literary shortcuts create a risky situation that is a known source of medication errors (Brunetti, Santell, & Hicks, 2007).

The Joint Commission has identified abbreviations, acronyms, symbols, and dose designations that should not be used for handwritten medication orders and other medication-related documentation. In our health care system, a list of not-to-be-used abbreviations was distributed to all clinicians (see Figure 15.5).

It is not enough to simply pass around a sheet of dangerous abbreviations. Resident and physician education should be conducted as well as clinical

FIGURE 15.5   Do-Not-Use Abbreviations

AVOID DANGEROUS PRESCRIPTION PRACTICES
Don't hold on to dangerous habits: *SPELL IT OUT*

DON'T USE		INSTEAD
U̸	The handwritten **U** after insulin, heparin, pitocin dose can be read as **a zero**, **a 4**, or **cc's**, causing dangerous overdoses	*Write "unit"*
μg̸	The handwritten **μg** is often mistaken as **mg**	*Write "microgram"*
q.d̸.	The handwritten **q.d.** can be misinterpreted as **"q.i.d."** if the middle period is raised or the tail of the **"q"** interferes	*Write "daily"*
q.o.d̸.	The handwritten **q.o.d.** can be interpreted as every day	*Write "every other day"*
q.i.d̸.	The handwritten **q.i.d.** can be interpreted as **daily** if the "I" is not written clearly	*Write "four times daily"*
x.0̸ or .̸x	Trailing zero (**x.0** mg) or lack of leading zero (**.x** mg) – decimal point can be missed	*Write "X mg"* *Write "0.X mg"*
MS̸	**MS** can mean morphine sulfate or magnesium sulfate – can be confused for one another	*Write "morphine sulfate"* *Write "magnesium sulfate"*

department informal sessions. Quality management staff should audit random charts to ensure that dangerous abbreviations are not being used. To reinforce appropriate behavior, pharmacists and nurses can serve as safeguards by asking that orders to be rewritten in an acceptable and safe form. Medical staff rules and regulations must incorporate this patient safety issue into performance expectations.

Create Redundant Processes

Redundancies act as safeguards to decrease errors. For example, physicians ordering high-risk medications may be required to write both the generic and brand names (if available). Both medication names provide the pharmacist with a double check to be sure the right drug is being dispensed. A beneficial redundant step in the medication ordering process is the read back of verbal or telephone orders by the person receiving the order. Ideally, the read back includes the product name, the spelling of the product name, and a statement of its indications.

The process of **medication reconciliation** is a redundant step that has proven useful at catching mistakes that might have otherwise caused patient harm (Barnsteiner, 2005; Rodehaver & Fearing, 2005). Medication reconciliation involves comparing a patient's current medications against the physician's admission, transfer, and discharge orders. Though this extra step takes time, medication errors due to omissions, duplications, dosing errors, or drug interactions can be avoided.

Process redundancies should be carefully selected as they can make a process more complex—leading to more rather than fewer errors. In addition, redundancies can have unintended consequences. For example, if people are aware that others are duplicating their efforts, redundancy can diffuse responsibility and lead individuals to overlook safety checks (Sagan, 2004).

Make Use of Independent Backups

Double checks are a form of redundancy. However, to be effective the double checks must be independent. Independent backups, though similar in nature to double-checking, are a different process. An independent backup involves two separate people checking independently of each other and then comparing their findings to see if they match. An independent backup is more effective in eliminating errors because it removes the bias produced by two people simultaneously sharing the same conclusion. Because independent backups can pose staffing challenges in most organizations, this redundant step is often reserved for prescribing, dispensing, and administering of select high-risk medications (Institute for Safe Medication Practices, 2003).

Technological Issues

With all the complexity involved in the medication delivery system, it is no wonder that new technologies are viewed as the answer for reducing the most prevalent process problems. Many technological changes have been suggested, some more sophisticated or costly than others. For example, by using prelabeled syringes nurses are less likely to mistakenly administer the wrong medication (Institute for Safe Medication Practices, 2008). The use of single-dose packaging rather than multidose containers for medications can reduce inadvertent overdosing (Carroll, 2003). Automated medication storage and dispensing cabinets on hospital units can improve the timeliness of medication delivery to units and, when specific safeguards are in place, can reduce medication administration errors (Institute for Safe Medication Practices, 2008).

The Food and Drug Administration (2004) proposes requiring bar codes on certain drug containers to ensure that the right drug in the right dose and route of administration is given to the right patient at the right time. For hospitalized patients, a bar-coded patient identification (ID) band can be scanned when medications are to be administered, with the information entered into a computer. If there is a mismatch between the patient ID and the medication ordered for the patient, a warning box pops up to alert staff of a possible error.

The CMS is encouraging adoption of electronic, computer-based technology to reduce medication errors through an electronic prescribing (e-prescribing) program that will ensure that pharmacists and physicians have appropriate patient information (Kaye, 2008). Electronic prescribing software should include reminders for correct dosages and drug interactions (IOM, 2006). Ideally, prescribers have electronic access to patient history and their current medications with pop-up screens that alert to potential problems. In-hospital medication ordering systems, such as CPOE, should include automated decision support systems.

Advocates of CPOE systems maintain that medication safety will be improved because the computer will help eliminate errors associated with the silos (caregivers not communicating with one another) and eliminate problems caused by handwriting illegibility, unsuspected drug-drug interactions, inappropriate dosage, and wrong route of administration (Kaushal, Shojania, & Bates, 2003). Because the physician's orders are electronically integrated with patient-specific information such as laboratory data and medication allergies, the CPOE system can check for possible **adverse drug reactions** due to allergies, dosage miscalculations, or drug interactions with other medications. Figure 15.6 compares the manual and computerized process of medication administration.

FIGURE 15.6 Medication Administration Process: Manual Versus Computerized

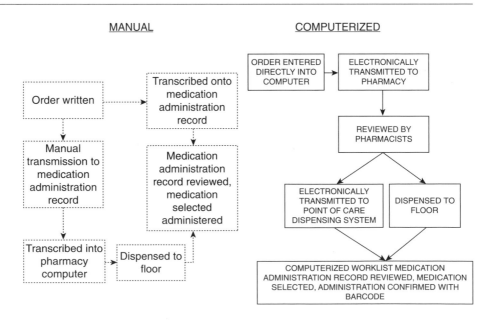

However, it should be noted that although technology is constantly improving, the computer cannot substitute for human intelligence, ingenuity, and spontaneity. Electronic health records and CPOE systems cannot evaluate the patient's reaction to the medication or ensure effective critical thinking and response to an adverse event. CPOE systems can contribute to medication errors if not adequately and appropriately programmed (Koppel et al., 2005). Even after adoption of technology-driven medication delivery improvements, leadership has to encourage HRO principles—a climate of vigilance, competence, and ongoing education.

Although the safety benefits of health information technology, such as CPOE, seem apparent, there are several obstacles to be addressed before such systems can be implemented by health care facilities. These obstacles and suggested solutions are covered in Chapter Thirteen.

Measuring and Improving the Quality of Medication Delivery

To reduce medication errors in institutional settings as well as private physician offices, data on medication errors must be collected and analyzed. This involves defining errors, developing appropriate measurements, and establishing a process to monitor and communicate results to relevant stakeholders (Dlugacz, 2006). Leadership commitment and resources are needed to support measurement efforts. The task of gathering and evaluating medication errors and near misses data may be assigned to the quality management department or in some institutions, the risk management department. Experienced professionals in these departments can assist in developing medication safety measurements (with appropriate numerators and denominators) and create an electronic database to capture and report results to various levels of the organization. Information needs to be gathered about the incidence of medication errors and near misses, the type of error (omission, route of administration, timing, wrong medication, wrong patient, wrong dosage) and also where and when the event occurred.

In addition, if there is a medication error or an adverse drug reaction, quality management can help to track processes and identify, through root cause analyses and failure mode and effects analyses, where in the process improvements are required. Most important, quality management databases that track and trend information over time can ensure the sustainability of improvements, once they are developed and communicated.

Table 15.2   Medication Measures

Drug Name / Category: (e.g.) Lipitor / Statin	Q1	Q2
Adverse Drug Reaction Rate[1] Reported Medication Error Rate[2] Medication Near Miss Rate[3]		

1. *Adverse Drug Reaction Rate*

$$\frac{\text{Number of patients with suspected drug reaction(s)}}{\text{Total discharges, } \textit{excluding} \text{ Psychiatry/Chemical Dependency, Newborns}}$$

2. *Reported Medication Error Rate*

$$\frac{\text{Number of Reported Medication Errors}}{\text{Total discharges, } \textit{excluding} \text{ Psychiatry/Chemical Dependency, Newborns}}$$

3. *Medication Near Miss Rate*

$$\frac{\text{Number of medication/therapeutic related events that were corrected/reported prior to administration}}{\text{Patient Care Days and Excluding Psychiatry/Chemical Dependency, Rehabilitation, Hospice, Newborns}}$$

In our health care system, several measurements are used to monitor performance variables associated with medication safety (see Table 15.2). The results are reported quarterly.

The measurement data illuminate aggregate processes and give decision-makers information from which to make knowledge-based decisions about medication safety improvement priorities (Dlugacz, 2010). Reporting measurement results has the further advantage of putting everyone involved in the complex process of medication delivery on the same page. When leadership sees variation in performance over time, they ask for further information to better understand the cause. If error rates are increasing, it is important for people to ask why.

Once improvements are made to the medication delivery system, the effectiveness of the changes must be measured to ensure sustainability. Monthly reports of performance results help to maintain oversight of improvements.

Medication Safety Infrastructure

It is a good idea to establish one or more multidisciplinary medication safety groups to monitor and improve the medication administration system. Some hospitals appoint a task group in each clinical service, whereas others rely on one committee (such as the pharmacy and therapeutics committee) to fulfill this role. These groups can help establish a nonpunitive incident and near-miss reporting system and select medication safety measures relevant to each clinical service.

When improvement opportunities are identified, the groups should spearhead process reviews and target inefficient practices for change. They can also evaluate new medication delivery technology to ascertain its impact on medication safety and suggest best practices for safe storage and dispensing of high-risk medications. These groups should ensure that staff are regularly informed of medication packaging, dosing, and prescribing problems and how to prevent them. The groups involved in the medication infrastructure must be focused on constantly improving processes and building awareness of medication safety throughout the organization.

Role of Patients in Medication Safety

Many patients do not understand their medication regimes; they do not know how to take their medication, the purpose of each medication, and the adverse symptoms that should be reported to their physician. Any initiative to improve medication safety must necessarily include patient education. The IOM recommends that patients be educated about medication safety to better protect themselves from harm. For instances, the IOM recommends (IOM, July 2006) that hospitalized patients:

- Ask their physician or nurse about drugs that they are given in the hospital

- Refuse to take a drug unless being told the purpose for doing so

- Have a surrogate present when receiving medication when patients are unable to monitor the medication process

- Before surgery, inquire as to what medications should be taken, and if any should be stopped

- Before discharge, ask for a list of medications to be taken at home, and have a provider review them to ensure appropriated administration

The ISMP advocates that drug information be simplified for consumers and that a national drug information hotline be established to answer consumer questions in real time. Also ISMP promotes drug information transparency—patients should have access to medication risk and benefit information as well as access to clinical outcome and effectiveness data.

Health literacy is a problem which goes largely unrecognized by the medical community; yet it has significant consequences for patients who don't understand their medication regime. The FDA recommends that consumers be well educated about medication safety, suggesting that patients be (Meadows, 2003):

- Made aware of the types of medication errors that occur

- Informed about what drug is being prescribed and for what reason

- Encouraged to ask their clinician to clearly explain drug regimens

- Informed on how to take medications (family members can help here)

- Encouraged to keep an accurate and up-to-date list of all medications and dosages, including over-the-counter drugs, supplements, and herbs

Our health care system developed patient-friendly guidelines to explain the process of care and to promote education, especially about discharge instructions including medications (see Figure 15.7). Discharge instructions are critical to safety because patients need to take their medications after leaving the hospital and comply with follow-up recommendations. Otherwise, their condition can easily deteriorate, requiring rehospitalization.

In addition to patient-friendly guidelines, our health care system provides patients with other instructive materials, such as medication safety videos and educational pamphlets. Our caregivers make it a practice to involve family members in medication administration education. In our experience, patients respond very well to memory aids such as telephone calls to explain medication regimens and repackaging of medication in one-dose-only packets to avoid overdosing. Better-educated patients are less likely to take their medication incorrectly.

Conclusion

Medication errors occur because human beings are fallible and medication delivery systems are complex and error-prone. Therefore, an understanding of human factors must be a component in medication error reduction strategies as

FIGURE 15.7   Patient Version of Pneumonia Guideline

PNEUMONIA GUIDELINE
Patient Version

This protocol is a general guideline and does not represent professional care standard governing provider's obligation to patients. Care is revised to meet the individual patient's needs.	
BLOOD DRAWING	A member of the Health Care Team may draw your blood as ordered by your doctor. It may be necessary to draw blood several times during the day in order to check your condition.
TESTS	You will have a chest x-ray and your oxygen level will be measured, additional tests may also be ordered by your doctor. The Health Care Team will explain any tests that are ordered.
TREATMENTS	You will have an intravenous line (I.V.). You may be given oxygen to help you
MEDICATIONS	*MEDICATIONS* *You will be given medication for your pain. The pain medication will be based on your needs, how it is given will be ordered by your doctor. Antibiotics will be given through your IV line and will be changed to an oral (by mouth) form before you go home. The Health Care Team will explain the medication you are taking and any side effects.*
DIET	
ACTIVITY	
TEAM ACTIVITIES	Members of the Health Care Team will go over your plan of care and answer any questions you or your family may have. Speak up if you have any questions or concerns and if you do not understand, ask again.
EDUCATION	You will be taught to use the pain scale. This will help the staff to understand and manage your pain. You will be taught safety precautions, which will include being asked your name and date of birth by the members of the Health Care Team before you receive any medications, treatments, procedures or tests. You will be taught about the medications you are taking and any possible side effects. You will also be given advice / counseling on not smoking and the effects of second hand smoke.
DISCHARGE PLANNING	Your discharge plan will be based on your needs. If you have questions about home care or were receiving home care services tell your nurse. A Social Worker / Case Manager may visit with you to talk about discharge planning. Your nurse will go over your discharge instructions with you and your family before you go home. Your recovery after leaving the hospital will depend on how active you are in your own care and how well you follow directions about the follow-up care and services you need.

well as identification of system-level flaws that address at-risk behaviors of professionals. Process redesign can help to alter behavior and improve safety. Technological advances, such as CPOE, and measurements that track medication errors can assist organizations with developing improved processes. Patient education can help patients protect themselves from harm.

Health care organizations are under pressure to adopt medication safety practices through understanding gaps in safety and implementing improvements. National agencies have targeted improvement strategies to address these problems, using financial incentives, threats of negative publicity, and accreditation standards. Yet with all the initiatives, efforts, incentives, and recommendations to improve medication safety, preventable errors still occur and organizations implement improvements slowly and often reluctantly. Financial, structural, and cultural barriers to adopting new processes have yet to be overcome. Through a combination of process improvements, cultural change, and organizational commitment, preventable medication errors can be reduced.

Discussion Questions

1. Discuss how adopting HRO principles will result in improvements in medication safety.

2. Identify measurements that could be used to evaluate medication safety performance in a hospital and in a physician private practice.

3. Search the literature related to medication safety improvement in a hospital to identify specific process redesign tactics in each of the following categories:

   - Standardize the process

   - Build decision and memory aids into the system

   - Make the desired action the default choice

   - Take advantage of people's usual habits, work patterns, and scheduling

   - Make process risks and actions to reduce risk known to caregivers

   - Create redundant processes

   - Make use of independent backups

4. Discuss the role of patients and consumer groups in reducing medication errors.

Key Terms

Accountable	Evidence-based medicine	Potential adverse drug event
Adverse drug event	Just culture	
Adverse drug reaction	Medication reconciliation	Risk points

References

Agency for Healthcare Research and Quality. (2008). *Becoming a high reliability organization: Operational advice for hospital leaders.* (AHRQ Publication No. 08–0022). Retrieved from http://www.ahrq.gov/qual/hroadvice/.

American Hospital Association, Health Research and Educational Trust, Institute for Safe Medication Practices (2002). Model strategic plan for medication safety. *Pathways for Medication Safety. Leading a strategic planning effort.* Section 1.2, p. 11. Retrieved from http://www.ismp.org/tools/pathwaysection1.pdf.

Barnsteiner, J. H. (2005). Medication reconciliation: Transfer of medication information across settings—keeping it free from error. *American Journal of Nursing, 105*(3 Suppl), 31–36.

Bates, D. W. (2002). Unexpected hypoglycemia in a critically ill patient. *Annals of Internal Medicine, 137*(2), 110–116.

Brunetti, L., Santell, J., & Hicks, R. (2007). Assessing the impact of abbreviations on patient safety. *Joint Commission Journal on Quality and Patient Safety, 33*(9), 576–583.

Callen, J., McIntosh, J., & Li, J. (2009). Accuracy of medication documentation in hospital discharge summaries: A retrospective analysis of medication transcription errors in manual and electronic discharge summaries. *International Journal of Medical Informatics*, (in press). doi:10.1016/j.ijmedinf.2009.09.002.

Carroll, P. (2003). Medication issues: The bigger picture. *RN, 66*(1), 52–58.

Cina, J., Gandhi, T., Churchill, W., Fanikos, J., McCrea, M., Mitton, P., …. Poon, F. (2006). How many hospital pharmacy medication dispensing errors go undetected? *Joint Commission Journal on Quality and Patient Safety, 32*(2), 73–80.

Davis, M. N., Toombs Smith, S., & Tyler, S. (2005). Improving transition and communication between acute care and long-term care: A system for better continuity of care. *Annals of Long-Term Care: Clinical Care and Aging, 13*(5), 25–32.

Desselle, S. P. (2005). Certified pharmacy technicians' views on their medication preparation errors and educational needs. *American Journal of Health-System Pharmacy, 62*(19), 1992–1997.

Dlugacz, Y. D. (2006). *Measuring health care: Using quality data for operational, financial and clinical improvement.* San Francisco: Jossey-Bass.

Dlugacz, Y. D. (2010). *Value based health care: Linking finance and quality.* San Francisco: Jossey-Bass.

DNV Healthcare (2009) *National Integrated Accreditation for Healthcare Organizations Accreditation Requirements* (Issue 307–8.0). Retrieved from http://www.dnv.com/binaries/NIAHO%20Accreditation%20Requirements-Rev%20307–8%200%282%29_tcm4–347543.pdf.

Feleke, R., Kalynych, C. J., Lundblom, B., Wears, R., Luten, R., & Kling, D. (2009). Color coded medication safety system reduces community pediatric emergency nursing medication errors. *Journal of Patient Safety, 5*(2), 79–85.

Food and Drug Administration. (2004). *HHS announces new requirements for bar codes on drugs and blood to reduce risks of medication errors.* Retrieved from http://www.fda.gov/NewsEvents/Newsroom/PressAnnouncements/2004/ucm108250.htm.

Galt, K. A. (2003). Interventions to improve medication safety in primary care practice. American Association of Family Practice. Conference presentation September 17, 2003.

Grasha, A. F. (2000). Into the abyss: Seven principles for identifying the causes of and preventing human error in complex systems. *American Journal of Health-System Pharmacists, 57*(6), 554–564.

Grasha, A. F. (2002). *Human factors annotated checklist, version 3.0.* Retrieved from http://www.pharmsafety.org/extras/HFChecklist.pdf.

Gurwitz, J., Field, T., Judge, J., Rochon, P., Harrold, L., Cadoret, C., …. Bates, D. (2005) The incidence of adverse drug events in two large academic long-term care facilities. *American Journal of Medicine, 118*(3), 251–258.

Hicks, R. W., Becker, S. C., & Chuo, J. (2007). A summary of NICU fat emulsion medication errors and nursing services: Data from MEDMARX. *Advances in Neonatal Care, 7*(6), 299–310.

Institute for Safe Medication Practices. (2003, March 6). The virtues of independent double checks—they really are worth your time! *ISMP Medication Safety Alert.* Retrieved from http://www.ismp.org/newsletters/acutecare/articles/20030306.asp.

Institute for Safe Medication Practices. (2008). Errors with injectable medications: Unlabeled syringes are surprisingly common! *Nurse Advisor—ERR, 6*(1), 1, 3.

Institute for Safe Medication Practices. (2009). ISMP's list of confused drug names. Retrieved from www.ismp.org/Tools/confuseddrugnames.pdf.

Institute of Medicine. (1999). *To err is human: Building a safer health system.* Washington, DC: National Academy Press.

Institute of Medicine. (2003). *Keeping patients safe: Transforming the work environment of nurses.* Washington, DC: National Academy Press.

Institute of Medicine. (2006). *Preventing medication errors: Quality chasm series.* Washington, DC: National Academy Press.

Institute of Medicine. (2006, July). What you can do to avoid medication errors. *Fact Sheet.* Retrieved from http://www.iom.edu/ /media/Files/Report%20Files/2006/Preventing-Medication-Errors-Quality-Chasm-Series/medicationerrorsfactsheet.ashx.

Jackson, R. (2005). From the editor … root causes of sentinel events. *Health Care Food & Nutrition Focus, 22*(7), 2.

Juarez, A., Gacki-Smith, J., Bauer, M. R., Jepsen, D., Paparella, S., VonGoerres, B., & MacLean, S. (2009). Barriers to emergency departments' adherence to four medication safety-related Joint Commission National Patient Safety Goals. *Joint Commission Journal on Quality and Safety, 35*(1), 49–59.

Kalisch, B. J., & Aebersold, M. (2006). Overcoming barriers to patient safety. *Nursing Economic$, 24*(3), 143–148.

Kaushal, R., Shojania, K. G., & Bates, D. W. (2003). Effects of computerized physician order entry and clinical decision support systems on medication safety: A systematic review. *Archives of Internal Medicine, 163*(12), 1409–1416.

Kaye, M. (2008, June). Mandating of electronic prescriptions for Medicare patients. *Online Journal of Nursing Informatics,* 12(2) [Online]. Available at http://ojni.org/12_2/kaye.html.

Kienle, P., & Uselton, J. P. (2008). Maintaining compliance with Joint Commission medication management standards. *Patient Safety and Quality Healthcare Newsletter.* Available at http://www.psqh.com/julaug08/medication.html.

Koppel, R., Metlay, J. P., Cohen, A., Abaluck, B., Localio, A. R., Kimmel, S. E., & Strom, B. L. (2005). Role of computerized physician order entry systems in facilitating medication errors. *Journal of the American Medical Association, 293*(1), 197–120.

Levine, R. L., Hergenroeder, G. W., Miller, C. C., & Davies, A. (2007). Venous thromboembolism prophylaxis in emergency department admissions. *Journal of Hospital Medicine, 2*(2), 79–85.

Meadows, M. (2003). Strategies to reduce medication errors: How the FDA is working to improve medication safety and what you can do to help. *FDA Consumer Magazine, 37*(3), 20–27.

National Coordinating Council for Medication Error Reporting and Prevention. (2005, December). *The first ten years: Defining the problem and developing solutions.* Retrieved from http://www.nccmerp.org/pdf/reportFinal2005–11–29.pdf.

Rodehaver, C., & Fearing, D. (2005). Medication reconciliation in acute care: Ensuring an accurate drug regimen on admission and discharge. *Joint Commission Journal on Quality and Safety, 31*(7), 406–413.

Sagan, S. D. (2004). The problem of redundancy problem: Why more nuclear security forces may produce less nuclear security. *Risk Analysis, 24*(4), 935–946.

Schyve, P. (2004). An interview with Lucian Leape. *Joint Commission Journal on Quality and Safety, 30*(12), 656.

Taxis, K., & Barber, N. (2003). Ethnographic study of the incidence and severity of intravenous medicine errors. *British Medical Journal, 326*(7391), 684–687.

Weick, K. E., & Sutcliffe. K. M. (2007). *Managing the unexpected: Resilient performance in an age of uncertainty* (2nd ed.). San Francisco: Jossey-Bass, 2007.

GLOSSARY

5S

A systematic approach for creating organization and standard work in the workplace.

5 Whys

An investigative tool used to find root causes by repeatedly asking the question, why?

Accident

Any unplanned event that results in injury or ill health to people, or damages equipment, property, or materials, but where there is risk of harm.

Accident trajectory

The series of events that led to a disastrous outcome, typically uncovered by a root cause analysis. Sometimes referred to as an error chain.

Accountable

Being held responsible.

Action plan

Strategies for improving a process or for preventing a problem from occurring or reoccurring. Sometimes referred to as improvement action, corrective action, or risk-reduction strategy.

Active failure

A human error or violation of safe practices.

Adverse drug event

An injury related to the use of a medication.

Adverse drug reaction

A subset of adverse drug event. It includes any undesirable, unintended, or unexpected clinical manifestation associated with use of a medication.

Adverse event

Any injury caused by medical care.

Adverse reaction

Unexpected harm resulting from a justified action where the correct process was followed for the context in which the event occurred.

Anticipatory failure analysis

Prospective risk assessment or hazard analysis.

Bar code scanning device

A mobile computer or personal digital assistant (PDA) used to scan bar-coded items (for example, medication containers, equipment, patient identification wristbands).

Barrier

Any measure taken to protect patients from hazards, including physical guards but also administrative measures such as rules and procedures. Sometimes referred to as safeguards or system defenses.

Catastrophic process

A process in which there is a high likelihood of patient death or severe injury immediately or within hours of a failure.

Check actions

The process of monitoring, intervening, and correcting errors or deviations in situation awareness among team members.

Checklist

Algorithmic listing of actions to be performed in a given clinical situation to ensure that, no mater how often performed by a given practitioner, no step will be forgotten.

Clinical pathway

A document that identifies and defines the tasks of the different patient care team members for a specific patient population.

Close call

An event or situation that did not produce patient injury, but only because of chance. Sometimes referred to as a *near miss*.

Collective mindfulness

An organizational trait that allows people to be better able to notice the unexpected in the making and halt its development.

Common cause variation

Variation in performance due to the process itself, not a disturbance in the process. If only common causes of variation are present, performance is expected to be stable and predictable over time.

Complex system

A system composed of interconnected parts that as a whole exhibit one or more properties not obvious from the properties of the individual parts.

Computerized physician/provider order entry (CPOE)

A computer-based system used by physicians and other providers to order medications, tests, or treatments for patients.

Confidence factor

A certainty or truth factor expressed as a numeric value. Used to describe the reliability of a piece of information whose truth is unclear or uncertain.

Constraining function

A system design that constrains some component from being able to lead to an error.

Contributing cause

A circumstance, action, or influence which is thought to have played a part in the origin or development of an incident or to increase the risk of an incident.

Control chart

A line graph that includes statistically calculated upper and lower control limits.

Control limits

Control limits define the area (set at one, two, or three standard deviations) on either side of the centerline, or mean, of data plotted on a control chart. Control limits reflect the expected variation in the data.

Crew resource management

Various approaches to training groups to function as teams, rather than as collections of individuals.

Dashboard

A special type of tabular report that uses symbols, colors, or both to draw people's attention to performance concerns.

DEB analysis (Deviation-Effect-Barrier)

A prospective analysis technique used to examine a health care system for design flaws before an incident happens.

Electronic health record (EHR) system

The portal through which clinicians access a patient's health record, order treatments or therapy, and document care delivered to patients.

Error

Failure to carry out a planned action as intended or application of an incorrect plan that leads to an undesirable outcome or significant potential for such an outcome. Includes an act of commission (doing something wrong) or omission (failing to do the right thing).

Error chain

See *accident trajectory*.

Error containment

Actions taken to limit adverse consequences once an incident happens.

Error elimination

The process is changed so an error is impossible to make.

Error management

Apply an understanding of the nature of human errors and the mechanisms behind them to design safer systems and processes.

Error-producing factor

See *red flag*.

Error reduction

Actions taken to limit the occurrence of errors.

Evidence-based medicine

A recommended treatment, the cause of some condition, or the best way to diagnose it that reflects the results of medical research, as opposed to, for example, a personal opinion.

Failure

Any event that has an impact on a system in a way that adversely affects the outcome.

Failure effect

The consequence a failure mode has on the patient.

Failure mode

The manner by which a failure is observed. Generally describes the way the failure occurs.

Failure mode and effect analysis

A team-based systematic and proactive approach for identifying the ways that a process or design can fail, why it might fail, the effects of that failure, and how it can be made safer.

Fatigue management

Activities designed to identify and control factors (environmental, organizational, and individual) that contribute to fatigue.

Fault tree analysis

A failure analysis method suited to anticipatory study of potential hazards.

Forcing function

An aspect of a design that prevents a target action from being performed or allows its performance only if another specific action is performed first.

Hand-off

Transition of patient care responsibilities from one provider to another.

Harm

Impairment of structure or function of the body or any deleterious effect arising there from. Harm includes disease, injury, suffering, disability, and death.

Hazard

A circumstance, action, or condition with the potential to cause patient harm.

Hazard and Operability Study (HAZOP)

A process hazard-seeking method popular in the chemical process industries.

Health information technology (HIT)

Any tool used in a health care organization to automate or mechanize clinical and administrative processes.

High-reliability organization (HRO)

Organization or system that operates in hazardous conditions but has fewer adverse events than would be expected.

High-risk process

A process with high potential for having an adverse impact on the safety of patients served.

Human factors analysis

The study of human abilities and characteristics as they affect the design and smooth operation of equipment, systems, and jobs. Sometimes referred to as *human factors engineering* or *reliability science*.

Human factors engineering

See human factors analysis.

Human root cause

A decision error.

Iatrogenic

Resulting from the activity of health care services.

Incident reporting

Identification of events or situations that could, or did, lead to an undesirable outcome.

Independent double check

When two people separately perform a task and compare the outcomes for validity.

Ishikawa diagram

A visual representation used to display the various factors that may be contributing to an undesirable effect. Sometimes referred to as a *fishbone diagram*.

Just culture

A culture in which frontline personnel feel comfortable disclosing errors, including their own, while maintaining accountability.

Kaizen

Continuous, incremental improvement.

Kanban

Japanese word for sign board.

Knowledge-based error

Errors in knowledge-based problem solving are also considered mistakes. When presented with new situations, the individual makes an error due to lack of knowledge.

Latent failure

The less obvious system or organizational reason for an incident. Sometimes referred to as a latent condition.

Latent root cause

See *latent failure*.

Lean

Absolute elimination of waste.

Medication error

Any preventable event that may cause or lead to inappropriate medication use or patient harm while the medication is in the control of the health care professional, patient, or consumer.

Medication reconciliation

The process of comparing a patient's current medication orders to all medications that the patient has been taking.

Misdiagnosis-related harm

Preventable harm that results from the delay or failure to treat a condition actually present (when the working diagnosis was wrong or unknown) or from treatment provided for a condition not actually present.

Mistake

When a person does what they meant to do, but should have done something else.

Mistake-proofing

Improving processes or system designs to prevent mistakes from being made or to make the mistake obvious at a glance.

Mode

The manifestation of a failure. Sometimes referred to as *failure modes*.

MTO analysis (Man-Technique Organization)

A technique derived from systems theory used to identify the underlying causes of accidents.

Near miss

An incident which did not reach the patient. Sometimes referred to as a *close call*.

Noncatastrophic process

A process that generally does not lead to patient death or severe injury within hours of a failure.

Operator

Staff working in the "sharp end" of the system (for example, doctors and nurses) in contrast to those working in the "blunt end" of the system (for example, hospital administrators).

Opportunity analysis

A data-driven technique used to identify specific failures that have occurred in a particular system.

Outcome measure

A statistical value that provides a measure of the results of performance.

Patient incident

Anything that happens involving a patient that is not consistent with the routine operation of the health care facility or the routine medical care of that particular individual.

Patient safety

The reduction of risk of unnecessary patient harm associated with health care to an acceptable minimum.

Patient safety culture

The product of individual and group values, attitudes, perceptions, competencies, and patterns of behavior that determine the commitment to, and the style and proficiency of, an organization's patient safety management.

Patient safety indicator

A statistical value that provides an indication of the safety performance of health care services.

Patient safety organization

An entity or a component of another organization that meets certain criteria established by the federal government to conduct activities to improve patient safety and health care quality.

Performance expectation

Desired performance. See also *performance goal*.

Performance gap

Difference between actual and expected performance.

Performance goal
> An operational definition of the desired state of performance. Sometimes referred to as a *performance target* or *expectation*.

Performance trend
> Pattern of gradual change in performance or an average or general tendency of performance data to move in a certain direction over time.

Physical root cause
> The observable consequences of decision errors.

Poka-yoke
> Japanese phrase meaning "to avoid errors."

Potential adverse drug event
> A hazardous situation that fails to cause injury by chance or because it is intercepted (caught) before the medication is administered to the patient. Sometimes referred to as a *near miss* or *close call*.

Preventable
> Accepted by the community as avoidable in the particular set of circumstances.

Proactive risk reduction
> Risk identification and control activities that take place before adverse consequences have occurred.

Process
> A goal-directed, interrelated series of actions, events, mechanisms, or steps.

Process flow diagram
> A flowchart listing the process steps in order.

Process measure
> A statistical value that provides a measure of the performance of a process.

Process owner
> Person who has the ultimate responsibility for the performance of a process in realizing its objectives and has the authority and ability to make necessary changes.

Prompt
> A cue as to what action should be taken next.

Prospective risk assessment
> An evaluation of the future risks of a system or process.

Red flag

Condition or circumstance that heightens the risk for a mistake.

Redundancy

In systems design, this refers to a backup mode or a secondary means of accomplishing what the primary system is supposed to do.

Reliability

Probability that a system or process will perform as expected without failure.

Reliability science

See *human factors analysis*.

Reliable process

One that performs as expected a high proportion of the time.

Resilience

The degree to which a system continuously prevents, detects, mitigates, or ameliorates hazards or incidents.

Risk

The likelihood of patient injury or death from a specified hazard.

Risk assessment

The process of assessing the risk of exposure to a particular hazard in a specified activity.

Risk management

Clinical and administrative activities to identify, evaluate, and reduce the risk of injury to patients, staff, visitors, and the organization itself.

Risk points

Areas of the process that are susceptible to failure.

Risk-reduction strategy

See *action plan*.

Root cause

Aspects of the process or the environment that are the basic reason for a failure or that initiate the problem that eventually leads to a failure. Sometimes referred to as *latent failures*.

Root cause analysis

A study undertaken to find the first or underlying cause of a problem. Root cause analysis involves the collection and study of data to determine a true cause to a problem.

Rule-based error

This type of error is often called a mistake. The intention is wrong because the operator applies a wrong rule.

Safety-critical task

A task that must be done properly all of the time.

Sentinel event

An adverse event in which death or serious harm to a patient has occurred.

Simulation training

A training technique used to replace or amplify real experiences with guided experiences that evoke or replicate substantial aspects of the real world in a fully interactive manner.

Situational factor

Unlucky circumstance that triggered the risk in the system.

Six sigma

A statistical approach to identifying and eliminating process variation.

Skill-based error

These errors are often labeled slips or lapses. The intention is right but the execution is wrong.

Socio-technical system

A system that comprises technical, psychological, and social elements.

Special cause variation

Variation in performance that is not due to a specific cause, but rather represents random variation inherent in the process being measured.

Standard work

A process that has been broken down into a series of clearly defined tasks, devoid of waste, and performed the same way every time by each individual involved in the process.

Statistical process control (SPC)

The use of statistics and control charts to measure key quality characteristics and control how the related process behaves. SPC separates special causes of variation from common causes.

Stop the line

Any member of the health care team can stop the process if it is determined that proceeding would be unsafe for the patient.

Swiss cheese model

A model of system failure developed by James Reason that illustrates how every step in a process has the potential for failure, to varying degrees. The ideal system is analogous to a stack of slices of Swiss cheese. The holes represent opportunities for the process to fail and each of the slices represent defensive layers in the process. An error may allow a problem to pass through a hole in one layer, but in the next layer the holes are in different places, and the problem should be caught.

System defense

See *barrier*.

System failure

A fault, breakdown, or dysfunction within an organization's operational methods, processes, or infrastructure.

Systems theory

A field of study designed to understand and describe the properties of complex systems such as biology (ecosystems), sociology, and organizations.

Task criticality

A procedure by which each potential failure mode is ranked according to the combined influence of severity and probability of occurrence.

Team

A group of health care workers who are members of different disciplines, each providing specific services to a patient.

Team dimensions

The optimal teamwork actions that ensure high quality patient care: (1) maintain team structure and climate; (2) plan and problem solve; (3) communicate with the team; (4) manage workload; and (5) improve team skills.

TeamSTEPPS® system

A teamwork system designed for health care professionals.

Teamwork

A distinguishable set of two or more people who interact, dynamically, interdependently, and adaptively toward a common and valued goal.

Tightly coupled process

One in which the steps follow one another so closely that a variation in the output of one step cannot be recognized and responded to before the next step is under way.

Time-out

A planned period of quiet or interdisciplinary discussion focused on ensuring that key procedural details have been addressed.

Total annual loss (TAL)

Frequency of failure (F) per year multiplied by the sum of all failure impacts (I). (F × I = TAL).

Unobstructed throughput

A balanced process free from bottlenecks.

Unreliable process

One that performs as expected a low proportion of the time.

User-friendly

Refers to anything made easy for people to use.

Value stream mapping

The use of symbols to create a map of patient or material movement through the organization.

Violation

Deliberate deviation from an operating procedure, standard, or rule.

Visual control

A simple and direct nonverbal method for relaying information to others.